Encyclopedia of Glaucoma: Clinical Theory

Volume II

Encyclopedia of Glaucoma: Clinical Theory
Volume II

Edited by **Abigail Gipe**

New Jersey

Published by Foster Academics,
61 Van Reypen Street,
Jersey City, NJ 07306, USA
www.fosteracademics.com

Encyclopedia of Glaucoma: Clinical Theory
Volume II
Edited by Abigail Gipe

International Standard Book Number: 978-1-63242-149-4 (Hardback)

Printed in the United States of America.

Contents

Preface

Every book is a source of knowledge and this one is no exception. The idea that led to the conceptualization of this book was the fact that the world is advancing rapidly; which makes it crucial to document the progress in every field. I am aware that a lot of data is already available, yet, there is a lot more to learn. Hence, I accepted the responsibility of editing this book and contributing my knowledge to the community.

Glaucoma is a disease that affects the optic nerve, visual field and is often followed by rising intraocular pressure. This book focuses on the fundamental and clinical science of glaucoma. It covers two important sections on Clinical Concepts – Glaucoma Evaluation and Management, and Specific Glaucoma Entities. It also showcases the latest advancements as well as future prospects in glaucoma. It is intended for experts in glaucoma, researchers, general ophthalmologists and amateurs to increase their knowledge and inspire further development in understanding and managing these complicated diseases.

While editing this book, I had multiple visions for it. Then I finally narrowed down to make every chapter a sole standing text explaining a particular topic, so that they can be used independently. However, the umbrella subject sinews them into a common theme. This makes the book a unique platform of knowledge.

I would like to give the major credit of this book to the experts from every corner of the world, who took the time to share their expertise with us. Also, I owe the completion of this book to the never-ending support of my family, who supported me throughout the project.

Editor

Part 1

Clinical Concepts – Glaucoma Evaluation and Management

1

Anterior Chamber Angle Assessment Techniques

Claudio Campa, Luisa Pierro, Paolo Bettin and Francesco Bandello
Department of Ophthalmology, University Vita-Salute, Scientific Institute San Raffaele
Milan,
Italy

1. Introduction

The anterior chamber angle is the actual anatomical angle created by the root of the iris and the peripheral corneal vault. Within it lie the structures involved in the outflow passage of the aqueous, namely the trabecular meshwork and the Schlemm's canal (figure 1).

The depth of the angle in a healthy eye is approximately 30°, with the superior part usually less deep than the inferior half. However the depth is influenced by gender, age and refractive error. Female gender has the greatest influence on iridocorneal angle reduction, followed by age and spherical equivalent (Rufer et al.).

The relationship of the iris plane to the cornea has a significant effect on the aqueous humor's accessibility to its outflow drainage system. In eyes where the iris and corneal endothelium are "closed"against one another, the aqueous will not be drained causing an increase of the intraocular pressure (angle closure glaucoma) (Lens, 2008).

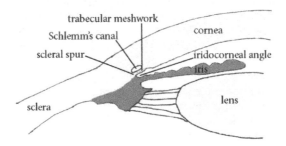

Fig. 1. Diagram of the anatomical structures forming the iridocorneal angle

Primary angle-closure glaucoma (PACG) is a leading cause of blindness worldwide (Quigley and Broman, 2006). Five overlapping conditions, not necessarily progressing in an orderly sequence, are usually described in this disease: angle closure suspect, intermittent (subacute) angle closure, acute angle closure, chronic angle closure and absolute angle closure (Kanski, 2007).

At the earliest stage (angle closure suspect), eyes have narrow or occludable angles without raised intraocular pressure (IOP) or glaucomatous optic neuropathy. It has been estimated that

22% of the eyes with angle closure suspect progress to acute angle closure (Thomas et al., 2003a) whereas 28.5% progress to chronic angle closure over 5–10 years (Thomas et al., 2003b). Prophylactic laser iridotomy performed in eyes with narrow angles may halt the progression of the angle closure process and prevent development of PACG (Nolan et al., 2003). Similarly peripheral iridoplasty, which may also be used to break an attack of acute angle-closure unresponsive to medical therapy or laser iridotomy, can be successfully employed in nonacute situations in patients with angle-closure when laser iridotomy fails to deepen the anterior chamber angle, i.e. particularly in case of plateau iris (Ritch et al., 2007, Ng et al., 2008).

Hence evaluation of anterior chamber angle (ACA) is of great importance to identify and treat those patients at risk for PACG.

It is well known that the depth and volume of the anterior chamber diminish with age and are related to the degree of ametropia. Male subjects have larger anterior chamber dimensions than female subjects. Although grading of limbal chamber depth using van Herick's technique (see below) is commonly used as a surrogate for measuring ACA, gonioscopy has represented for many years the only method able to adequately quantify ACA. However this technique has a subjective and semi-quantitative nature, is hardly reportable due to the difficulty of obtaining good images and requires a good training to be performed properly.

Moreover, in some circumstances such as plateau iris, the angle can be narrow despite a deep anterior chamber. For these reasons, with technology advancements, several new techniques have been proposed with the aim of providing a better imaging of the anterior segment. In this chapter we will show the clinical findings of each method reviewing the strengths and limitations of each approach.

2. van Herick test

Performed on the slit lamp without any additional aids, the van Herick test allows quick, not invasive assessment of anterior angle width. The technique was originally described by van Herich (Van Herick et al., 1969): a narrow slit of light is projected onto the peripheral nasal or temporal cornea at an angle of 60° as near as possible to the limbus. This results in a slit image on the surface of the cornea the width of which is compared with the peripheral anterior chamber depth ("black space") (figure 2). A four-point scale is then used, with each grade indicating the probability of angle closure. In grade 4 the anterior chamber depth (ACD) is ≥100% corneal thickness and the angle is wide open; in grade 3 it is > 25 to 50% and the angle is incapable of closure; in grade 2 it is 25% and the angle closure is possible; in grade 1 is < 25% and the angle closure is likely.

Studies have shown suboptimal results when using van Herick test to screen for primary angle closure (Alsbirk, 1986), (Congdon et al., 1997), (Thomas et al., 1996): particularly it has been found that measurements performed at the nasal limbus tend to overestimate the angle width. To improve precision in quantification of ACD, Foster (Foster et al., 2000a) proposed a modified scheme in which the original grade 1 was sub-divided into 0%, 5%, and 15% corneal thickness, and a grade of 75% corneal thickness was added to compensate for the gap between the original grades 3 and 4. This seven-point grading system resulted in 99% sensitivity compared to gonioscopic evaluation; the interobserver agreement for this augmented grading scheme was good (weighted kappa 0.76). However it is hardly reproducible in clinical practice.

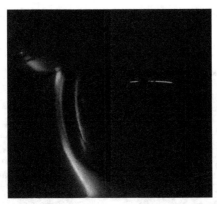

Fig. 2. An example of van Herick technique for assessing anterior chamber depth (a grade 4 is shown, see text)

3. Smith method

Another optical technique used to determine ACD is Smith's slit-length method (Smith, 1979). It is performed using a standard slit-lamp. The illumination system is located in the subject's temporal field at an angle of 60° and the slit-beam is projected horizontally. If measuring the patient's right eye the right ocular of the slit lamp is used and vice versa for the left eye. A beam of approximately 1.5 mm thickness, with its orientation horizontal, is placed across the cornea. The procedure involves focusing the slit-beam on the corneal surface while an out of focus image of the slit-beam is observed on the iris/lens surface. The length of the slit-beam when the two corneal and iris/lens images are just touching is multiplied by a constant to give the ACD in millimetres (figure 3). In the original description of the method by Smith the constant was 1.40, while others (Barrett et al., 1996) have proposed more recently 1.31. Both constants have been determined using an optical pachymetry.

The Smith method has been validated by a number of authors (Barrett et al., 1996) (Douthwaite and Spence, 1986). It allows the clinician to obtain reliable estimates of axial ACD, without any attachments to the slit-lamp biomicroscope. The axial ACD estimates are accurate to within ± 0.25 mm (Smith, 1979), ± 0.2 mm (Jacobs, 1979) and ± 0.33 mm (Barrett et al., 1996) as compared to pachymetry and to within ± 0.42 mm, as compared to ultrasonography. There is no effect of the central corneal thickness on the ACD estimate made using this method (Osuobeni et al., 2003), which has also a minimum inter and intra observer variation (Osuobeni et al., 2000).

From birth to the age of 13 years, the mean value of ACD increases from 2.37 to 3.70 mm for Northern European boys, and from 2.39 to 3.62 mm for girls (Larsen, 1971). There is very little change in the mean anterior chamber depth from the teenage years to about 30 years, while there is a decline in the mean anterior chamber depth from 30 to 60 years, probably because of the increase of lens thickness (Fontana and Brubaker, 1980). Between this age range the typical value is around 2.5 mm. The depth and volume of the anterior chamber are also related to the degree of ametropia. Male subjects usually have larger anterior chamber dimensions than female subjects. There is a direct association between narrow anterior chamber angle and shallow anterior chamber depth (Wishart and Batterbury, 1992).

Consequently, the ACD quantification represents an indirect means of assessing the anterior chamber angle and identifying patients who are more likely to develop PACG. Usually eyes with ACD <2 mm are considered at risk (Wishart and Batterbury, 1992).

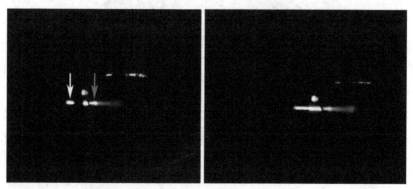

Fig. 3. Measurement of the anterior chamber depth using Smith's method. Yellow arrow indicates the focused horizontal corneal-imaged slit and red arrow the out-of-focus iris/lens-imaged slit (see text for details)

4. Gonioscopy

Gonioscopy still represents the gold standard for assessment of the angle. This technique was first developed by Trantas in the late 1800s and subsequently modified by Koeppe and Barkan to allow a direct visualization of the structure of the anterior chamber angle with a contact lens (Friedman and He, 2008). Nowadays however indirect gonioscopy (which relies on mirrors or prisms to reflect light from the angle to the viewer) is usually preferred because of several advantages over direct gonioscopy: the patient can be examined at the slit lamp using a variable magnification and there is no astigmatic aberration. Two lenses are commonly employed: the Zeiss-type and the Goldmann-type. The Zeiss-type lens has a 9-mm diameter corneal surface (radius of curvature 7.72 mm) and doesn't require a coupling agent. The Goldmann-type has larger base diameter (corneal surface 12 mm and radius of curvature 7.38 mm) and requires a coupling agent (thick artificial tears or hydroxypropyl methylcellulose) when placed on the cornea. Although use of Zeiss-type lens needs more training and expertise, it has undoubted advantages because leaves the anterior segment clear for later viewing of the posterior pole and compresses the cornea centrally, which in turns allows for greater dynamic assessment of the angle structures.

Moreover pressure on the larger base lenses can lead to compression over Schwalbe's line with a consequent alteration of angle's morphology.

Since illumination conditions and degree of pupil dilation may dramatically alter angle configuration, a strict assessment protocol should be followed: the patient should look straight ahead and should be examined in a dark room, using a 1-mm beam with adequate illumination to visualize angle structures (Weinreb and Friedman, as cited in (Friedman and He, 2008).

Three grading systems have been proposed for documenting angle findings seen in gonioscopy: Scheie (Scheie, 1957), Schaffer (Shaffer, 1960) and Spaeth (Spaeth, 1971) classification (table 1).

Scheie		Schaffer			Spaeth		
Classification	Findings	Classification	Findings	Angle width (deg.)	Classification		Findings
Wide open	All structures visible	Grade 4	Ciliary body is visible	35-45	Iris insertion	A B C D E	Anterior Behind In sclera Deep angle recess Extremely deep recess
Grade I	Iris root not visible	Grade 3	Scleral spur is visible	20-35	Width of angle recess		0, 10, 20, 30 and 40 degrees
Grade II	Ciliary body not visible	Grade 2	Only trabecular meshwork is visible	20	Peripheral iris configuration	S R Q	Steep Regular Queer
Grade III	Posterior trabecular meshwork not visible	Grade 1	Only Schwalbe's line is visible	≤ 10	12 o'clock pigmentation	0 1+ 2+ 3+ 4+	None Just visible Mild Moderately dense Dense
Grade IV	None of angle structures visible	Grade 0	Angle is closed	0			

Table 1. Angle grading systems

In the Scheie scheme grade zero represents a wide open angle. Grade 1 is a "slightly narrow" angle and the iris root is not visible; grade 2 means that the ciliary body is not visible while grade 3 means that the posterior (pigmented) trabecular meshwork is not visible. Grade 4 is a closed angle and therefore no angle structures are visible. Scheie believed that persons with grade 3 and grade 4 angles were at greatest risk of PACG.

The Shaffer system is currently the most popular grading system. It uses both angle width and angle structures to classify angle grade: this is confusing because sometimes width and structures seen may place an angle into different categories. In this grading system angles between 35 and 45 degrees are classified as grade 4, those between 20 and 35 as grade 3, those between 10 and 20 as grade 2 and those ≤10 as grade 1, with a closed angle (zero degrees) classified as grade 0. Angle width is often preferred to angle depth in the description of ACA, because the latter may differ in different locations. Taking into consideration the angle structures, Shaffer classification's grade 4 comprises all structures, grade 3 the structures up to the scleral spur, grade 2 up to the trabecular meshwork, in grade 1 only the Schwalbe's line is visible and in grade 0 none of the angle structures are visible.

Spaeth classification provides the most comprehensive approach to angle assessment. This classification includes three components: angular width of angle recess, configuration of the peripheral iris, insertion site of the iris root. The width of the angle recess is graded from 10 to 40 degrees. The iris configuration is reported as "r" (regular), "s" (steep, as in plateau iris configuration), or "q" (queer, or backward, bowing as may occur in pigment dispersion syndrome). The insertion of iris root ranges from A – anterior to the Schwalbe's line, B - behind Schwalbe's line, but anterior to scleral spur, C - posterior to scleral spur (i.e., scleral spur visible, but not ciliary body), D - ciliary body visible, and E - large amount of ciliary body visible. When the iris is appositional with the angle, the "apparent" iris insertion, seen without indentation, is noted as a letter placed in parenthesis, while the "actual" insertion is noted with a letter not placed in parenthesis. Finally the Spaeth system rates also the pigment of the posterior trabecular meshwork at 12 o'clock from 0 to 4+ (black pigmented meshwork) and the presence or absence of peripheral anterior synechiae (PAS). An example of wide open angle is given in figure 4.

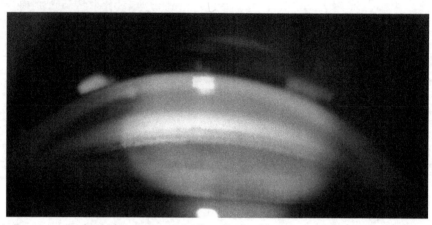

Fig. 4. Gonioscopy of a wide open angle. All angle structures are visible. From down to top: ciliary body band with some iris processes reaching the trabecular meshwork, scleral spur, pigmented (posterior) trabecular meshwork, nonpigmented (anterior) trabecular meshwork and Schwalbe's line delineated by some scattered pigment

Not many studies have been published on the reliability of the angle grading systems. Some authors have reported a weighted k values for inter-observer reproducibility of Shaffer classification in the ranges of 0.6 using a Goldmann-style lens (Foster et al., 2000b) (Aung et al., 2005). The Spaeth system has shown high reproducibility and comparability to UBM in 22 patients (Spaeth et al., 1995).

A quantitative grading of the angle has been proposed by some authors (Cockburn, 1980, Congdon et al., 1999), but has not gained popularity in clinical practice.

Once an angle is viewed and it is determined that there is iridotrabecular contact, it is necessary to determine whether the angle is appositionally closed or if there are permanent PAS. To pursue this task a gentle indentation with the goniolens is performed ("dynamic gonioscopy"). By indenting the central cornea (usually with a Zeiss-type lens) the aqueous is displaced into the peripheral anterior chamber where it bows the iris posteriorly and widens the chamber angle. This widening differentiates areas where the peripheral iris is permanently adherent to the peripheral cornea (i.e. PAS) from areas where the iris is merely reversibly apposed to the peripheral cornea.

Caution must be taken in distinguishing PAS from iris processes. Iris processes, either plastered across the surface of the angle or bridging from the peripheral iris to the angle structures, are pigmented strands continuous with and histologically identical to the iris. These are a normal variant and have no effect upon aqueous outflow. On the contrary PAS are abnormal adhesions of the peripheral iris to the angle structure that, if extensive enough, can eventually reduce trabecular outflow. Usually PAS tend to be wider (at least half of 1 clock hour in width) and are present to the level of the trabecular meshwork or higher.

Examples of PAS include the fibrovascular membrane formed in neovascular glaucoma, proliferating abnormal endothelial cells in the iridocorneal endothelial (ICE) syndromes, epithelialization of the angle due to epithelial ingrowth, or inflammatory trabecular and keratic precipitates in contact with an inflamed iris in uveitis.

The gonioscopic criteria for an occludable angle usually include: 1) trabecular meshwork invisible in 270° or more of the entire angle in the primary position of gaze without indentation and / or 2) angular width less than 20 degrees by the Shaffer grading (Kim and Jung, 1997). Often these criteria are used to identify angles that require treatment (i.e. iridotomy), although there is still no unanimous consensus (Friedman, 2001, Foster et al., 2002).

5. Pentacam

The Pentacam (Oculus, Inc., Lynnwood, WA, USA) is a rotating Scheimpflug camera with a short-wavelength slit light (475 nm, blue light-emitting diode laser) that is able to take 25 slit images of the anterior segment of the eye in 2 seconds with 500 true elevation points in each image. Any eye movement is detected (and the results corrected) by a second camera. A three-dimensional model of the anterior segment can therefore be built with the obtained data including the corneal thickness, corneal topographic parameters, central ACD, anterior chamber angle (ACA), anterior chamber volume (ACV) and other parameters. Interestingly the software doesn't require any manual initiation. Two chamber angles for each chosen meridian are provided. It is noteworthy to mention that ACA is calculated by lengthening the posterior cornea and the iris contour to compute the chamber angle using an interpolation method, because Pentacam cannot image the angle recess and scleral spur. Several studies have investigated the reliability of Pentacam (and other Scheimpflug cameras) in measuring ACA. Lam (Lam et al., 2002) found on 25 healthy subjects with open angles that the 95% limit of agreement on repeat measurements of angle width was 5°, and inter-observer agreement was 6°. Rabsilber showed good reliability of Pentacam in assessing ACA in 76 healthy volunteers (Rabsilber et al., 2006). Although measurement of the ACA obtained with the Pentacam seem to correlate significantly with Shaffer's grade determined by gonioscopy, a certain discrepancy has been reported between ACA and ACD measured by Pentacam and ultrasound biomicroscopy (UBM) or anterior-segment optical coherence tomography (AS-OCT) in eyes with a narrow angle (Liang et al.) (Kurita et al., 2009) (Mou et al.). This may be due to the inability of the Pentacam to visualize the most peripheral part of the iris. Alternatively the placement of an eye cup, which is necessary for UBM examination, may be responsible of a flattening of the cornea which in turns leads to an artificial reduction of the ACD. Hence ACV seems to be the most efficient parameter to screen patients with POAG or POAG suspect using the Pentacam (Kurita et al., 2009). However although Pentacam non-contact approach to angle assessment is highly appealing for screening purposes, it is limited to visualization of only the angle recess. Scheimpflug photography indeed does not display the retroiridal structures or the ciliary body, which are of great interest in glaucoma diagnosis.

6. Ultrasound Biomicroscopy (UBM)

Ultrasound-based diagnostic imaging uses a probe containing a piezoelectric transducer to emit a sound wave which propagates through tissues and is partially reflected –echoes-from anatomic structures differing in acoustic impedance (density × speed of sound). Some of the echoes return to the transducer and are converted back into voltages and amplified. The range of each echo is proportional to the time delay between sound wave emission and echo return, specifically, $r = ct/2$, where r is the range, c is the speed of sound (1532 m/s at 37°C in normal saline) and t is the time (Ursea and Silverman).

Each pulse/echo event thus provides information along one line of sight. By mechanically scanning the probe, information along an ordered series of lines is obtained. By converting echo amplitude into pixel intensity, a 2D cross-sectional B-scan image is then produced.

Ultrasonic imaging resolution improves by increasing the frequency of the transducer. However higher frequencies produce a correspondingly smaller wavelength which is less able to penetrate the tissues.

Ultrasound systems utilizing probes of approximately 35 MHz or more have come to be known as "ultrasound biomicroscopy" (UBM) or 'very high-frequency ultrasound systems'. Such systems have a tissue penetration of only 5 mm but provide lateral and axial resolutions approximately of 40 and 20 microns, respectively. They allow therefore for a more detailed assessment of the anterior ocular structures than was available using traditional B-scan ultrasound.

UBM systems are now produced by numerous companies, with probes ranging from 50 to 80 MHz. Handheld UBM probes are now often equipped with acoustically transparent, fluid-filled 'bubble tips' that can be placed directly onto the globe. These obviate the use of water-baths or scleral shells for acoustic coupling, greatly simplifying the examination and allowing the patient to be examined in a sitting position.

UBM provides both quantitative and qualitative information on the anterior segment of the eye. Pavlin and coworkers carried out the first clinical UBM study of the ocular structures in glaucomatous patients in the early 1990s (Pavlin et al., 1992). Subsequently many authors proposed different biometric parameters to characterize the angle and anterior segment. The most common include: angle-opening distance (AOD), trabecular-iris angle (TIA), trabecular–ciliary process distance (TCPD), iris thickness (ID), angle-recess area (ARA), iris ciliary process distance (ICPD), iris-lens contact distance (ILCD) (see Table 2 and figure 5 for details).

AOD and ARA can be measured at various distances from the sclera spur. Theoretically, 500 μm is the appropriate distance because it approximates the length of the trabecular meshwork. However, a longer measurement distance of 750 μm uses information from a large region of the image and may be more robust, especially for ARA, since it is less affected by local iris surface undulations. Henzan and coworkers studied the performance of the UBM parameters in differentiating primary angle closure/primary angle closure suspect from non-occludable angle eyes through the receiver operating characteristic (ROC) curve and the area under the curve (AUC). They found that AOD_{500} and TIA under light conditions had the greatest AUC of 0.94. The ideal cutoff values for the AOD_{500} and TIA under light conditions determined with the Youden index (=sensitivity - [1 - specificity]) were 0.17 mm (sensitivity, 0.82; specificity, 0.96) and 15.2 degrees (sensitivity, 0.83; specificity, 0.93), respectively (Henzan et al.).

A limitation of these findings is that UBM measurements of angle structures can be influenced by a number of variables including patient's age and gender (Friedman et al., 2008), direction of gaze, accommodation, room illumination, variation in image acquisition (position of the probe, meridians scanned) (Friedman and He, 2008).

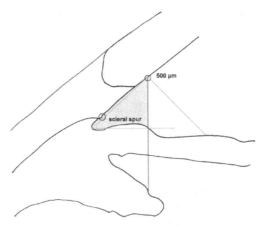

Fig. 5. Diagram illustrating several biometric descriptors of the angle, including angle-opening distance (blue line), iris thickness (yellow line), trabecular-iris angle (red line), trabecular-ciliary process distance (green line) and angle recess area (light blue area). In this example measurements are made 500 μm from the sclera spur

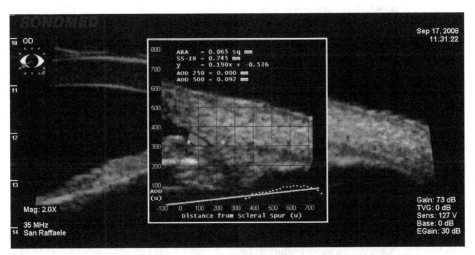

Fig. 6. Screen shot of the analysis software from the UBM Pro 2000 (UBM Pro 2000, Paradigm Medical Industries, Salt Lake City, UT, USA)

One would expect high variability in the measurements because of the partly subjective nature of the caliper placement on visualized anatomic landmarks. On the contrary the reported reproducibility of analyses on single UBM images seems to be pretty good.

Marchini showed high reproducibility in a paper comparing UBM parameters in angle closure patients (range of coefficient of variation 1.4 -16%) (Marchini et al., 1998).

Even better reproducibility was reported by Gohdo when measuring the ciliary body thickness (CBT) one and two millimeters posterior to the scleral spur (coefficient of variation < 2.5%) (Gohdo et al., 2000).

In any case image analysis using calipers to mark each structure takes a large amount of time due to the need to place a cursor at each point for any given measurement.

To overcome this issue, Ishikawa and colleagues created a semi-automated program (UBM Pro 2000, Paradigm Medical Industries, Salt Lake City, UT, USA) that provides several important parameters once the scleral spur is identified (figure 6) (Ishikawa et al., 2000).

Parameter	Description	Range*		References
		Occludable angle (OA)	Nonoccludable angle (NOA)	
AOD_{500}	Distance from cornea to iris at 500 µm from the scleral spur	0.11± 0.04	0.29 ± 0.13	(Henzan et al.)
TIA	Angle formed from angle recess to points 500 µm from scleral spur on corneal endothelium and perpendicular on surface of iris	10.3±3.9	24.2± 9.3	(Henzan et al.)
TCPD	Measured from point on endothelium 500 µm from scleral spur perpendicularly through iris to ciliary process	0.62 ± 0.11	0.77±0.16	(Henzan et al.)
ID	Measured from perpendicular 500 µm from scleral spur	0.40 ±0.05	0.41±0.05	(Henzan et al.)
ARA_{750}	Area of triangle between angle recess, iris and cornea 750 µm from scleral spur	0.10±0.08	0.13 ±0.01	(Friedman et al., 2003) for NOA (Yoo et al., 2007) for OA
ICPD	Distance from the posterior iris surface to the ciliary process perpendicular 500 µm from scleral spur	0.39± 0.21	0.40± 0.10	(Sihota et al., 2005)
ILCD	Length of contact between surfaces of lens and iris	0.79±0.22	0.98± 0.41	(Sihota et al., 2005)

*All values (mean±standard deviation) are in mm except TIA which is in degrees and ARA_{500} which is in mm².

Abbreviations: AOD=angle-opening distance; TIA=trabecular-iris angle; TCPD=trabecular–ciliary process distance; ID:iris thickness; ARA=angle-recess area; ICPD=iris ciliary process distance; ILCD=iris-lens contact distance;

Table 2. Biometric parameters used in UBM for characterizing the angle and anterior segment in subjects with an occludable/nonoccludable angle

The software calculates AOD_{250}, AOD_{500}, ARA_{750} and performs linear regression analysis of consecutive AODs, producing two figures: the acceleration and the y-intercept. Acceleration tells how rapidly the angle is getting deeper, using the tangent of the angle instead of degrees as the unit. The y-intercept refers to the distance between the scleral spur and the iris surface along the perpendicular to the trabecular meshwork plane.

Acceleration and the y-intercept can be negative numbers. A negative number for acceleration means that the angle has an almost normal configuration at its peripheral part and becomes very shallow or is attached to the cornea at its central part. A negative y-intercept means that the angle recess is very shallow or is attached to the cornea at its periphery, whereas it is relatively wide centrally. According to Ishikawa and colleagues this software dramatically improves the overall reproducibility, with a coefficient of variation ranging between 7.3 and 2.5 for the various parameters (Ishikawa et al., 2000).

UBM gives also valuable qualitative information which helps in the diagnosis and in the management of several ocular diseases. In plateau iris syndrome UBM well demonstrates the ciliary body anteriorly positioned compressing the iridocorneal angle and placing the peripheral iris in apposition to the trabecular meshwork (figure 7).

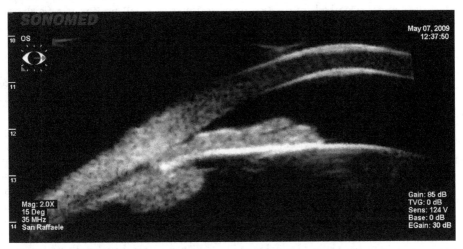

Fig. 7. Ultrasound biomicroscopy view of an eye with plateau iris syndrome

In pigment dispersion syndrome UBM shows an open angle, a characteristic concave iris and a ciliary body rotated posteriorly (figure 8).

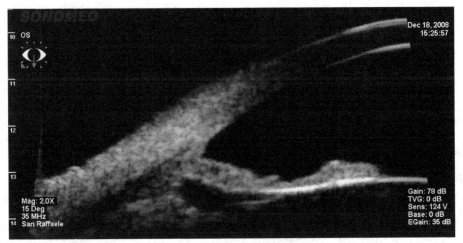

Fig. 8. Ultrasound biomicroscopy view of an eye with pigment dispersion syndrome

Angle recession, intraocular foreign bodies, ciliary body cysts are also easily detectable by UBM. Lastly UBM may represent a useful tool for the planning and guidance of glaucoma surgery, including the evaluation of filtering blebs, sclerectomy and canaloplasty, as well as the diagnosis and evaluation of postoperative complications.

7. Anterior segment optical coherence tomography (AS-OCT)

Optical coherence tomography (OCT) of the eye was first described by Huang and coworkers at the Massachusetts Institute of Technology (Boston, MA, USA) in 1991 (Huang et al., 1991). OCT uses a near-infrared light that is directed throughout ocular tissues. While most of the light is absorbed by the tissues or scattered, a small portion is reflected and collected by an interferometer in order to produce an image. In time-domain OCT, the reference mirror is mechanically scanned in the range axis, and this allows determination of the range to optical reflections along the tissue path, which are represented by interference fringes in the OCT signal.

OCT was initially developed only for retinal imaging; in 1994 Izatt et al. (Izatt et al., 1994) for the first time used it also for imaging the anterior chamber (anterior segment OCT, AS-OCT). Since then, AS-OCT has rapidly become popular for ACA assessment.

Originally anterior and posterior segment imaging used the same wavelength (830 nm). Subsequently a longer wavelength of 1310 nm was preferred for AS-OCT. This increases the depth of penetration by reducing the amount of light scattered by the sclera and limbus, allowing for visualization of the ACA morphology in greater detail. In addition, the 1310 nm light incident on the cornea is strongly absorbed by water in the ocular media, with only 10% reaching the retina. This enables the AS-OCT to utilize higher power, enhancing imaging speed and eliminating motion artifacts (Quek et al.). The Visante™ OCT (Carl Zeiss Meditec, Dublin, CA, USA) and the SL-OCT (Heidelberg Engineering, GmbH, Dossenheim, Germany) are 2 commercially available devices which use this wavelength providing an axial and transverse resolution of 18 μm and 60 μm, respectively, for the Visante and <25 μm and 20–100 μm for the SL-OCT (Quek et al.). SL-OCT incorporates OCT technology into a modified slit-lamp biomicroscopy system: this requires slower image acquisition speed and more operator skills.

More recently the new frequency (Fourier) domain OCTs have been developed, where the broadband signal is broken into a spectrum using a grating or linear detector array (i.e. sensitive detectors arranged in grating or single row), and depth is determined from the Fourier transform of the spectrum without motion along the reference arm (Ursea and Silverman). The fast readout speed of the detectors (typically tens of kilohertz) allows acquisition at video frame rates (30 fps) while the multiplexed scheme provides a signal-to-noise ratio (SNR) advantage over time domain OCT (TD-OCT). Fourier (also called Spectral) domain OCTs (SD-OCTs) allows scans at a rate of 26,000 A-scans per second and more images to be taken in a single pass. These devices produce therefore detailed cross-sectional images of structures at an axial resolution of 5 μm and a transverse resolution of 15 μm.

The RTVue (Optovue Inc.,Fremont, CA, USA), the Cirrus high-definition OCT (HD-OCT) 4.0 (Cirrus; Carl Zeiss Meditec Inc.) and the OPKO Spectral OCT SLO (OPKO Health, Inc.) are all SD-OCT systems that can be used for either retinal or anterior segment imaging (when used with a corneal adaptor module).

AS-OCTs provide same type of ACA measurements of UBM, with the same advantages and limitations (i.e. they are influenced by patient's age and gender, direction of gaze, accommodation, room illumination, meridians scanned). Furthermore, likewise UBM, some AS-OCTS have a built-in semi-automated software which offers the most common biometric parameters of ACA after the manual localization of the scleral spur (figure 9) (table 3). Contradictory results are present in literature on the agreement between UBM and AS-OCT in quantitative ACA measurement and detection of narrow angles. Some authors have found the two methods to be quite similar (Radhakrishnan et al., 2005, Dada et al., 2007); others have shown poor agreement (Mansouri et al.). In a study including 32 patients Wang et al. have reported that low-resolution OCT is similar to UBM for most of the studied angle measurements, while high-resolution OCT tends to give higher measurements than both low-resolution OCT and UBM. Furthermore AS-OCT measurements seem more reproducible than those from UBM (Wang et al., 2009). Likewise UBM, AS-OCT may be used for qualitative evaluation of ACA in a variety of ocular diseases (plateau iris syndrome, pigment dispersion syndrome, etc.) and it is undoubtedly safer than UBM in the evaluation of filtering blebs because AS-OCT is non-contact technique.

Parameter	Description	Range*		References
		Occludable angle (OA)	Nonoccludable angle (NOA)	
AOD$_{500\ nasal}$	Distance from cornea to iris at 500 μm from the scleral spur	0.33±0.14	0.50±0.21	(Grewal et al.)
AOD$_{500}$ temporal	See above	0.30±0.11	0.51±0.22	(Grewal et al.)
TISA $_{500nasal}$	Trapezoidal area with the following boundaries: anteriorly, AOD500; posteriorly, a line drawn from the scleral spur perpendicular to the plane of the inner scleral wall to the opposing iris; superiorly, the inner corneo-scleral wall; and inferiorly, the iris surface.	0.23±0.14	0.34±0.11	(Grewal et al.)
TISA 500temporal	See above	0.23 ±0.14	0.33±0.12	(Grewal et al.)
ARA$_{750\ nasal}$	Area of triangle between angle recess, iris and cornea 750 μm from scleral spur	0.08	0.29	(Pekmezci et al., 2009)
ARA$_{750temporal}$	See above	0.09	0.28	(Pekmezci et al., 2009)

*All values (mean±standard deviation) are in mm except ARA and TISA which are in mm².
Abbreviations: AOD=angle-opening distance; TISA=trabecular-iris space area; ARA=angle recess area;

Table 3. Most common biometric parameters used in AS-OCT for characterizing the angle and anterior segment in subjects with an occludable/non-occludable angle

Compared to UBM, AS-OCT is a technique more rapid, more easily practiced by a technician, better tolerated because requires no contact. A limitation of AS-OCT is that it doesn't allow visualizing the ciliary body and the supra-choroidal space. Using gonioscopy as reference standard several authors have shown sensitivities of AS-OCT in detecting narrow angles up to 98%, although often the specificity was significantly lower (between 55 and 85%) (Nolan et al., 2007, See et al., 2007) (Pekmezci et al., 2009). AS-OCT tends indeed to detect more closed ACAs than gonioscopy, particularly in the superior and inferior quadrants (Nolan et al., 2007, Sakata et al., 2008a).

Angle recess area at 750 μm from scleral spur (ARA$_{750}$) and angle-opening distance at 500 μm from the scleral spur (AOD$_{500}$) seem to have the highest correlation with gonioscopy (Pekmezci et al., 2009).

Radhakrishnan indicated an AOD 500 cutoff of 190 μm for detecting occludable angles (Radhakrishnan et al., 2005).

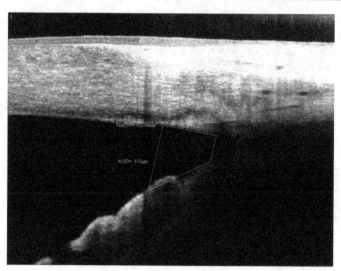

Fig. 9. Screen shot of the ACA measurements (angle-opening distance and trabecular-iris space area at 500) provided by the analysis software of RTVue OCT (Optovue Inc., Fremont, CA, USA)

As for UBM, also for AS-OCT angle classification hinges on accurate localization of the scleral spur, as it is used as the reference point for all the other quantitative measurements. However, this localization is not always easy to be found possibly generating non-negligible intra- and inter-observer variance.

The sclera spur can be defined as the point where there is a change in curvature of the inner surface of the angle wall, often appearing as an inward protrusion of the sclera.

Studies investigating the visibility of the sclera spur with AS-OCT showed a visualization between 70% and 78.9% of analyzed images (Sakata et al., 2008b) (Wong et al., 2009). Most of the cases in which the scleral spur could not be detected occurred in images in which the internal surface of the sclera formed a smooth continuous line (with no inward protrusion of the sclera or change in its curvature) or in images with suboptimal quality. Less frequently, the scleral spur was difficult to identify owing to an atypical contour of the inner corneoscleral wall.

Despite the possible difficulty in localization of sclera spur, several studies have shown low intra- and inter-observer variability of AS-OCT ACA measurements, which tends to increase only when AS-OCT image acquisitions are performed by less-experienced operators (Khor et al., Tan et al., Muller et al., 2006, Li et al., 2007) In a recent study the range of intra-observer variability in image analysis was from 9.4% to 12.5% in the experts and from 4.2% to 17.4% in the non-experts. Inter-observer variability was 10.7% in the experts and 10.2% in the non-experts. The reproducibility was high, 0.875 and 0.942 in the experts and 0.906 in the non-experts (Tan et al.).

8. Conclusions

Several new technologies are becoming more and more popular for the assessment of the angle and anterior segment. They can provide useful additional qualitative information to those obtained with the traditional tools (slit-lamp and gonioscopy). Furthermore they can offer also precise ACA measurements which however are often not comparable each other. Hence we believe that one should build its normative data - using gonioscopy as reference standard- to use them for screening for angle closure purposes.

However, as technologies evolve, it is likely that the diagnostic performance of different techniques/instruments may soon reach acceptable specificity and sensitivity levels for mass screening for angle closure.

9. References

Alsbirk, P.H. (1986). Limbal and axial chamber depth variations. A population study in Eskimos. *Acta Ophthalmol (Copenh)*, Vol. 64, No. 6, (Dec 1986) pp. (593-600), 0001-639X (Print)

Aung, T., Lim, M.C., Chan, Y.H., Rojanapongpun, P. & Chew, P.T. (2005). Configuration of the drainage angle, intraocular pressure, and optic disc cupping in subjects with chronic angle-closure glaucoma. *Ophthalmology*, Vol. 112, No. 1, (Jan 2005) pp. (28-32), 1549-4713 (Electronic)

Barrett, B.T., McGraw, P.V., Murray, L.A. & Murgatroyd, P. (1996). Anterior chamber depth measurement in clinical practice. *Optom Vis Sci*, Vol. 73, No. 7, (Jul 1996) pp. (482-486), 1040-5488 (Print)

Cockburn, D.M. (1980). A new method for gonioscopic grading of the anterior chamber angle. *Am J Optom Physiol Opt*, Vol. 57, No. 4, (Apr 1980) pp. (258-261), 0093-7002 (Print)

Congdon, N.G., Spaeth, G.L., Augsburger, J., Klancnik, J., Jr., Patel, K. & Hunter, D.G. (1999). proposed simple method for measurement in the anterior chamber angle: biometric gonioscopy. *Ophthalmology*, Vol. 106, No. 11, (Nov 1999) pp. (2161-2167), 0161-6420 (Print)

Congdon, N.G., Youlin, Q., Quigley, H., Hung, P.T., Wang, T.H., Ho, T.C. & Tielsch, J.M. (1997). Biometry and primary angle-closure glaucoma among Chinese, white, and black populations. *Ophthalmology*, Vol. 104, No. 9, (Sep 1997) pp. (1489-1495), 0161-6420 (Print)

Dada, T., Sihota, R., Gadia, R., Aggarwal, A., Mandal, S. & Gupta, V. (2007). Comparison of anterior segment optical coherence tomography and ultrasound biomicroscopy for assessment of the anterior segment. *J Cataract Refract Surg*, Vol. 33, No. 5, (May 2007) pp. (837-840), 0886-3350 (Print)

Douthwaite, W.A. & Spence, D. (1986). Slit-lamp measurement of the anterior chamber depth. *Br J Ophthalmol*, Vol. 70, No. 3, (Mar 1986) pp. (205-208), 0007-1161 (Print)

Fontana, S.T. & Brubaker, R.F. (1980). Volume and depth of the anterior chamber in the normal aging human eye. *Arch Ophthalmol*, Vol. 98, No. 10, (Oct 1980) pp. (1803-1808), 0003-9950 (Print)

Foster, P.J., Buhrmann, R., Quigley, H.A. & Johnson, G.J. (2002). The definition and classification of glaucoma in prevalence surveys. *Br J Ophthalmol*, Vol. 86, No. 2, (Feb 2002) pp. (238-242), 0007-1161 (Print)

Foster, P.J., Devereux, J.G., Alsbirk, P.H., Lee, P.S., Uranchimeg, D., Machin, D., Johnson, G.J. & Baasanhu, J. (2000a). Detection of gonioscopically occludable angles and primary angle closure glaucoma by estimation of limbal chamber depth in Asians: modified grading scheme. *Br J Ophthalmol*, Vol. 84, No. 2, (Feb 2000a) pp. (186-192), 0007-1161 (Print)

Foster, P.J., Oen, F.T., Machin, D., Ng, T.P., Devereux, J.G., Johnson, G.J., Khaw, P.T. & Seah, S.K. (2000b). The prevalence of glaucoma in Chinese residents of Singapore: a cross-sectional population survey of the Tanjong Pagar district. *Arch Ophthalmol,* Vol. 118, No. 8, (Aug 2000b) pp. (1105-1111), 0003-9950 (Print)

Friedman, D.S. (2001). Who needs an iridotomy? *Br J Ophthalmol,* Vol. 85, No. 9, (Sep 2001) pp. (1019-1021), 0007-1161 (Print)

Friedman, D.S., Gazzard, G., Foster, P., Devereux, J., Broman, A., Quigley, H., Tielsch, J. & Seah, S. (2003). Ultrasonographic biomicroscopy, Scheimpflug photography, and novel provocative tests in contralateral eyes of Chinese patients initially seen with acute angle closure. *Arch Ophthalmol,* Vol. 121, No. 5, (May 2003) pp. (633-642), 0003-9950 (Print)

Friedman, D.S., Gazzard, G., Min, C.B., Broman, A.T., Quigley, H., Tielsch, J., Seah, S. & Foster, P.J. (2008). Age and sex variation in angle findings among normal Chinese subjects: a comparison of UBM, Scheimpflug, and gonioscopic assessment of the anterior chamber angle. *J Glaucoma,* Vol. 17, No. 1, (Jan-Feb 2008) pp. (5-10), 1057-0829 (Print)

Friedman, D.S. & He, M. (2008). Anterior chamber angle assessment techniques. *Surv Ophthalmol,* Vol. 53, No. 3, (May-Jun 2008) pp. (250-273), 0039-6257 (Print)

Gohdo, T., Tsumura, T., Iijima, H., Kashiwagi, K. & Tsukahara, S. (2000). Ultrasound biomicroscopic study of ciliary body thickness in eyes with narrow angles. *Am J Ophthalmol,* Vol. 129, No. 3, (Mar 2000) pp. (342-346), 0002-9394 (Print)

Grewal, D.S., Brar, G.S., Jain, R. & Grewal, S.P. Comparison of scheimpflug imaging and spectral domain anterior segment optical coherence tomography for detection of narrow anterior chamber angles. *Eye (Lond),* (Feb 18, 1476-5454 (Electronic)

Henzan, I.M., Tomidokoro, A., Uejo, C., Sakai, H., Sawaguchi, S., Iwase, A. & Araie, M. Comparison of Ultrasound Biomicroscopic Configurations Among Primary Angle Closure, Its Suspects, and Nonoccludable Angles: The Kumejima Study. *Am J Ophthalmol,* (Mar 28, 1879-1891 (Electronic)

Huang, D., Swanson, E.A., Lin, C.P., Schuman, J.S., Stinson, W.G., Chang, W., Hee, M.R., Flotte, T., Gregory, K., Puliafito, C.A. & et al. (1991). Optical coherence tomography. *Science,* Vol. 254, No. 5035, (Nov 22 1991) pp. (1178-1181), 0036-8075 (Print)

Ishikawa, H., Liebmann, J.M. & Ritch, R. (2000). Quantitative assessment of the anterior segment using ultrasound biomicroscopy. *Curr Opin Ophthalmol,* Vol. 11, No. 2, (Apr 2000) pp. (133-139), 1040-8738 (Print)

Izatt, J.A., Hee, M.R., Swanson, E.A., Lin, C.P., Huang, D., Schuman, J.S., Puliafito, C.A. & Fujimoto, J.G. (1994). Micrometer-scale resolution imaging of the anterior eye in vivo with optical coherence tomography. *Arch Ophthalmol,* Vol. 112, No. 12, (Dec 1994) pp. (1584-1589), 0003-9950 (Print)

Jacobs, I.H. (1979). Anterior chamber depth measurement using the split-lamp microscope. *Am J Ophthalmol,* Vol. 88, No. 2, (Aug 1979) pp. (236-238), 0002-9394 (Print)

Kanski, J.J. (2007). *Clinical ophthalmology: a systematic approach,* (6th), Butterworth Heinemann Elsevier, 9780080449692 (hbk.)

Khor, W.B., Sakata, L.M., Friedman, D.S., Narayanaswamy, A., Lavanya, R., Perera, S.A. & Aung, T. Evaluation of scanning protocols for imaging the anterior chamber angle with anterior segment-optical coherence tomography. *J Glaucoma,* Vol. 19, No. 6, (Aug 365-368), 1536-481X (Electronic)

Kim, Y.Y. & Jung, H.R. (1997). Clarifying the nomenclature for primary angle-closure glaucoma. *Surv Ophthalmol*, Vol. 42, No. 2, (Sep-Oct 1997) pp. (125-136), 0039-6257 (Print)

Kurita, N., Mayama, C., Tomidokoro, A., Aihara, M. & Araie, M. (2009). Potential of the pentacam in screening for primary angle closure and primary angle closure suspect. *J Glaucoma*, Vol. 18, No. 7, (Sep 2009) pp. (506-512), 1536-481X (Electronic)

Lam, A.K., Chan, R., Woo, G.C., Pang, P.C. & Chiu, R. (2002). Intra-observer and inter-observer repeatability of anterior eye segment analysis system (EAS-1000) in anterior chamber configuration. *Ophthalmic Physiol Opt*, Vol. 22, No. 6, (Nov 2002) pp. (552-559), 0275-5408 (Print)

Larsen, J.S. (1971). The sagittal growth of the eye. 1. Ultrasonic measurement of the depth of the anterior chamber from birth to puberty. *Acta Ophthalmol (Copenh)*, Vol. 49, No. 2, 1971) pp. (239-262), 0001-639X (Print)

Lens, A., Nemeth, S.C., Ledford, J.K. (2008). *Ocular Anatomy and Physiology*, (Second Edition), Slack Incorporated, 978-1-55642-792-3,

Li, H., Leung, C.K., Cheung, C.Y., Wong, L., Pang, C.P., Weinreb, R.N. & Lam, D.S. (2007). Repeatability and reproducibility of anterior chamber angle measurement with anterior segment optical coherence tomography. *Br J Ophthalmol*, Vol. 91, No. 11, (Nov 2007) pp. (1490-1492), 0007-1161 (Print)

Liang, J., Liu, W., Xing, X., Liu, H., Zhao, S. & Ji, J. Evaluation of the agreement between Pentacam and ultrasound biomicroscopy measurements of anterior chamber depth in Chinese patients with primary angle-closure glaucoma. *Jpn J Ophthalmol*, Vol. 54, No. 4, (Jul 361-362), 1613-2246 (Electronic)

Mansouri, K., Sommerhalder, J. & Shaarawy, T. Prospective comparison of ultrasound biomicroscopy and anterior segment optical coherence tomography for evaluation of anterior chamber dimensions in European eyes with primary angle closure. *Eye (Lond)*, Vol. 24, No. 2, (Feb 233-239), 1476-5454 (Electronic)

Marchini, G., Pagliarusco, A., Toscano, A., Tosi, R., Brunelli, C. & Bonomi, L. (1998). Ultrasound biomicroscopic and conventional ultrasonographic study of ocular dimensions in primary angle-closure glaucoma. *Ophthalmology*, Vol. 105, No. 11, (Nov 1998) pp. (2091-2098), 0161-6420 (Print)

Mou, D., Fu, J., Li, S., Wang, L., Wang, X., Wu, G., Qing, G., Peng, Y. & Wang, N. Narrow- and open-angle measurements with anterior-segment optical coherence tomography and Pentacam. *Ophthalmic Surg Lasers Imaging*, Vol. 41, No. 6, (Nov 1 622-628), 1938-2375 (Electronic)

Muller, M., Dahmen, G., Porksen, E., Geerling, G., Laqua, H., Ziegler, A. & Hoerauf, H. (2006). Anterior chamber angle measurement with optical coherence tomography: intraobserver and interobserver variability. *J Cataract Refract Surg*, Vol. 32, No. 11, (Nov 2006) pp. (1803-1808), 0886-3350 (Print)

Ng, W.S., Ang, G.S. & Azuara-Blanco, A. (2008). Laser peripheral iridoplasty for angle-closure. *Cochrane Database Syst Rev*, No. 3, 2008) pp. (CD006746), 1469-493X (Electronic)

Nolan, W.P., Baasanhu, J., Undraa, A., Uranchimeg, D., Ganzorig, S. & Johnson, G.J. (2003). Screening for primary angle closure in Mongolia: a randomised controlled trial to determine whether screening and prophylactic treatment will reduce the incidence of primary angle closure glaucoma in an east Asian population. *Br J Ophthalmol*, Vol. 87, No. 3, (Mar 2003) pp. (271-274), 0007-1161 (Print)

Nolan, W.P., See, J.L., Chew, P.T., Friedman, D.S., Smith, S.D., Radhakrishnan, S., Zheng, C., Foster, P.J. & Aung, T. (2007). Detection of primary angle closure using anterior segment optical coherence tomography in Asian eyes. *Ophthalmology*, Vol. 114, No. 1, (Jan 2007) pp. (33-39), 1549-4713 (Electronic)

Osuobeni, E.P., Hegarty, C. & Gunvant, P. (2003). The effect of central corneal thickness on estimates of the anterior chamber depth. *Clin Exp Optom*, Vol. 86, No. 6, (Nov 2003) pp. (371-375), 0816-4622 (Print)

Osuobeni, E.P., Oduwaiye, K.A. & Ogbuehi, K.C. (2000). Intra-observer repeatability and inter-observer agreement of the Smith method of measuring the anterior chamber depth. *Ophthalmic Physiol Opt*, Vol. 20, No. 2, (Mar 2000) pp. (153-159), 0275-5408 (Print)

Pavlin, C.J., Harasiewicz, K. & Foster, F.S. (1992). Ultrasound biomicroscopy of anterior segment structures in normal and glaucomatous eyes. *Am J Ophthalmol*, Vol. 113, No. 4, (Apr 15 1992) pp. (381-389), 0002-9394 (Print)

Pekmezci, M., Porco, T.C. & Lin, S.C. (2009). Anterior segment optical coherence tomography as a screening tool for the assessment of the anterior segment angle. *Ophthalmic Surg Lasers Imaging*, Vol. 40, No. 4, (Jul-Aug 2009) pp. (389-398), 1542-8877 (Print)

Quek, D.T., Nongpiur, M.E., Perera, S.A. & Aung, T. Angle imaging: advances and challenges. *Indian J Ophthalmol*, Vol. 59 Suppl, (Jan S69-75), 1998-3689 (Electronic)

Quigley, H.A. & Broman, A.T. (2006). The number of people with glaucoma worldwide in 2010 and 2020. *Br J Ophthalmol*, Vol. 90, No. 3, (Mar 2006) pp. (262-267), 0007-1161 (Print)

Rabsilber, T.M., Khoramnia, R. & Auffarth, G.U. (2006). Anterior chamber measurements using Pentacam rotating Scheimpflug camera. *J Cataract Refract Surg*, Vol. 32, No. 3, (Mar 2006) pp. (456-459), 0886-3350 (Print)

Radhakrishnan, S., Goldsmith, J., Huang, D., Westphal, V., Dueker, D.K., Rollins, A.M., Izatt, J.A. & Smith, S.D. (2005). Comparison of optical coherence tomography and ultrasound biomicroscopy for detection of narrow anterior chamber angles. *Arch Ophthalmol*, Vol. 123, No. 8, (Aug 2005) pp. (1053-1059), 0003-9950 (Print)

Ritch, R., Tham, C.C. & Lam, D.S. (2007). Argon laser peripheral iridoplasty (ALPI): an update. *Surv Ophthalmol*, Vol. 52, No. 3, (May-Jun 2007) pp. (279-288), 0039-6257 (Print)

Rufer, F., Schroder, A., Klettner, A., Frimpong-Boateng, A., Roider, J.B. & Erb, C. Anterior chamber depth and iridocorneal angle in healthy White subjects: effects of age, gender and refraction. *Acta Ophthalmol*, Vol. 88, No. 8, (Dec 885-890), 1755-3768 (Electronic)

Sakata, L.M., Lavanya, R., Friedman, D.S., Aung, H.T., Gao, H., Kumar, R.S., Foster, P.J. & Aung, T. (2008a). Comparison of gonioscopy and anterior segment ocular coherence tomography in detecting angle closure in different quadrants of the anterior chamber angle. *Ophthalmology*, Vol. 115, No. 5, (May 2008a) pp. (769-774), 1549-4713 (Electronic)

Sakata, L.M., Lavanya, R., Friedman, D.S., Aung, H.T., Seah, S.K., Foster, P.J. & Aung, T. (2008b). Assessment of the scleral spur in anterior segment optical coherence tomography images. *Arch Ophthalmol*, Vol. 126, No. 2, (Feb 2008b) pp. (181-185), 0003-9950 (Print)

Scheie, H.G. (1957). Width and pigmentation of the angle of the anterior chamber; a system of grading by gonioscopy. *AMA Arch Ophthalmol,* Vol. 58, No. 4, (Oct 1957) pp. (510-512), 0096-6339 (Print)

See, J.L., Chew, P.T., Smith, S.D., Nolan, W.P., Chan, Y.H., Huang, D., Zheng, C., Foster, P.J., Aung, T. & Friedman, D.S. (2007). Changes in anterior segment morphology in response to illumination and after laser iridotomy in Asian eyes: an anterior segment OCT study. *Br J Ophthalmol,* Vol. 91, No. 11, (Nov 2007) pp. (1485-1489), 0007-1161 (Print)

Shaffer, R.N. (1960). Primary glaucomas. Gonioscopy, ophthalmoscopy and perimetry. *Trans Am Acad Ophthalmol Otolaryngol,* Vol. 64, (Mar-Apr 1960) pp. (112-127), 0002-7154 (Print)

Sihota, R., Dada, T., Gupta, R., Lakshminarayan, P. & Pandey, R.M. (2005). Ultrasound biomicroscopy in the subtypes of primary angle closure glaucoma. *J Glaucoma,* Vol. 14, No. 5, (Oct 2005) pp. (387-391), 1057-0829 (Print)

Smith, R.J. (1979). A new method of estimating the depth of the anterior chamber. *Br J Ophthalmol,* Vol. 63, No. 4, (Apr 1979) pp. (215-220), 0007-1161 (Print)

Spaeth, G.L. (1971). The normal development of the human anterior chamber angle: a new system of descriptive grading. *Trans Ophthalmol Soc U K,* Vol. 91, 1971) pp. (709-739), 0078-5334 (Print)

Spaeth, G.L., Aruajo, S. & Azuara, A. (1995). Comparison of the configuration of the human anterior chamber angle, as determined by the Spaeth gonioscopic grading system and ultrasound biomicroscopy. *Trans Am Ophthalmol Soc,* Vol. 93, 1995) pp. (337-347; discussion 347-351), 0065-9533 (Print)

Tan, A.N., Sauren, L.D., de Brabander, J., Berendschot, T.T., Passos, V.L., Webers, C.A., Nuijts, R.M. & Beckers, H.J. Reproducibility of anterior chamber angle measurements with anterior segment optical coherence tomography. *Invest Ophthalmol Vis Sci,* Vol. 52, No. 5, 2095-2099), 1552-5783 (Electronic)

Thomas, R., George, R., Parikh, R., Muliyil, J. & Jacob, A. (2003a). Five year risk of progression of primary angle closure suspects to primary angle closure: a population based study. *Br J Ophthalmol,* Vol. 87, No. 4, (Apr 2003a) pp. (450-454), 0007-1161 (Print)

Thomas, R., George, T., Braganza, A. & Muliyil, J. (1996). The flashlight test and van Herick's test are poor predictors for occludable angles. *Aust N Z J Ophthalmol,* Vol. 24, No. 3, (Aug 1996) pp. (251-256), 0814-9763 (Print)

Thomas, R., Parikh, R., Muliyil, J. & Kumar, R.S. (2003b). Five-year risk of progression of primary angle closure to primary angle closure glaucoma: a population-based study. *Acta Ophthalmol Scand,* Vol. 81, No. 5, (Oct 2003b) pp. (480-485), 1395-3907 (Print)

Ursea, R. & Silverman, R.H. Anterior-segment imaging for assessment of glaucoma. *Expert Rev Ophthalmol,* Vol. 5, No. 1, (Feb 1 59-74), 1746-9899 (Electronic)

Van Herick, W., Shaffer, R.N. & Schwartz, A. (1969). Estimation of width of angle of anterior chamber. Incidence and significance of the narrow angle. *Am J Ophthalmol,* Vol. 68, No. 4, (Oct 1969) pp. (626-629), 0002-9394 (Print)

Wang, D., Pekmezci, M., Basham, R.P., He, M., Seider, M.I. & Lin, S.C. (2009). Comparison of different modes in optical coherence tomography and ultrasound biomicroscopy in anterior chamber angle assessment. *J Glaucoma,* Vol. 18, No. 6, (Aug 2009) pp. (472-478), 1536-481X (Electronic)

Wishart, P.K. & Batterbury, M. (1992). Ocular hypertension: correlation of anterior chamber angle width and risk of progression to glaucoma. *Eye (Lond)*, Vol. 6 (Pt 3), 1992) pp. (248-256), 0950-222X (Print)

Wong, H.T., Lim, M.C., Sakata, L.M., Aung, H.T., Amerasinghe, N., Friedman, D.S. & Aung, T. (2009). High-definition optical coherence tomography imaging of the iridocorneal angle of the eye. *Arch Ophthalmol*, Vol. 127, No. 3, (Mar 2009) pp. (256-260), 1538-3601 (Electronic)

Yoo, C., Oh, J.H., Kim, Y.Y. & Jung, H.R. (2007). Peripheral anterior synechiae and ultrasound biomicroscopic parameters in angle-closure glaucoma suspects. *Korean J Ophthalmol*, Vol. 21, No. 2, (Jun 2007) pp. (106-110), 1011-8942 (Print)

2

Management of Glaucoma in the Era of Modern Imaging and Diagnostics

Anurag Shrivastava and Umar Mian
Montefiore Medical Center: Albert Einstein COM
U.S.A.

1. Introduction

In light of a rapidly expanding geriatric demographic worldwide, and the concomitant increased prevalence of glaucoma, the need for reliable and reproducible methods for disease progression has become increasingly necessary. Given the high costs and morbidity of treatment, whether medical, laser, or incisional, the ability to detect disease and to further demonstrate progression allows glaucoma specialists to make more informed decisions regarding both the initiation, and advancement of therapeutic modalities. Furthermore, our ability to image both the anterior segment and the optic nerve head has allowed for better elucidation of anatomic variants and mechanisms of secondary glaucomas, along with better detection of subtle glaucomatous optic neuropathies and progression of nerve fiber layer defects.

The treatment of glaucoma has advanced rapidly over the past decades, yet remains a chronic disease requiring life long control. The expansion of the armamentarium of interventions possible to help retard progression of disease has allowed us to cater treatments to the specific needs of an individual patient. As glaucomatous damage is essentially irreversible, the holy grail of glaucoma treatment, regardless of etiology, is early detection of a progressive disease state. Intraocular pressure (IOP) remains the only modifiable risk factor for glaucoma patients, and continues to serve as the metric by which the success of therapeutic intervention is judged. The need for accuracy of these measurements has led to a better understanding of ocular tissue properties, and potentially their relative effects on disease progression.

In terms of diagnosis and management of glaucoma, progress has been made since the days when visual field testing remained the only option for the detection and documentation of disease and its progression. As traditional perimetry provides a functional assessment of a patient's disease state, the need for reliable structural measurements has resulted in the development of a multitude of technologies. The relationship between structural damage and functional loss, however, is often complicated, and much remains to be elucidated at the current time. Since structural and functional assessments give us different information, both are often used in conjunction for the detection and treatment of glaucoma. Understanding the limitations of both assessments is tantamount when considering various therapeutic algorithms. Ultimately, it remains the role of the clinician to determine an individual patient's risk of progression. This is optimally achieved by determining the level of intervention necessary to prevent functional loss, balancing the risks, side effects, and costs of treatment.

2. Assessment and measurement of intraocular pressure

As intraocular pressure (IOP) remains the only modifiable risk factor for glaucoma, the importance of consistent and accurate measurements cannot be overstated. Reduction of IOP remains the cornerstone for the treatment of glaucoma, as adequate and reproducible data on neuroprotective agents is currently lacking. Given that all forms of tonometry have limitations, the reference standard for IOP assessment continues to be Goldmann applanation tonometry (GAT). A brief review of the principle behind IOP measurement is provided here. GAT relies on the Imbert-Fick principle, and is in part based upon a standardized GAT applanation diameter of 3.06mm. The IOP is inferred from the force needed to flatten this standardized area of the central cornea. Therefore, it is intuitive that central corneal pathologies and properties will affect these IOP measurements.

For patients with high corneal astigmatism, it is important to take the average of two measurements 90 degrees apart by adjusting the applanation tip accordingly. GAT measurements need to be furthermore adjusted according to standard corneal pachymetry nomograms, although no one nomogram that exists that is universally accepted. A range of IOP correction from 1.1 to 7.14mm Hg/100 microns of corneal thickness exists in the current literature[1]. It is of interest that the clinical utility of these adjustments remains somewhat controversial, and that other corneal biomechanical properties may be of higher utility (See Ocular Response Analyzer below). Regardless, it is likely that corneal pachymetry measurements below 500 microns underestimate IOP, and those over 600 microns overestimate the measurement. A variety of tonometers have been developed in response to these properties, and some are discussed within this section.

2.1 Tonopen (Reichert technologies depew, NY)

The Tonopen is a modified Mackay-Marg tonometer, and is commercially sold as the Tonopen XL, and more recently, the Tonopen Avia. Mackay-Marg tonometers work on the principle that the applanating force to flatten a cornea (transuducer with a 1.5 mm applanation tip) must be equivalent to the counteracting force from within the eye. The transducer only measures the pressures at the center of the applanator, in contrast to the GAT, and is theorized to be less dependent on intrinsic corneal properties. The Tonopen contains a micro strain gauge attached to a 1.0 mm transducer, sampling at a rate of 500 measurements per second. This high sampling rate allows the Tonopen to provide accurate and reproducible IOP measurements. The Tonopen has several major advantages over GAT. It does not require a slit lamp, and is therefore not dependent on patient positioning, allowing for easy use outside the examnination room setting.. It further provides objective results, and requires less skill and training than GAT to perform. The Tonopen is particularly useful in children and non-cooperative patients. The surface area of applanation is one-third that of the GAT, and the ability to measure IOP from a non-central location may be an advantage in patients with certain corneal pathologies.

A study done in the earlier years of the Tonopen on 15 eyes which needed corneal glue, or had band keratopathy, demonstrated that the Tonopen was equivalent to the GAT when the unaffected area was applanated The study further concluded that the Tonopen grossly overestimated the IOP when the affected area was tested[2]. A large cross-sectional study of over 2000 primary care patients who were screened for ocular hypertension (OHTN) with the Tonopen described no adverse effects of tonometry, and further determined the incidence of OHTN and primary open angle glaucoma (POAG) to be 4.89% and 1.04%

respectively. Broman, et al.[3], examined 230 glaucomatous eyes with the Tonopen, GAT, Ocular Response Analyzer (ORA- see below), and further obtained measurements of central corneal thickness (CCT), axial length, corneal curvature, corneal astigmatism, central visual acuity, and refractive error. The IOP measured was noted to be lowest by the Tonopen, and highest by the ORA. Interestingly, it was found that the GAT was least affected by corneal pachymetry, and corneal hysteresis (see ORA below) was correlated with CCT. The authors concluded that corneal parameters affect tonometers in different ways. Lester, et al.[4] in an analysis of 104 patients found that the Tonopen XL gave similar results to GAT in only 62% of patients, and in subgroup analysis, found that the Tonopen XL underestimates IOP when GAT was above 20mm Hg.

2.2 Ocular Response Analyzer (ORA: Reichert instruments, depew, NY)

The Ocular Response Analyzer is a modified non-contact tonometer, which measures previously un-recordable corneal biomechanical properties. These properties are thought to be the result of viscous damping of corneal tissue. The ORA utilizes a rapid air impulse, combined with a highly sensitive optical system, to record applanation pressures when the cornea is both maximally deformed inwards, and then once again on reformation. The *average* of the two IOP measurements is termed IOPg, to denote the fact that it is the equivalent of the correlated GAT. The *difference* between the two IOP measurements is termed corneal hysteresis (CH) (Figure 1-2). The ability to measure hysteresis allows for further derivations of other newer metrics, such as corneal-corrected IOP (IOPcc) and the corneal resistance factor (CRF). These derived metrics eliminate the need for corneal pachymetry compensation of IOP. The IOPcc is derived from a normative database of patients undergoing keratorefractive surgery, and "compensates" the IOP based on corneal properties, not corneal thickness. CRF is a measurement of the cumulative effects of both the viscous and elastic resistance encountered by the air jet while deforming the corneal surface, and is derived from CH measurements using various algorithms. ORA measurements have proven to be particularly useful in patients with corneal edema and some secondary glaucomas, where IOPg can serve as a surrogate for GAT when it is not possible. Patients with abnormal ORA hysteresis measurements may be at higher risk for corneal ectasia and possibly post keratorefractive surgery complications as well[5].

A study of 90 eyes (30 normal, 30 with POAG, 30 pseudoexfoliative) was recently performed with the ORA, and corneal hysteresis was found to be significantly lower in pseudoexfoliatives when compared to the controls and POAG patients[6]. Another recent review of 108 POAG patients demonstrated both lower corneal hysteresis and resistance factor measurements when compared to those of ocular hypertensives and controls[7]. In a prospective cross-sectional study of 117 POAG patients with asymmetric visual fields, Anand et al[8] demonstrated that abnormal ORA parameters were significantly associated with the eye with the greater visual field defect. Neither corneal pachymetry, nor GAT, were significantly different between the eyes. These findings suggest that the ORA is able to detect subtle differences in asymmetric glaucoma, when GAT and CCT measurements are symmetric.

Lastly, Ang et al performed a prospective comparative analysis of 40 patients with normal tension glaucoma (NTG) with 41 diagnosed with POAG, demonstrating higher hysteresis measurements in the NTG group. The highest recorded GAT measurement was also statistically significantly correlated with lower hysteresis and higher resistance factor values. These findings suggest that alterations in corneal biomechanical properties may occur in response to chronically elevated IOP[9]. It is clear that the ORA is able to distinguish corneal biomechanical properties that were previously undetectable. As our understanding of the clinical relevance of these parameters improves, the predictive and diagnostic utility of ORA will likely lead to a greater adoption of this technology.

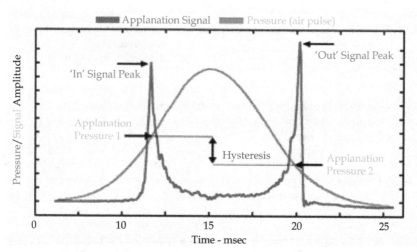

Ocular Response Analyzer(ocularresponseanalyzer.com), Reichert Industries website, 2011

Fig. 1. Ocular Response Analyzer (ORA). The ORA results from both eyes are displayed in graphical form, and are referred to as the "Signal Time Response" curves. The dynamic air puff to the cornea leads to two applanation events (inward and outwards), and the delays in these events are due to intrinsic corneal biomechanical properties. The Y-axis is the "Pressure/Signal Amplitude", and the X-axis is time in msec. The solid curve which peaks in the center of the plot is the pressure (air pulse). The bimodal peaked line represents the applanation signal. The first peak represents the "in-signal", when the cornea is flattened inwards by the air-puff. The second peak represents the "out-signal", when the cornea essentially "unflattens" back to its original state. The intersection of the pressure and signal plots at both peaks represents the two applanation measurements respectively. The average of the two pressures is the calculated IOPg, or Goldmann-correlated IOP. The difference between the two pressures is termed corneal hysteresis (CH), and is thought to be due to the viscous damping effects of the corneal tissue. The normal range of CH varies significantly from 8-16mm Hg, with the value of 11mm Hg considered normal. The IOPcc and CRF are derived from the CH. The IOPcc is the estimated IOP given the CH of a cornea, and is considered to be independent of pachymetry, etc. The CRF provides an estimate of the overall resistance of the cornea, and normal values range similar to the CH

2.3 Pascal dynamic contour tonomoter (DCT)
The Pascal DCT (Zeimer Ophthalmics, Port, Switzerland) was developed in response to the large degree of variability of IOP measurements obtained by GAT, with respect to various corneal properties and biomechanics. It further eliminates the subjective nature of GAT by providing a slit-lamp mounted digital readout of the IOP. The advantages of the digital readout, along with the resultant reductions in intra-observer variability, are intuitive in a

busy clinical setting. Measurement of the ocular pulse amplitude (OPA) , a metric estimating the quality of ocular blood flow, is further displayed digitally. The SensorTip™ of the DCT is a concave applanator which houses a piezo resistant pressure sensor able to take approximately 100 measurements per second. A spring loaded Cantilever maintains a constant applanation force of 1 gram, reducing the likelihood of iatrogenic corneal injury as well. A major theoretical advantage of DCT, when compared to GAT, is that IOP measurements from DCT are not affected by corneal pachymetry. This difference is especially useful for keratorefractive and keratoconic[10]patients, where thin corneas and astigmatism greatly affect GAT measurements. The DCT clearly addresses many of the major shortcomings of standard GAT. DCT likely will play a larger role in glaucoma

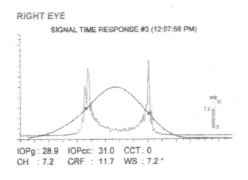

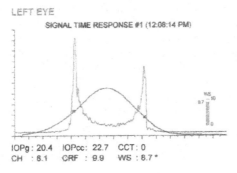

Fig. 2. ORA of glaucoma patient

The ORA scans of a patient show extremely an extremely high IOPg in both eyes, with the right eye being significantly higher than the Left (28.9 mm Hg, 20.4 mm Hg). CH values are low in both eyes, with an IOPcc even higher than IOPg (31.0 mm Hg OD, 22.7 mm Hg OS). The intraocular pressures of this patient by GAT have ranged from 12m Hg-18mm Hg on medical therapy, significantly lower than the measurements by the ORA. It is likely that the ORA is demonstrating a gross underestimation of this patient's IOP control. If functional and structural analysis continues to show progression, it is likely that this patient will need more aggressive IOP management than that being demonstrated by serial GAT. As with all testing, it is important to reproduce abnormal results prior to advancing to any therapeutic intervention management, especially given that data generated from the DCT can be wirelessly integrated into many electronic medical record (EMR) systems. A hand-held DCT has been developed recently, and results have been shown to be consistent with the slit-lamp mounted model[11].

The DCT has been widely studied, and the current body of literature supports its use clinically. A retrospective review of 200 patients by Ang, et al.[9] demonstrated poor correlation of DCT with GAT measurements that had been corrected with six different pachymetry compensation formulae. Gunvant, et al[12] examined 120 eyes, and demonstrated that the Ehlers formula for GAT correction actually reduced agreement with DCT measurements. This study demonstrates that simple GAT corneal correction factors may be inadequate to compensate for complex corneal biomechanics. Kotecha, et al[13], examined 100 patients with GAT, ORA, and DCT, and concluded that the DCT demonstrated the best repeatability and reproducibility. Interestingly, ORA and DCT generally measured the IOP to be 2 mm higher than GAT in this study. Sullivan-Mee, et al[14] performed a similar analysis on 126 eyes, and found that all three forms of tonometry (GAT, ORA, and DCT) had similar repeatability and reproducibility, concluding from their data that the ORA and DCT are acceptable alternatives to GAT in routine clinical practice.

2.4 Icare® rebound tonometry (IRT)

Rebound tonometry, commercially available as the Icare tonometer TA01i (Tiolat Oy, Helsinki, Finland), has shown tremendous promise in the realm of pediatric ophthalmology and community screenings in particular. The Icare tonometer does not require topical anesthesia, and is able to provide rapid digital IOP measurements painlessly. The handheld device is first stabilized on the patient's forehead, and a small disposable rebounding probe briefly applanates the cornea. It is able to measure the IOP in microseconds, obviating the need for anesthesia and prolonged measurements, making the technology especially useful for children and special needs patients. The probe is briefly magnetized by an induction coil prior to firing, and the tonometer calculates and digitally displays the IOP from the generated induction current. It is important to note that IRT is likely subject to the same constraints as GAT with respect to various corneal parameters.

Flemmons et al[15]collected GAT and IRT measurements from 71 pediatric glaucoma patients, and found that the IRT measurements were within 3mm Hg of GAT in 63% of patients. It was further noted that the IOP was higher by IRT than GAT in 75% of patients measured. Scuderi, et al,[16] in a clinical study of 93 patients, examined the validity and limitations of IRT. They concluded that IRT was comparable to other nonconventional tonometers, and can replace GAT when it is not available. Munkwitz, et al[17] similarly examined 75 patients with GAT and IRT, and found that the IRT performed well within 3mm Hg for normotensive patients. However, in patients with IOPs ranging from 22-60 mm Hg, the IRT was shown to have larger variability than the GAT. This result potentially reduces the validity of IRT measurements in ocular hypertensive patients.

One of the most challenging aspects of glaucoma management is an absence of IOP data between office visits. Compliance rates likely change in the days preceding office visits, and extrapolating IOP over time from limited data points has serious limitations. In diabetic and hypertensive patients, inter-visit monitoring of blood pressure and blood glucose offers internists a great deal of information regarding the efficacy of treatment for these diseases. The possibility of home monitoring of IOP by IRT was addressed in a recent study by Asrani, et al. They observed excellent inter- and intra-observer variability (less than 3mm Hg) in 100 patients that performed IRT on themselves, compared with IRT and GAT performed by a technician[18]. The possibility of home monitoring of IOP may have particular significance for patients where large diurnal IOP variability is suspected given normal measurements at office visits.

3. Standard automated perimetry (SAP) and short wavelength automated perimetry (SWAP) – Functional assessment of the glaucoma patient

SAP, or static perimetry, is most commonly performed by the Humphrey or Octopus perimeter. Alternately, manual (kinetic) perimetry, is most commonly performed with the Goldmann perimeter, although it is important to note that some automated perimeters do have kinetic testing functionality. SAP serves as a nonspecific assessment of visual function, and is designed to detect loss of sensitivity to light perception. This is traditionally done with a white stimulus on a standardized white background of uniform luminescence. However, newer testing paradigms which isolate specific wavelengths of light (see SWAP testing below) have been introduced for certain clinical indications. SAP serves as a global metric of functional loss. In clinical practice, this means that visual field deficits may represent a disease process anywhere from the ocular surface to the visual cortex. Characteristic patterns of deficit allow the practitioner to anatomically localize the site of injury, and are tremendously useful in the diagnosis and monitoring of many disease states. It is important to note that any visual field defect that is suspected to obey the vertical midline warrants further neurological assessment. The temporality and congruity of the field deficits further provide useful clues to the etiology of the defects. Bitemporal lesions generally localize pathology to the sella turcica adjacent to the optic chiasm, whereas homonomous defects are generally post-chiasmal. Highly congruous homonomous defects, especially with macular sparing, often localize to occipital pathology.

SAP testing relies on a variety of strategies, which ultimately determine the threshold necessary to reliably detect the presence of a stimulus in predetermined locations within the visual field. Algorithms and testing strategies have been constantly advancing to maximize sensitivity and specificity, while reducing test time and patient fatigue. Given the wide variety of options, it is imperative that the clinician not only chooses the correct test, but also furthermore accounts for an individual patient's ability to reliably perform that test.

The decision to advance treatment based on visual field analysis is inherently fraught with confounding factors. While the advent of structural analysis (see below) have allowed for some quantification of glaucomatous defect, the necessity for analysis and documentation of functional disease progression with perimetry remains a vital component of glaucoma management. This is especially the case when there are disparities between clinical examination, perimetry, and structural analysis. An improved understanding of the limitations of standard perimetry and structural analysis allows the astute clinician to avoid treatment errors. This is particularly important given the high levels of morbidity associated with many of the interventions presently available. The following sections aim to highlight the strengths and weaknesses of the wide range of testing modalities currently available.

3.1 Humphrey field analyzer (HFA)

One of the most commonly utilized perimetry devices is the HFA, with over 35,000 units in use currently worldwide. Indeed, many of the landmark glaucoma trials such as the Ocular Hypertensive Trial (OHTS)[19], Advanced Glaucoma Intervention Study (AGIS)[20], and Collaborative Initial Glaucoma Treatment Study (CIGTS)[21]to name a few, used this form of perimetry to diagnose and detect functional glaucomatous progression. HFA analysis is the current gold standard for clinical trials, allowing for older studies to be appropriately compared. Recent advancements in progression analysis software by multiple vendors have increased the clinical utility of serial SAP testing by allowing for greater detection of subtle changes.

The choice of the most appropriate HVF should be based upon a wide variety of considerations. Some of these considerations include the extent of the visual field that needs to be tested, the intensity and size of the stimulus needed, and the best suited testing strategy for the clinical question being analyzed (i.e. screening vs. monitoring progression, etc.). An important caveat is that once a reliable visual field is obtained, it is advisable to utilize the same testing strategy as much as possible to reliably detect disease progression over time.

3.1.1 Degrees of visual field tested

The major options on standard HVF perimetry are 10-2, 24-2, 30-2, and the less commonly performed 60-2. The first number refers to the number of degrees around the fovea that will be tested (i.e. a 10-2 test 10 degrees of the visual field centered at the fovea). The second digit which is currently always "2", refers to the protocol type which tests points on either side of the horizontal and vertical meridians, as opposed to points on the meridians themselves. Testing points directly on the meridia is denoted with a "1" as the second digit. The "1" strategy is particularly useful in neuro-ophthalmic evaluation, to highlight the presence of vertical midline defects, for example. In general, the use of 10-2 testing is reserved for patients with very advanced glaucoma to detect subtle progression in an extremely constricted field, and for patients with suspected maculopathy. The 60-2 strategy can be applied in patients where peripheral defects detected by smaller field analyses require further confirmation, however patient fatigue and artifacts may limit the clinical utility of this strategy.

The choice between 24-2 and 30-2 is somewhat variable between practitioners, and there are advantages and disadvantages to each test. Many glaucoma specialists follow patients with 24-2 testing in lieu of full 30-2 testing as it has been demonstrated that both tests have approximately equal sensitivity and specificity[19] in the detection of glaucomatous field damage. The 30-2 paradigm can lead to significantly more fatigue for patients given the additional test spots in the periphery of the visual field. The 30-2 tests one more row of points in the peripheral visual field compared to the 24-2. This area of the field is most sensitive to rim, lid, and other artifacts, thereby reducing its clinical utility in some cases. As the detection of subtle field changes necessitates accurate testing (see below: reliability indices), the choice of a 24-2 paradigm may allow for improved reliability and more clinically meaningful data. Some clinicians choose to order a 30-2 test as the baseline, and assuming that it is normal, will follow patients with 24-2 testing. It is important to note that often multiple tests need to be performed to set a reliable baseline, as field testing accuracy generally improves along a variable learning curve. In patients having difficulty with increased test time, it is appropriate to set a baseline with the most extensive test that a patient can reasonably tolerate (see below: testing strategies) Important testing specifications are reviewed below:

- 10-2: The points adjacent to the horizontal and vertical meridians test 1 degree of the visual field; points tested peripheral to these points are 2 degrees apart

- 24-2 and 30-2: The points adjacent to the horizontal and vertical meridians test 3 degrees of the visual field; points tested peripheral to these points are 6 degrees apart

In a patient with a subtle maculopathy, affecting only a few degrees of the central visual field, defects can easily be missed by the 24-2 and 30-2 based on the aforementioned testing specifications, as the scotoma could fall in the region between the tested points. Alternately, dense paracentral/arcuate scotomas characteristic of glaucomatous optic neuropathies can "blacken" out an entire 10-2 field, and the 24-2 or 30-2 paradigms are far better suited.

a. Screening considerations

Screening protocols are variable amongst practitioners and practices. Large volume screenings for glaucoma are often performed with Humphrey Matrix Analyzers/ (FDT) based on the test time needed to perform the analysis. It is appropriate for "high risk" patients being screened (eg Strong family history of glaucoma, ocular hypertensives, IOP/cup-to-disc asymmetry, etc.) to perform more extensive perimetry with SITA-fast protocols (see below). Patients with positive screening tests warrant further work-up, often with structural and corneal biomechanical analyses.

b. Other considerations

As HFA analyses are based on age-matched controls, it is imperative that the correct birth date is entered prior to testing. The age groups of patients in the database are stratified into 10 year increments. For example, a 59 year old patient will be compared to age matched controls between the ages of 50-60. It is common, therefore, for patients to have deterioration of their visual field as they progress through each decade of life. Alternately, "improvements" in the visual field can be seen immediately after the patient's age increases to the next decade stratification. Furthermore, assessment of the mental and physical status of an elderly patient to determine whether they will be able to tolerate the high levels of concentration required to perform the test.

Refractive errors, especially presbyopic errors, need to be neutralized with the appropriate loose lenses, and vertex distances/head positioning optimized. Astigmatic correction over 1.25D should be neutralized along with spherical aberration. The HVF will determine the optimal neutralization from manifest refractions accounting for a target distance of 30cm. Reassessing head position relative to refractive neutralization is critical during testing, as rim artifacts can be generated by the lenses if head positioning is not adequately monitored. Furthermore, prismatic deviation caused by high power lenses need to be accounted for when testing is analyzed, and peripheral rim defects discounted appropriately in these cases. Pupil size is able to be measured by HFA, and is displayed with the results. Pupil size generally less than 2-3mm can lead to artifactual loss of threshold sensitivity of both central and peripheral fields[22]. This is of particular importance in following patients on miotic therapy for glaucoma. Pharmacological dilation of the pupil in these cases may help limit the effects of the miotic pupil. Patients should be consistently dilated for subsequent fields if this strategy is employed. Changes in the refractive error secondary to pharmacological dilation are likely negligible in the largely non-presbyopic patient demographic that commonly undergo perimetric evaluation.

A standard background light intensity of 31.5 asb (apostilbs) is used for the HVF, to match the scotopic light conditions outlined by Goldmann perimetry standards. HVF targets come in sizes ranging from 0.25 mm^2 to 64.00 mm^2 represented by Roman numerals I through V (see Goldmann Visual Fields below). Typically, a size III stimulus (4 mm^2) is used in patients with good visual acuity (usually at least 20/200 or better). In these cases of decreased visual acuity, the use of larger size V (64 mm²) test stimulus may be helpful, although many clinicians will opt for Goldmann Visual Fields for these low vision patients. Stimulus intensity, color, and duration can furthermore be varied by the operator based upon clinical needs.

Gaze tracking is possible with all HVF machines, and the reliability of an individual test can be further analyzed beyond the reliability indices calculated for each field. A real time fixation monitor is displayed at the bottom of each visual field printout. Upward deflections represent the moment a patient saccades away from a target, and downward deflections represent a tracking failure commonly secondary to blinking.

3.1.2 Testing algorithms – Swedish interactive testing algorithm (SITA)

SITA testing was designed to optimize visual field accuracy while reducing testing time. It is based on the concept of "threshold", which is a term that is defined as the intensity of light that a patient can detect 50% of the time. The threshold represents the minimal amount of light intensity that can be reliably detected. SITA testing determines this threshold by presenting points with varying intensities using a "bracketing" technique. Specifically, this technique involves measuring intensities above and below the threshold, as defined above. This technique is much more efficient than full threshold protocols, and generally is able to maintain a high degree of concordance in a much shorter time period. The SITA algorithm is dynamic, and the stimuli are timed based on an individual patient's response time. Algorithms are age-matched, so proper patient data entry is imperative. SITA-Fast and SITA standard algorithms remain options that can reduce test time by about 70% and 50%[23], respectively, when compared with full threshold tests. The differences between the protocols lies in the variability in response allowed when determining threshold values, with the SITA standard being more rigorous in repetition of points. In other words, the SITA-FAST strategy has a lower level of confidence needed to be achieved at each point relative to SITA-Standard. The SITA-fast protocol utilizes the expected thresholds based on normative population databases. The utilization of these normative assumptions increases the efficiency of the test, but is limited by the fact that it does not account for threshold variability at the individual level. The SITA fast protocol is generally more than adequate for screening examinations and for those patients who cannot perform SITA standard secondary to fatigue. Most glaucoma specialists rely on SITA standard testing to monitor for subtle changes indicating progression. This is particularly critical in the regions of the visual field surrounding an existing scotoma. A study by Budenz, et al demonstrated an overall sensitivity of 98% and 95% for SITA standard and SITA fast protocols when compared to full threshold testing. The same study demonstrated sensitivity in patients with mild glaucomatous damage as 92% and 85% respectively[24]. Specificity was determined to be 96% for both algorithms.

3.1.3 Short wavelength automated perimetry (SWAP) – Blue-on-yellow perimetry

SWAP testing is based upon the concept that glaucoma is characterized by damage to cells in the visual pathway that are more sensitive to blue light, with a peak activity at 440 nanometers. Blue cones in the photoreceptor layer of the retina eventually synapse in the koniocellular layers of the lateral geniculate body, via small bistratified retinal ganglion cells. The fact that SWAP testing isolates one type of ganglion cell should not imply that these cells are necessarily the first to be affected by glaucomatous injury. Moreover, SWAP testing avoids the masking effects of inherent redundancies within the visual pathways by isolating one particular system.[25,26]

SWAP testing is generally more fatiguing than SAP, and is also much more affected by lens opacification and drusen in patients with macular degeneration. Recent development of SITA-SWAP testing has helped reduce test duration while maintaining sensitivity. The stimulus size for the blue target in SWAP testing is larger than that of SAP (equivalent to Goldmann V vs. III sized targets, respectively). More light is needed to activate the blue cone system[27], and although the blue target is generally less bright, the larger test stimulus size partially compensates for it. The caveat is, that a larger test stimulus can over estimate fixation losses in patients with relatively small blind spots, even though fixation maybe maintained.

Many studies have demonstrated the ability of SWAP testing to detect visual field abnormalities earlier than SAP testing[28,29]. A recent publication demonstrated less persuasive results regarding the early predictive abilities of SWAP testing. However, methodological differences between Johnson's original data from the prior decade may help explain the varied results[30]. Other reports indicate that patients with visual field defects on SAP demonstrate dramatically larger defects when tested with SWAP[31-33]. As data is continually being collected regarding SWAP testing in glaucoma patients, a better understanding of the protocol's benefits and limitations will help elucidate the role of SWAP testing in functional assessment of the glaucoma patient. At the time of this publication, SWAP testing largely remains the test most commonly used in younger patients with high clinical suspicion for glaucoma. This is especially the case in patients with previous normal SAP testing.

3.1.4 Reliability indices

In order to make determinations about clinically significant functional progression, it is imperative that visual fields are as reliable and reproducible as possible. Assessment of a glaucomatous scotoma by *reliable* perimetry is expected to fluctuate given the natural history of the disease and the manner in which we quantify defects. Alternately stated, seemingly progressive visual field loss can often "reverse" with serial testing, indicating that the etiology of the deterioration may indeed be non-physiological. The establishment of a blind spot corresponding to the position of the optic nerve is accomplished by placing testing points within this region during reliable fixation. It is even more challenging to separate fluctuation from progression when analyzing visual fields that are considered "unreliable". The establishment of an adequate baseline is important clinically, and essential if progression analysis is desired (see GPA below).

Fixation losses are measured by introducing stimuli into the physiological blind spot, and monitoring whether patients are able to detect them. A fixation loss indicates that the blind spot has moved (i.e. the patient has refixated to an alternate location within the perimeter). False positives are defined as patient responses when no stimulus is present. False negative responses are defined as a lack of detection of a suprathreshold stimulus (i.e. not being able to detect a more intense stimulus after the threshold is determined).

Reliable fields generally are recommended to have false positive and negative rates fewer than 35%, and fixation losses less than 20%. In clinical practice, many patients are not able to adequately perform the testing regardless of algorithm, and alternate means of documenting functional progression are necessary. Birt, et al.,[33] demonstrated in a review of 768 visual field test from 106 glaucoma patients, that only 59.5% of test were considered reliable by the aforementioned criterion. Elevating the fixation loss threshold criterion from 20% to 33% increased the number of fields meeting reliability standards to over 75%. Newkirk[34], et al further demonstrated that artificially introducing false positives of 33% to a visual field improved the calculated mean deviation (MD) by 6dB; an amount that can easily mask progressive damage. Vingrys et al[35]demonstrated similar results, suggesting that the cutoffs for reliability of false positive results be reduced to 20% or less. Bengtsson, et al.[36], hve shown that false positive rates are the least variable in test-retest paradigms, and are likely to be the most reliable index of visual field accuracy based on the SITA algorithms.

3.1.5 Glaucoma Hemifield test/analysis (GHT)
The GHT was developed by Asman, et al in the early 1990s to measure asymmetries in threshold sensitivity around the horizontal meridian. It functionally analyzes five corresponding pairs of mirror image sectors in the superior and inferior horizontal fields, corresponding to the normal anatomy of the retinal nerve fiber layer. Outer edge, temporal, and blind spot points are excluded from the analysis, and can be used with either the 30- or 24-2 protocols. Abnormal GHT values indicate asymmetry around the horizontal meridian, and allows for rapid evaluation of zone defects that affect the superior or inferior hemifields in particular[37] The results are further stratified into 5 categories: "Outside Normal Limits", "Borderline", "Generalized Reduction of Sensitivity", "Abnormally High Sensitivity", and "Within Normal Limits". The definition of "Outside Normal Limits" is based upon defects between the respective upper and lower paired sectors greater than what would be expected in 1% of the normative database, or a sum difference at 0.5% normal population level. "Borderline" results indicate the same criterion at the 3% normal population level. Katz, et al analyzed the rate of incident field loss after one abnormal GHT, and found that GHT is not a consistent criterion for defining incident field loss. They further concluded that the use of two or three consecutive abnormal fields to define incident field loss makes it more likely that subsequent test results will be abnormal[38]. Susanna, et al. further analyzed the ability of the GHT to detect early glaucomatous changes, and found the sensitivity, specificity, and reproducibility of the GHT to be 100,100, and 83.3% respectively[39]. Johnson, et al more recently concluded that the GHT, GHT hemifield cluster, and Pattern Deviation plots provided the highest sensitivity and specificity of all the visual field metrics[40]

3.1.6 Glaucoma progression analysis (GPA)
Given the often large amounts of data provided by serial perimetry, the absolute need for automated detection of progressive visual field loss has lead to advancements in software that efficiently summarize function over time. This capability allows clinicians to rapidly detect areas of the visual field that have deteriorated from baseline threshold values. These are defined by the user as the first reliable field or fields (full threshold or SITA). The data output of GPA analysis summarizes the probability of the presence of glaucomatous progression. It factors in normal fluctuation from a large database, and subtracts out deficits secondary to media opacification as well. The data is summarized in probability plots, demonstrating the likelihood of functional progression with variably darkened triangular symbols. Triangles that are darker represent a portion of the visual field that has consistently worsened over multiple tests. A minimum of five examinations over at least three years must be included in GPA 2 for the linear regression results to be presented. The

open triangles represent deterioration from baseline with a 0.5 confidence interval, the half-shaded triangles represent deterioration at the same point on 2 visual fields, and finally the darkened triangle represents deterioration at the same location on 3 visual fields. Deterioration is defined as greater than that of the normal fluctuation that occurs within a normative database. Again, the lack of a uniform definition of deterioration is a severe limitation when comparing progression analyses. Consensus regarding this definition continues to be the source of much debate. Furthermore, the clinical relevance of any defined progression must be evaluated on an individual case basis to avoid errors in treatment strategy. Regardless of the definition of progression, it is widely accepted that the accuracy of progression rates is vastly improved with additional data points. This functionally translates into establishing a reliable baseline, repeating visual fields often, and using a longitudinal analysis to determine the rate of progression. In this manner, the likelihood of clinically relevant deterioration can be most accurately assessed.

As the assessment of glaucoma progression involves some degree of subjectivity, there are often discrepancies in patients who demonstrate mild changes in function. A recent review of 510 Humphrey visual fields of 83 eyes by 3 examiners demonstrated that clinician agreement of progression on sequential fields was actually better without the GPA analysis[41]. Clinician agreement (inter-observer reliability) obviously may not be an appropriate reference standard for the determination of disease progression given the subjective nature of the analysis. Another review of 90 eyes with greater than 5 reliable visual fields demonstrated that the GPA performed better in the detection of progression, when compared to a pattern deviation based visual field index (VFI)[42]. Another retrospective review of 93 glaucoma patients with 5 reliable fields concluded that there is a strong correlation between GPA identification of glaucomatous progression and a thorough objective clinical assessment of the visual fields. They further concluded that GPA could be a useful test to aid clinicians in the detection of glaucomatous progression, with high specificity, strong positive likelihood ratio, good sensitivity and negative likelihood ratio[43]. Diaz-Aleman, et al[44] examined 56 eyes of 42 patients with at least 7 reliable fields, and compared threshold noiseless trend (TNT) to GPA, and showed that TNT had a higher specificity and concordance with clinical examiners than GPA.

It is important to note that no universal definition of glaucoma, whether via a statistical package or point-by-point analysis, has been universally accepted. The optimal characterization of glaucomatous progression is the source of much of the research on perimetry that is currently being performed. Furthermore, as the perimetric definitions of progression vary significantly amongst many of the major landmark glaucoma studies, comparisons of results between the major trials has been limited. Clinically relevant models derived from these studies lack reproducibility, and no one index has been shown to be superior at the time of this publication (Figures 3-8).

While a useful adjunctive tool, GPA has had variable success when compared to other methodologies. It is our opinion that GPA serves as a useful tool in conjunction with other standard examination techniques when compared to grossly comparing serial HVF examinations without point by point analysis. The software will unlikely replace careful clinical examination utilizing a gestalt technique in its current clinical application. Monitoring the rate of visual field deterioration by multiple metrics, while accurately predicting the onset of functional loss with particular regard to projected life expectancy, is likely the optimal strategy in determining optimal treatment.

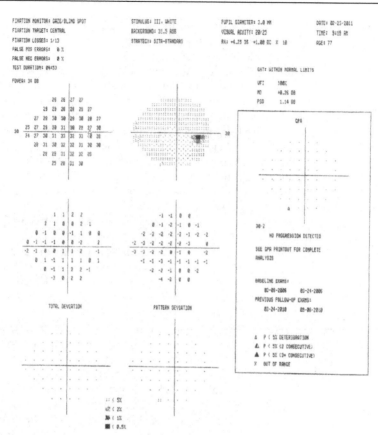

Fig. 3. HVF single field analysis with progression analysis summary: OD

This HVF is an example of the normal scan of the right eye of a patient being followed as a glaucoma suspect. Important demographic information is included at the top of the printout, including the date of birth. The type of visual field, in this case, Central 24-2 Threshold Test, is listed directly below. The type of Fixation Monitor (Gaze/Blind Spot), Stimulus Size (III) and Color (White stimulus on White Background), and the pupil diameter in mm (3.0 mm) is displayed in the next line, along with the date of the examination. The standard background intensity of 31.5 asb is used for this test, and the BCVA is further inputted from the chart. Reliability indices including Fixation Losses, False Positive and False Negative Errors, are displayed as a ratio and percentage respectively. The testing strategy is also displayed (SITA-Standard). Making clinical assessments of progression based upon serial analysis of fields utilizing different strategies should be avoided. The optimal refractive correction for the 30cm test distance is displayed, and it is one of the essential roles of the perimetrist to accurately correct the patient with large diameter loose lenses. The test duration is also recorded, and can give insight into a patient's performance. Longer test durations are likely to be prone to errors secondary to fatigue, and may have poorer reliability indices as well. Often the second eye tested will have lower test times, indicating the possibility of a learning curve effect during that perimetry session. Alternating the first eye tested for subsequent fields may "reverse" this phenomenon when unexplained asymmetry is found. The threshold sensitivities, along with mean and pattern deviations are plotted along with probability analysis for a given defect. Darker shaded boxes within the field indicate a higher probability that the defect is valid compared to age-matched controls (range from 0.5% - 5%). The glaucoma hemifield test (GHT) is displayed in the upper right hand corner of this scan, indicating in this case that no asymmetry was found between the upper and lower sectors analyzed. Finally, the GPA summary plot is found in the boxed results section. In this case, no progression was detected. Symbols are placed at any test point location that has changed from baseline by more than the variability you would see in 19 out of 20 stable glaucoma patients at the approximately the same stage of the disease. The dates of the baseline and previous fields, used by the software to determine the likelihood of progression, are further displayed. The accuracy of the progression analysis improves dramatically with both a reliable baseline, and a larger number of follow-up fields.

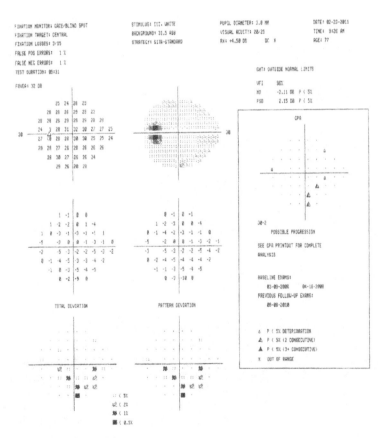

Fig. 4. Single field analysis: OS

In contrast to the right eye of the same patient, the left eye is demonstrating early changes in the pattern deviation of the inferior field (indicated by variably shaded boxes). The GHT is considered "Outside Normal Limits", and the GPA has determined the presence of "Possible Progression". The half-shaded triangles indicate p-values < 5% on 2 consecutive fields.

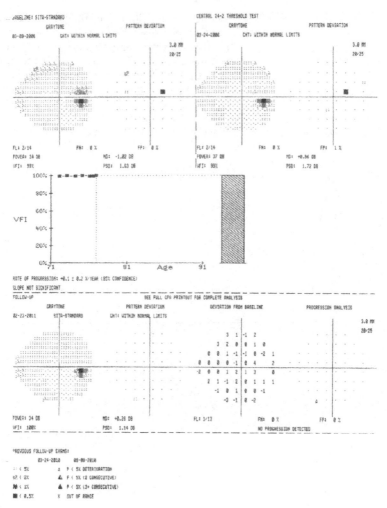

Fig. 5. GPA Summary OD

The GPA summary displays the grey scale for the baseline test, along with some of the indices for each of the tests displayed, including MD, PSD, GHT, Reliability Indices, Pupil size, and BCVA. The rate of change is also plotted over time (patient's age in years) against a visual field index (VFI). A VFI score of 100% represents a normal visual field, and 0% represents completely blackened perimetry. The VFI is calculated from pattern deviation plots, and was developed in response to the effects of media opacity on previous metrics. The rate of progression as a percentage is further displayed and analyzed. In this case, a +0.1 ± 0.2%/year was determined to be a normal slope. The shaded box at the far right of the plots is the extrapolated final VFI given a life expectancy of approximately 100 years old and the calculated rate of progression. The bottom half of the printout displays the results of the most recent exam, and provides probability plots for point-by-point likelihood of progression compared to baseline and prior follow-up examinations.

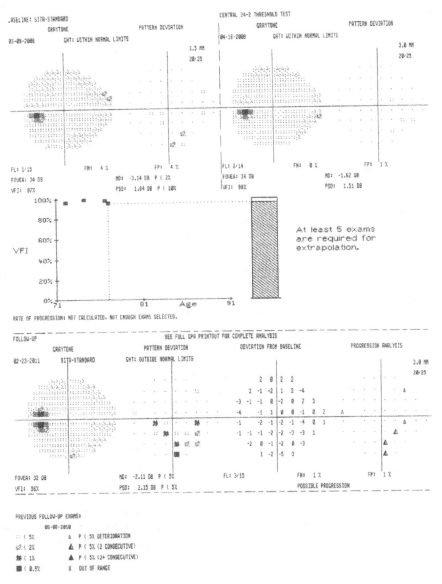

Fig. 6. GPA summary OS

In this case, it is demonstrated that the VFI extrapolation requires at least 5 consecutive tests to be considered reliable (only 4 visual fields are inputted), and a rate to be accurately calculated. The accuracy of this progression software significantly improves over time as additional fields are added to the analysis. The baseline visual fields in this patient are normal, in contrast to the defects noted in the most previous field detailed at the bottom of the printout. This patient is considered clinically to be at moderate risk of functional progression in this eye.

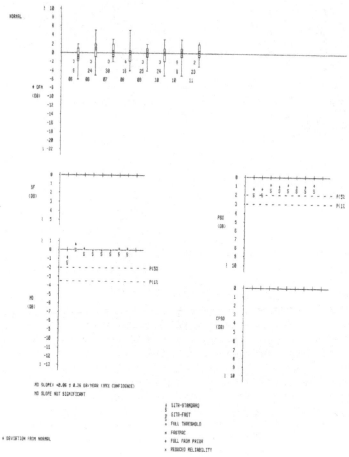

Fig. 7. Change analysis OD

The Change Analysis box plots display a variety of visual field metrics in the form of frequency distributions. The Y-axis is valued in Db, and represents the difference between the observed values relative to a normative database. The actual values observed are displayed in a chronological fashion centered on the 0 dB point (ie no deviation from normal). Positive deflections (above 0 db) indicate a "better than normal" threshold, and negative deflections indicate "worse than normal" threshold values. In this manner, the highest point (top of the "T") for each field represents the point with the highest threshold relative to normal. The shaded boxes for each data set indicate the percentile rank within each field. The highest value of the uppermost box for each data set is the 85th percentile, the middle represents the 50th percentile (ie half of the thresholds are above, and the other half below), and the bottom value represents the 15th percentile. The slope of the line for each visual field index is graphically displayed and then analyzed. In this example, the MD slope is calculated as +0.06 ± 0.26dB/year, indicating that no progression is noted during the testing interval. It is important to note that other diagnoses besides glaucoma can adversely affect the indices as well. Clinical correlation is always imperative.

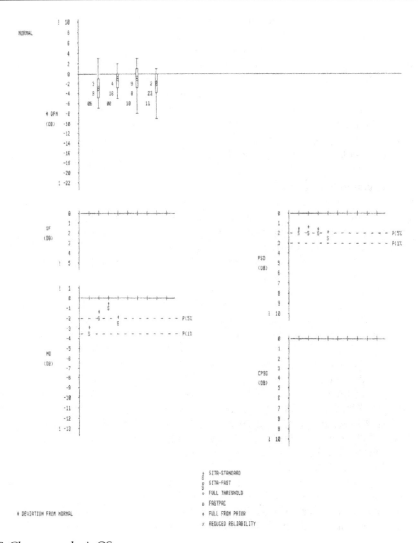

Fig. 8. Change analysis OS

In contrast to the right eye, the median values for the fields included are below the 0db line. The highest threshold points for each field (top of the "T") are above normal limits, however the range of percentile rankings tend to be below the 0 dB mark. The PSD plot further demonstrates possible worsening of the visual field, particularly in the latest examination.

3.2 Alternate functional assessment

When a patient is determined by multiple attempts and strategies to be a poor test taker by conventional SAP, alternate strategies may need to be employed to measure the visual field and establish an adequate baseline. As therapeutic algorithms are often advanced (ie topical therapy, laser, incisional surgery) based upon demonstration of functional progression of disease, it is optimal for the clinician to exhaust any and all options available to determine the functional status of a patient. The Octopus perimeter is an alternative to the HVF, and offers many advantages in these patients. The Goldmann kinetic perimeter is an also relatively commonly used option in these patients for multiple reasons. As fixation can be manually monitored, patients are able to take breaks during testing, and receive coaching and encouragement on a point by point basis. Frequency Doubling Technology (FDT), Matrix analyzers, while much faster than traditional SAP, may not necessarily be appropriate as an alternate testing protocol for many patients. Simple confrontational visual fields provide only a gross estimate of visual function, and are clearly not an appropriate way to follow patients with, or at risk for glaucoma.

3.2.1 Octopus visual field analyzer

The Octopus visual field analyzer (Haag-Streit International, Koeniz, Switzerland) has had major advancements over the past decade, which largely developed in response to many of the limitations of the HVF. One of the key advancements in the technology is an improved fixation/blink monitor which continually tracks and accounts for fixation losses and eye blinking, along with automatic adjustments based on head and eye positioning relative to the perimeter. This additional functionality can dramatically improve the accuracy of the test, and further limit lens/rim artifacts that may occur with traditional SAP. Furthermore, the Tendency Oriented Perimeter (TOP) strategy employed by the Octopus reduces test duration for threshold analysis to an average of 2.5 minutes per eye, significantly reducing patient fatigue. The Octopus' EyeSuite™ Progression software offers intuitive plots demonstrating both global and cluster progression, and has the ability to integrate structural assessment as well. The Octopus test stimuli and background intensities are matched to those of Humphrey and Goldmann perimeters (See HFA above and GVF below).

Studies comparing the Octopus and Humphrey visual field analyzers have demonstrated variable results. King, et al[45] demonstrated that the SITA Fast and TOP strategies were highly correlated in a study of 76 glaucoma patients. They did note that although the TOP strategy was faster than the SITA protocol, it tended to underestimate the focal visual field defects. A recent analysis by Lan, et al[46] demonstrated a similar finding when comparing the Octopus to FDT (see below). Often times, the establishment of newer baselines with an alternate protocol proves to be a major barrier to adaptation. As with many technologies, ease of integration into electronic medical records has proven to be a driving force for changes in clinical practice. The utility of testing patients with multiple functional assessments remains to be determined given the likelihood of discordance.

3.2.2 Goldmann visual field (GVF)

The major difference between SAP and Goldmann visual field testing is that the SAP is a static visual field, whereas Goldmann visual field testing is kinetic, defined as perimetry utilizing a moving stimulus (3-5 degrees/second)[47]. It is important to note that the GVF may be used as a manual static perimeter as well, and is generally reserved for improved isolation of an existing scotoma. In the case of kinetic Goldmann perimetry, the moving stimulus is controlled by a skilled operator. This subjectivity is a major drawback, as subtle changes in the visual field can easily be missed given the summative variability of both the patient and operator[48]. However, given that each patient response can be carefully monitored, the added reliability of GVF testing makes the test clinically useful in patients who are unable to perform SAP. This is especially true in patients with poor central visual acuity who are unable to reliably fixate for automated perimetry. This is indeed one of the most common reasons that GVF testing is ordered for glaucoma patients.

An additional advantage of the GVF is that it is it the only form of perimetry that is able to test the entire visual field. This encompasses 60 degrees superiorly and nasally, 75 degrees inferiorly, and 110 degrees temporally, although there are few clinical indications that demand testing far peripheral points. Neuro-ophthamic evaluation for functional visual loss and other central processes remains another common indication for GVF testing.

Definitions of stimuli and target sizes are summarized below.

Stimulus size	Stimulus Intensity
0 = 1/16 mm²	1 – 4 : represent 5dB increments
I = 1/4 mm²	a - e : represent 1 dB increments
II = 1 mm²	
III = 4mm²	
IV= 16mm²	
V= 64 mm²	

3.2.3 Frequency doubling technology (FDT) and the Matrix™ perimeter

FDT perimetry is based on a phenomenon that when an achromatic sinusoidal grating ,with low spatial frequency, flickers at a high temporal frequency, the apparent spatial frequency of the grating appears to be doubled[49]. Glaucoma is thought to preferentially effect cells in the magnocellular pathway, which have been demonstrated to be more sensitive to motion and flicker detection[50]. On the other hand, theories contend that the FDT illusion is based on higher cortical processing, and no retinal substrate exists to account for the phenomenon[51]. Regardless, the appeal of a technology that is theoretically able to preferentially detect damage to this visual pathway is obvious, and the clinical utility of FDT has advanced remarkably over the past decades. Current screening and full threshold strategies can be performed in minutes, reducing the inaccuracies of testing patients that are easily fatigued by the duration of SAP and similar strategies (Figures 9-10). Reproducibility of FDT results has further been demonstrated in multiple studies[52,53]. The reported sensitivity of FDT ranged from 0.51 to 1.00, and specificity from 0.58 to 1.00 determined by a meta-analysis of pooled data in 2006, with similar findings in more recent data.[54,55]

Nakagawa, et al.[56] recently examined 39 open angle glaucoma patients with low to moderate IOP, comparing FDT to SAP. With almost 5 years of follow-up, they determined that FDT was useful for monitoring defects detected in the SAP-normal hemifield in OAG eyes with low-to-normal IOP. A detailed study of 60 eyes with normal SAP ("pre-perimetric glaucoma") found that FDT testing was able to detect abnormalities in an astounding 65% of patients, of which 51% later developed defects by SAP over 4-27 months[57], a clear demonstration of the clinical utility of FDT in early detection of disease processes. Ferraras, et al[58] examined 278 subjects with pre-perimetric glaucoma by SAP, but with structural abnormalities by HRT, GDx-VCC, and OCT (see below). This study demonstrated that 20% of patients with structural loss had abnormalities on SWAP and FDT testing when SAP was found to be normal.

The Humphrey Matrix perimeter (Carl Zeiss Meditec, Dublin, Calif) was introduced in 2005, as a newer generation FDT perimetry option with the implementation of multiple efficiency measurements to reduce test taking duration. Fixation monitoring technology has been implemented, as have a wide variety of testing options ranging from screening to full threshold algorithms. The option of smaller stimuli able to resolve subtle maculopathies, etc. is a further advancement from older generation FDT perimeters.

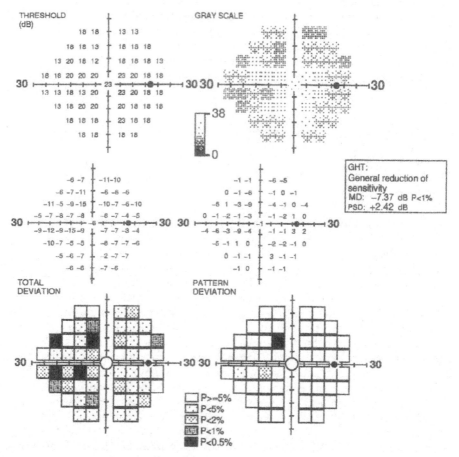

Fig. 9. Frequency doubling technology (FDT): Right eye of same patient on same day as HVF

The FDT plots of the right eye of the same patient show similar metrics to the HVF single field analysis (See Figure 1). The total deviation plot demonstrates more damage than the pattern deviation plot, likely indicating the presence of a media opacity in this patient. The pattern deviation plot demonstrates one point , in the superior field close to the vertical meridian, with a p<0.5 value not detected by the HVF. The significance of this point of visual field loss, as with any finding, needs to be correlated clinically with structural examination and careful ophthalmoscopy. This may indicate a false positive value, or possibly an early defect that the FDT was able to resolve prior to HVF change.

A recent prospective study of 115 glaucomatous eyes examined with the Humprey Matrix perimeterand SITA-SWAP demonstrated sensitivity of 87% for early glaucoma (pattern standard deviation was 94% and mean deviation was 91%); and nearly 100% sensitivity and specificity for moderate to advanced glaucoma when compared to SAP[59]. Another study comparing FDT to SAP in 50 patients with confirmed glaucoma by SAP demonstrated excellent sensitivities of greater than 90%, and demonstrated that FDT had greater specificity than SAP in detecting more severe defects.[60] These recent results certainly demonstrate that FDT is a technology that likely will play an increasing role in the functional assessment of glaucoma patients.

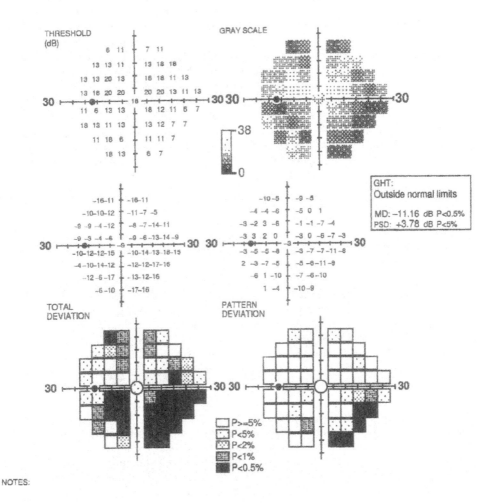

Fig. 10. Frequency doubling technology: Left eye of same patient on same day as HVF

The FDT plot clearly demonstrates a focal defect in the inferonasal field that corresponds to the HVF defects (See Figures 4-6). It is interesting to note that the MD is significantly lower (-11.16 dB) than that calculated from a HVF the same day (-2.11 dB). This large discrepancy may be indicative of the FDT's ability to detect disease at an earlier state. However, the rate of change demonstrated in subsequent FDT evaluations will provide more insight into the likelihood of clinical relevant progression.

4. Structural assessment of the glaucoma patient

The assessment of structural abnormalities of the anterior segment and the optic nerve can be performed utilizing a variety of technologies. Each of these diagnostic modalities offers a range of imaging resolutions, and the latest iterations offer extremely detailed images. Arguably, the largest advantage of adjunctive structural assessment is the fact that the measurements are purely objective (ie not subject to the inherent variability seen in all forms of subjective functional assessment). Another important ramification of these advancements is the ability to detect structural abnormalities prior to functional loss. In patients with documented functional loss, structural assessment further allows for quantification of the magnitude of defects. The detailed summary images rendered allow clinicians to actively engage patients in their diagnosis and treatment with simple color coded plots of the relevant anatomy. A great deal of research has been done utilizing these technologies, and it has clearly changed the manner in which clinicians diagnose, treat, and monitor disease progression. Furthermore, objective measurements are inherently less likely to be subject to test taking environments, and are therefore more translatable between practitioners. As structural assessments are not without limitations, it is the role of the clinician to reconcile discordant data, and make the most appropriate recommendations based on the totality of information available.

Prior to the modern imaging techniques further described below, clinicians relied on careful fundoscopic examination and red-free photography to visualize the retinal nerve fiber layer. A recent study by Suh, et al analyzed progressing normal tension glaucoma patients with red-free photography, visual fields, and stereo disc photography[61]. Four characteristic progression patterns were noted including: widening of the existing defect towards the macula, deepening of the defect without expansion, appearance of a new defect, and finally widening of a defect away from the macula. It was noted that almost 95% of these patients exhibited widening of the defect towards the macula, and deepening of the existing defect. Interestingly, no progression was clinically observed on the disc stereo photographs (n=65) or in the visual fields (n=55) in 64 eyes (98.5%) and 46 eyes (83.6%), respectively[61]. Although useful, reproducible high quality red-free images are often difficult and expensive to obtain. Serial red-free photography has largely been supplanted by the newer diagnostic modalities presented below for more routine cases.

4.1 Ocular coherence tomography (OCT)

OCT is one of the technologies that has absolutely revolutionized the field of ophthalmology. Clinicians are now able to resolve, at the micrometer level, exceptional three dimensional images of ocular tissues *in vivo*. These detailed images have allowed us to follow a variety of disease states with incredible accuracy, and help monitor the efficacy of therapeutic interventions. OCT is based upon the principle of interferometry, and provides a non-invasive "optical biopsy" of almost every aspect of the ocular anatomy. OCT is powered by low-coherence near infrared light (820nm), and renders images of microstructures based upon reflected signals. The light source at this wavelength offers excellent tissue penetration and has an exceptional safety profile. The super luminescent diode light source is split, simultaneously illuminating the ocular tissue specified, along with an internal reference mirror. The interference patterns of the backscattered light is detected by photo detectors, and then graphically interpreted into a standardized output format.

4.1.1 Time-domain OCT

This technology is used by the Stratus® OCT (Carl Zeiss Meditec, Dublin, CA), allowing for approximately 10 micrometer resolution at an acquisition rate of approximately 400 scans/second. This technology has recently been somewhat supplanted by higher generation OCT scanners in many practices. (see Spectral Domain OCT below). The most commonly used protocol for glaucoma management is the Fast Retinal Nerve Fiber (RNFL) scan, with thinning of the RNFL serving as a surrogate for the measurement of ganglion cell loss. The optic nerve head can be further analyzed to determine rim volume, depth, and cup to disc ratio, amongst other parameters. The Fast RNFL protocol measures the thickness of the RNFL in a circumferential fashion around the optic nerve at around a 3.4mm diameter. The thicknesses of the RNFL from both eyes are then compared to an age-matched normative database. The results are displayed in graphical form with a color coding system designed to represent the severity of the thinning. The average RNFL thickness is calculated from the thicknesses of individually displayed measurements from all four quadrants of the optic nerve. Time-domain OCT has limitations with regards to resolution and data acquisition speeds. This is based on the fact that the technology is limited by the velocity of movement of-a mirror-interferometer Kanamori, et al.[62] compared the RNFL scans and mean deviation (MD) from SAP of 237 glaucomatous eyes versus 160 controls, and found a significant correlation between RNFL thinning and greater MD. Furthermore, the average RNFL thickness proved to be the most reliable parameter in monitoring glaucomatous progression. Gupta, et al.[63] in a recent review in the neuro-ophthalmic literature, demonstrated that patients with non-glaucomatous optic neuropathies had a thinner RNFL thickness than patients with glaucomatous optic neuropathy. Leung, et al.[64] conducted a large study of 137 eyes obtaining 1373 Fast RNFL scans, 1373 normal RFNL scans, and 1236 visual fields over a median period of 4 years, and determined that the Fast RNFL protocol was the most reliable Stratus OCT protocol to detect and follow progression in glaucomatous eyes.

Given the objective nature of OCT scans, there is a tendency amongst clinicians to rely on these examinations more than functional assessment with perimetry. While this may be deemed appropriate in patients unable to perform perimetric evaluation reliably, the limitations of OCT must be taken into account as well. Reliable OCTs are often impossible in patients with severe surface disease, miotic pupils, dense media opacification, high axial length with associated peripapillary atrophy, and vitreous disease. Correlations should routinely be performed between OCT results and the clinical appearance of the optic nerve, as the scans may underestimate cupping when there is glaucomatous undermining under the rim tissue.

Our group[65] recently published a study further demonstrating the confounding effects of vitreous traction on the retinal nerve fiber layer. Approximately 110 eyes of patients were examined with Stratus OCT. Those noted to have partial vitreous detachments at the optic nerve head were found to have artifactually elevated RNFL measurements when matched to controls. Given the relatively high incidence of partial posterior vitreous detachments in the glaucoma group, it was hypothesized that RNFL damage from glaucoma may be masked by the effects of the vitreo-retinal interface. It was concluded from these results that both structural and functional assessments are imperative to determine the presence of glaucomatous damage in these patients in particular. Further investigation of the natural history of PVD, along with changes in the measured retinal nerve fiber layer by OCT, is currently underway. A corollary analysis of the effects of aging on vitreous separation is furthermore being investigated The vitreoretinal interface has been extensively examined by

OCT, particularly in diabetics. Ophir et al, amongst others, have performed multiple analyses utilizing 3-D SD-OCT (see below) to demonstrate that the subtleties of the vitreoretinal interface can be resolved accurately[66,67].

4.1.2 Spectral domain (SD) OCT

SD-OCT, also known as Fourier Domain OCT or High Definition OCT (HD-OCT), is the latest commercially available iteration of the OCT technology at the time of this publication. The commercially available Cirrus® OCT (Carl Zeiss Meditec, Inc.) has tremendous advantages over the Stratus OCT in the evaluation and management of many eye conditions. SD-OCT measures the cross-spectral density, a Fourier transformation aimed to estimate the spectral density from a sequence of time samples. The measurements are performed at the detection arm of the interferometer[68]. This allows for much higher resolution and lower test times, as there are no "moving-part" limitations within the interferometer. Furthermore, the ability of the SD-OCT to capture approximately 20,000 axial scans per second, compared to 400 scans/sec for the Stratus OCT, allows for significantly more accurate imaging. This further translates into scans that are less subject to micro-saccadic eye movements during data acquisition. The resultant axial resolution of the scans can be less than 6 micrometers. The Cirrus OCT is furthermore able to match anatomical landmarks from prior scans, minimizing the errors associated with scan misalignment. Misalignment errors are indeed an important source of confounding data with previous versions of the OCT. This is especially the case when longitudinal progression analysis is performed. Lastly the ability to render 3-Dimensional imaging of complex ocular anatomy is yet another major advancement.

Many ophthalmic practices have updated the Stratus OCT to one of the SD-OCT modules in the recent past. It is important to note that the aforementioned differences do not easily allow clinicians to compare RNFL measurements between the two technologies, and accurate correction factors are currently lacking. The re-establishment of a new baseline RNFL thickness with the SD-OCT is quite commonly done in many of these cases. Knight, et al.[69] compared the Stratus OCT to the Cirrus OCT RNFL measurements of 130 eyes with glaucoma relative to normal controls. They demonstrated that the RNFL thickness measured by the Stratus OCT tended to be higher than that of the Cirrus OCT. Sung, et al[70], performed a similar comparative study of 60 normals, 48 glaucoma suspects, and 55 glaucoma patients, They demonstrated that the Cirrus OCT had better sensitivity and specificity for disease than the Stratus OCT, and classified a significantly higher proportion of patients as abnormal. Specifically, Cirrus OCT demonstrated higher sensitivity and specificity (63.6% and 100%) than the Stratus OCT (40.0% and 96.7%) Leung, et al.[64], in a study of 128 glaucomatous eyes over 2 years, similarly concluded that the Cirrus OCT detected glaucomatous changes earlier and more often that the Stratus OCT. A portion of this difference can be attributed to decreased measurement variability with the Cirrus OCT.

Newer versions being developed will likely offer even greater sensitivity and specificity, improved resolution, and clinical progression analysis. Incorporation and evaluation of perimetry in the analysis will likely help bridge the current gap that exists between structural damage and functional loss These advancements will likely be in part possible with the exponentially growing adoption of electronic medical record (EMR) systems. At the time of this publication, significant barriers exist with respect to the interface between EMR, and the variety of functional and structural assessment tools that were traditionally designed as stand-alone technologies.

4.2 Confocal scanning laser ophthalmoscopy (SLO)

Retinal imaging with a confocal scanning laser ophthalmoscope (cSLO) involves scanning a small laser beam over the retina, and constructing an image from the descanned reflected light. By applying the confocal principle, tomographic images can be produced[71]. The confocal principle involves measurement of reflected laser light which is concentrated through a pinhole. SLO is based upon acquiring point-by-point images from a series of depths, and then reconstructing them into three-dimensional topographic images.. The Heidelberg Retinal Tomography (HRT) unit scans the fundus with a 670-nm diode laser, creating a three-dimensional map of the fundus and optic nerve. This is accomplished by obtaining multiple optical sections at different depths using a confocal aperture[72] The commercially available (HRT) unit has undergone advancements since the advent of the technology, to its current form as the HRT-III. HRT is used clinically in a similar manner to OCT scans in the evaluation and management of glaucoma. Exceptional imaging quality and newer iterations of progression analysis have made the HRT one of the leading structural analysis tools in practice today. HRT scans further employ eye tracking technology to improve the validity and reproducibility of serial examination. The analysis of the optic nerve head further includes a variety of metrics designed to document morphological variants (Figure 11). The clinical and predictive utility of these parameters continues to be the subject of a great deal of research and subsequent debate. As with any testing modality, data from the HRT needs to be correlated to an individual patient's clinical picture to determine its validity.

Kalabhoukhava, et al.[72], analyzed 59 subjects with ocular hypertension and glaucoma over 50 months with HRT, perimetry, and stereo disk photography. After expert review of the patients at the 50 month time point, subjects were grouped as either progressive or non-progressive. HRT parameters (cup shape measurement, classification index, the third moment in contour, cup/disc ratio, cup area, rim area, and area below reference) showed statistically significant morphological changes in only the progressive group (ie no change from baseline in the "stable" group). These results effectively demonstrate the high diagnostic utility of HRT testing as an adjunctive assessment tool for glaucoma evaluation. Kilintizis, et al[73], demonstrated that changes in HRT parameters of "length of contour" (LC) and "standard deviation of contour" (SDC) were of particular significance when comparing almost 100 glaucoma patients to controls. Balasubramanian, et al.[74] compared HRT I and II parameters in 380 eyes, and concluded that the stereometric parameters were not significantly altered by the newer generation scans. Another study by this same group performed an observational cohort study of 246 eyes followed with HRT, topographic change analysis (TCA), SAP, and stereo photography. It was concluded from the variability in results that there is a great deal of discordance in the detection of longitudinal change[75] between these modalities. Somewhat conflicting assessments of the utility of the HRT, as with all of the aforementioned diagnostic modalities, reminds us that the clinical utility of any data collected greatly relies on the clinician's subjective correlations.

4.3 Scanning laser polarimetry (SLP)

The original GDx (Laser Diagnostic Technologies, San Diego, CA), and newer versions with variable corneal compensation GDx-VCC (Carl Zeiss Meditec, Dublin, CA), analyze RNFL thickness with a different method than the OCT and HRT. The RNFL is birifringent secondary to the highly ordered microtubule arrays of the axon microtubules. As the near infrared laser light (780 nm) is split by the birifringent tissue, a phase shift phenomenon

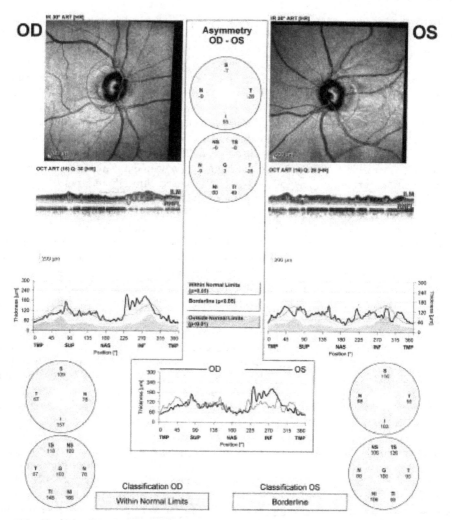

Fig. 11. Heidelberg retinal tomography (HRT) summary of RNFL of same patient on same day as HVF and FDT

Structural analysis may demonstrate an anatomical correlate to demonstrable visual field loss. The digital images are rendered at the top of the summary slide. The green circle demonstrates the limits of the area that is being examined. Centration is optimal in this case, and the newest generation HRT scanners are able to register and match previous scans to improve the reliability of progression analysis. The difference, or calculated asymmetry, between the two eyes is displayed in the top center of the summary printout. The difference in measure RNFL (OD – OS) is graphically displayed by location in the circumpapillary region with S= Superior, N= Nasal, I=Inferior, T=temporal, along with combinations in between the regions (ie TS = Temporal Superior, etc.). Negative values indicate that the left eye has a thicker RNFL, and positive values indicate the opposite. The circumpapillary RNFL.

occurs given the difference in velocity of the reflected light. RNFL thickness can be calculated based on the magnitude of this phase shift. As the anterior segment structures also demonstrate the property of biriferigence, it is necessary to subtract these effects, and newer versions with customized corneal compensation have proven to be much more accurate than prior versions utilizing a fixed compensation algorithm[76]. While the newest generation SLP is far more accurate than earlier versions, the technology is subject to some degree of variability in eyes that show so called "atypical birefringence patterns". Normal patterns of birefringence are generally characterized by the presence of high peripapillary retardation superiorly and inferiorly. This pattern corresponds histologically to the distribution of the superior and inferior arcuate nerve fiber bundles.[77] Abnormal patterns, that are considered normal variants, could therefore confound the data analysis and subsequent detection of disease.

Kim, et al.[78] measured the RNFL of 60 normal patients to 60 glaucoma patients with GDx VCCand Stratus OCT. The results demonstrated no significant differences between the instruments, with high correlations in the superior and inferior quadrants in particular. Pablo, et al[79]analyzed 181 eyes diagnosed with OHTN with GDx-VCC and Stratus OCT, and also found similar diagnostic accuracy between the two. Aptel, et al.[80], compared 120 eyes with Cirrus OCT and GDx-VCC (40 normals, 40 glaucoma suspects, 40 glaucoma) compared with visual field sensitivity, and found that the Cirrus OCT had a stronger correlation to function than the GDx-VCC. Lopez-Pena[81] performed a prospective study of 423 eyes 87 normal eyes, 192 ocular hypertensive eyes, 70 pre-perimetric glaucomas and 74 glaucomatous eyes) to compare SAP with GDx-VCC. The results of this large study showed only weak to moderate correlations with RNFL measurements and visual field defects in the glaucoma group. The relationship between HRT structural defects with functional visual field changes is clearly yet to be well defined.

5. Conclusions

The management of glaucoma in the modern era, despite the advent of a host of technologies, remains more of an art than a science in many respects. Improvements in tonometry will continue to improve the accuracy of IOP measurement, especially as the effects of corneal biomechanical properties continue to be elucidated. The potential for accurate home monitoring will allow for better assessment of diurnal and inter-visit IOP control. Similarly, improved imaging techniques will allow for earlier detection of disease with continually improving resolution and reproducibility. It is important to consider that early detection of glaucoma inherently carries the risk of over-diagnosis and subsequent overtreatment. Rates of progression, with all of the modalities described, need to be established prior to the initiation or advancement of therapy. Understanding the limitations of the testing is imperative when making assessments regarding both structure and function. A gestalt approach to glaucoma management allows the specialist to amalgamate a host of information, and effectively cater therapies based on the information available. The modern age of glaucoma care has had notable advancements, and the future of glaucoma management will allow for the optimal care of this globally disabling disease.

6. References

[1] Yeshigeta, G. et al. The Influence of Central Corneal Thickness on Intraocular Pressure Measured by Goldmann Applanation Tonometry Among Selected Ethiopian

Communities J Glaucoma: October/November 2010 - Volume 19 - Issue 8 - p 514–518

[2] Azuara-Blanco, T. Bhojani, A. Sarhan, C Pillai, H. Dua Tono-Pen determination of intraocular pressure in patients with band keratopathy or glued cornea *Br J Ophthalmol.* 1998 June; 82(6): 634–636.

[3] Broman AT, Congdon NG, Bandeen-Roche K, Quigley HA. Influence of corneal structure, corneal responsiveness, and other ocular parameters on tonometric measurement of intraocular pressure. *J Glaucoma.* 2007 Oct-Nov;16(7):581-8.3.

[4] Lester M, Mermoud A, Achache F, Roy S. New Tonopen XL: comparison with the Goldmann tonometer. *Eye* (Lond). 2001 Feb;15(Pt 1):52-8.

[5] Kirwan C, O'Keefe M. Corneal hysteresis using the Reichert ocular response analyser: findings pre- and post-LASIK and LASEK. *Acta* Ophthalmol. 2008 Mar;86(2):215-8.

[6] Ayala M. Corneal Hysteresis in Normal Subjects and in Patients with Primary Open-Angle Glaucoma and Pseudoexfoliation Glaucoma. *Ophthalmic Res.* 2011 Apr 6;46(4):187-191.

[7] Detry-Morel M, Jamart J, Pourjavan S. Evaluation of corneal biomechanical properties with the Reichert Ocular Response Analyzer. *Eur J Ophthalmol.* 2011 Mar-Apr;21(2):138-48.

[8] Anand A, De Moraes CG, Teng CC, Tello C, et al. Corneal hysteresis and visual field asymmetry in open angle glaucoma. *Invest Ophthalmol Vis Sci.* 2010 Dec;51(12):6514-8.

[9] Ang GS, Bochmann F, Townend J, Azuara-Blanco A. Corneal biomechanical properties in primary open angle glaucoma and normal tension glaucoma. *J Glaucoma.* 2008 Jun-Jul;17(4):259-62.

[10] Mollan SP, Wolffsohn JS, Nessim M, Laiquzzaman M, Sivakumar S, Hartley S, Shah S. Accuracy of Goldmann, ocular response analyser, Pascal and TonoPen XL tonometry in keratoconic and normal eyes. *Br J Ophthalmol* 2008;92:1661-1665.

[11] Knecht PB, Schmid U, Romppainen T, Hediger A, Funk J, Kanngiesser H, Kniestedt C. Hand-held dynamic contour tonometry. *Acta Ophthalmologica* Volume 89, Issue 2, pages 132–137, March 2011

[12] Gunvant P, Newcomb RD, Kirstein EM, Malinovsky VE, Madonna RJ Meetz RE Measuring accurate IOPs: Does correction factor help or hurt? 2010. *OPTH* 4:611-6

[13] Kotecha A, White E, Schlottmann PG, Garway-Heath DF. Intraocular pressure measurement precision with the Goldmann applanation, dynamic contour, and ocular response analyzer tonometers. *Ophthalmology.* 2010 Apr;117(4):730-7.

[14] Sullivan-Mee M, Gerhardt G, Halverson KD, Qualls C. Repeatability and reproducibility for intraocular pressure measurement by dynamic contour, ocular response analyzer, and goldmann applanation tonometry. *J Glaucoma.* 2009 Dec;18(9):666-73.

[15] Flemmons MS, Hsiao YC, Dzau J, Asrani S, Jones S, Freedman SF. Icare rebound tonometry in children with known and suspected glaucoma. *J AAPOS.* 2011 Apr;15(2):153-7.

[16] Scuderi GL, Cascone NC, Regine F, Perdicchi A, Cerulli A, Recupero SM. Validity and limits of the rebound tonometer (ICare®): clinical study. *Eur J Ophthalmol.* 2011 May-Jun;21(3):251-7.

[17] Munkwitz S, Elkarmouty A, Hoffmann EM, Pfeiffer N, Thieme H. Comparison of the iCare rebound tonometer and the Goldmann applanation tonometer over a wide IOP range. Graefes Arch Clin Exp Ophthalmol. 2008 Jun;246(6):875-9.

[18] Asrani S, Chatterjee A, Wallace DK, Santiago-Turla C, Stinnett S. Evaluation of the ICare rebound tonometer as a home intraocular pressure monitoring device. J Glaucoma. 2011 Feb;20(2):74-9.

[19] Kass MA, Heuer DK, Higginbotham EJ, et al. Ocular Hypertension Treatment Study Group. The Ocular Hypertension Treatment Study (OHTS): a randomized trial determines that topical ocular hypotensive medication delays or prevents the onset of primary open-angle glaucoma. *Arch Ophthalmol.* 2002;120:701–13

[20] The AGIS Investigators. The Advanced Glaucoma Intervention Study (AGIS):11. Risk factors for failure of trabeculectomy and argon laser trabeculoplasty in advanced glaucoma patients. *Am J Ophthalmol.* 2002;134:481–498

[21] Musch DC, Lichter PR, Guire KE, Standardi CL CIGTS Study Group. The Collaborative Initial Glaucoma Treatment Study: study design, methods, and baseline characteristics of enrolled patients. *Ophthalmology.* 1999;106:653–662

[22] Lindenmuth KA, Skuta GL, Rabbani R, Musch DC. Effects of pupillary constriction on automated perimetry in normal eyes. *Ophthalmology.* 1989 Sep;96(9):1298–1301.

[23] Nordmann JP, Brion F, Hamard P, Mouton-Chopin D. Evaluation of the Humphrey perimetry programs SITA Standard and SITA Fast in normal probands and patients with glaucoma. *J Fr Ophthalmol.* 1998 Oct;21(8):549-54

[24] Budenz DL, Rhee P, Feuer WJ, McSoley J, et al. Sensitivity and specificity of the Swedish interactive threshold algorithm for glaucomatous visual field defects. *Ophthalmology.* 2002 Jun;109(6):1052-8

[25] Martin PR, White AJ, Goodchild AK, et al. Evidence that blue-on cells are part of the third geniculocortical pathway in primates. *Eur J Neurosci.* 1997 Jul;9(7):1536-41.

[26] Dacey DM, Lee BB. The 'blue-on' opponent pathway in primate retina originates from a distinct bistratified ganglion cell type. *Nature.* 1994 Feb 24;367(6465):731-5.

[27] Tarek Shaarawy, Mark B. Sherwood, Roger A. Hitchings, Jonathan G. Crowston Glaucoma: Expert Consult Premium Edition Volume 2.

[28] Johnson CA, Adams AJ, Casson EJ, Brandt JD. Blue-on-yellow Perimetry can predict the development of glaucomatous visual field loss. *Arch Ophthalmol* 1993;111:645-50.

[29] Johnson CA, Adams AJ, Casson EJ, Brandt JD. Progression of early glaucomatous visual field loss as detected by blue-on-yellow and standard white-on-white automated Perimetry. *Arch Ophthalmol* 1993;111:651-6.

[30] Van Der Schoot J, Reus NJ, Colen TP, Lemij HG. The ability of short-wavelength automated perimetry to predict conversion to glaucoma. *Ophthalmology.* 2010; 117(1):30-34.

[31] Bengtsson B. A New Rapid Threshold Algorithm for Short-Wavelength Automated Perimetry Invest. *Ophthalmol. Vis. Sci.* March 2003 vol. 44 no. 3 1388-1394

[32] Bengtsson B, Heijl A. Diagnostic Sensitivity of Fast Blue–Yellow and Standard Automated Perimetry in Early Glaucoma:A Comparison between Different Test Programs. *Ophthalmology* July 2006; 113(7) 1092-1097

[33] Birt CM, Shin DH, Samudrala V, et al. Analysis of reliability indices from Humphrey visual field tests in an urban glaucoma population. *Ophthalmology.* 1997 Jul; 104(7):1126-30.

[34] Newkirk MR, Gardiner SK, Demirel S, Johnson CA. Assessment of False Positives with the Humphrey Field Analyzer II Perimeter with the SITA Algorithm. *Invest. Ophthalmol. Vis. Sci.* Oct 2006: 47(10) 4632-4637

[35] Vingrys AJ, Demirel S. False-response monitoring during automated perimetry. *Optom Vis Sci.* 1998 Jul;75(7):513-7.

[36] Bengtsson B, Olsson J, Heijl A, Rootze'n H. A new generation of algorithms for computerized threshold perimetry, SITA. *Acta Ophthalmol Scand.* 1997;75:368-375.

[37] Åsman P, Heijl A. Glaucoma Hemifield Test: Automated Visual Field Evaluation *Arch Ophthalmol.* 1992;110(6):812-819.

[38] Katz J, Quigley HA, Sommer A. Detection of incident field loss using the glaucoma hemifield test. *Ophthalmology.* 1996 Apr;103(4):657-63.

[39] Susanna R Jr, Nicolela MT, Soriano DS, Carvalho C. Automated perimetry: a study of the glaucoma hemifield test for the detection of early glaucomatous visual field loss. *J Glaucoma.* 1994 Spring;3(1):12-6.

[40] Johnson CA, Sample PA, Cioffi GA, et al. Structure and Function Evaluation (SAFE) (I. Criteria for glaucomatous visual field loss using standard automated perimetry (SAP) and short wavelength automated perimetry (SWAP). *Am J Ophthalmol.* 2002;134:177-185

[41] Lester M, Corallo G, Capris E, Capris P. Agreement in detecting glaucomatous visual field progression by using guided progression analysis and Humphrey overview printout. *Eur J Ophthalmol.* Feb 2011: 21(5): 6-6.

[42] Casas-Llera P, Rebolleda G, Muñoz-Negrete FJ, et al. Visual field index rate and event-based glaucoma progression analysis: comparison in a glaucoma population. *Br J Ophthalmol.* 2009 Dec;93(12):1576-9. Epub 2009 Jun 16.

[43] Arnalich-Montiel F, Casas-Llera P, Muñoz-Negrete FJ, Rebolleda G. Performance of glaucoma progression analysis software in a glaucoma population. *Graefes Arch Clin Exp Ophthalmol.* 2009 Mar;247(3):391-7. Epub 2008 Nov 4.

[44] Diaz-Aleman VT, Anton A, de la Rosa MG, Johnson ZK, et al. Detection of visual-field deterioration by Glaucoma Progression Analysis and Threshold Noiseless Trend programs. *Br J Ophthalmol.* 2009 Mar;93(3):322-8. Epub 2008 Jul 11.

[45] King AJ, Taguri A, Wadood AC, Azuara-Blanco A. Comparison of two fast strategies, SITA Fast and TOP, for the assessment of visual fields in glaucoma patients. *Graefes Arch Clin Exp Ophthalmol.* 2002 Jun;240(6):481-7. Epub 2002 May 15.

[46] Lan YW, Hsieh JW, Sun FJ. Comparison of matrix perimetry with octopus perimetry for assessing glaucomatous visual field defects. *J Glaucoma.* 2011 Feb;20(2):126-32.

[47] Alward, W. Krachmer, J editor; Glaucoma the requisites in Ophthalmology. *Mosby*, St Louis; 2000; p57-61.

[48] Katz J, Tielsch JM, Quigley HA, Sommer A. Automated perimetry detects visual field loss before manual Goldmann perimetry. *Ophthalmology* 1995;102(1):21-6.

[49] Kelly DH. Frequency doubling in visual responses. J Opt Soc Am 1966;56:1628-33.

[50] Maddess T, Severt WL. Testing for glaucoma with the frequency-doubling illusion in the whole, macular and eccentric visual fields. *Aust N Z J Ophthalmol* 1999;27:194-6.43.

[51] White AJ, Sun H, Swanson WH, Lee BB. An examination of physiological mechanisms underlying the frequency-doubling illusion. *Invest Ophthalmol Vis Sci* 2002; 43:3590-9.

[52] Anderson AJ, Johnson CA. Frequency-doubling technology perimetry. *Ophthalmol Clin North Am.* 2003;16:213-25

[53] Spry PG, Johnson CA, McKendrick AM, Turpin A. Variability components of standard automated perimetry and frequency-doubling technology perimetry. *Invest Ophthalmol Vis Sci* 2001;42:1404-10.

[54] Paczka JA, Friedman DS, Quigley HA, et al. Diagnostic capabilities of frequency-doubling technology, scanning laser polarimetry, and nerve fiber layer photographs to distinguish glaucomatous damage. *Am J Ophthalmol* 2001;131:188-97.

[55] Cello KE, Nelson-Quigg JM, Johnson CA. Frequency doubling technology perimetry for detection of glaucomatous visual field loss. *Am J Ophthalmol* 2000;129:314-22.

[56] Nakagawa S, Murata H, Saito H, et al. Frequency Doubling Technology for Earlier Detection of Functional Damage in Standard Automated Perimetry-Normal Hemifield in Glaucoma With Low-to-Normal Pressure. *J Glaucoma.* 2011 May 3. [Epub ahead of print]

[57] Fan X, Wu LL, Ma ZZ, et al. Usefulness of frequency-doubling technology for perimetrically normal eyes of open-angle glaucoma patients with unilateral field loss. *Ophthalmology.* 2010 Aug;117(8):1530-7, 1537.

[58] Ferreras A, Polo V, Larrosa JM, Pablo LE, Pajarin AB, Pueyo V, Honrubia FM. Can frequency-doubling technology and short-wavelength automated perimetries detect visual field defects before standard automated perimetry in patients with preperimetric glaucoma? *J Glaucoma.* 2007 Jun-Jul;16(4):372-83.

[59] Clement CI, Goldberg I, Healey PR, Graham S. Humphrey matrix frequency doubling perimetry for detection of visual-field defects in open-angle glaucoma. *Br J Ophthalmol.* 2009 May;93(5):582-8.

[60] Leeprechanon N, Giangiacomo A, Fontana H, et al. Frequency-doubling perimetry: comparison with standard automated perimetry to detect glaucoma. *Am J Ophthalmol.* 2007 Feb;143(2):263-271.

[61] Suh MH, Kim DM, Kim YK, Kim TW, Park KH. Patterns of progression of localized retinal nerve fibre layer defect on red-free fundus photographs in normal-tension glaucoma. *Eye (Lond).* 2010 May;24(5):857-63.

[62] Kanamori A, Nakamura M, Escano MF, et al. Evaluation of the glaucomatous damage on retinal nerve fiber layer thickness measured by optical coherence tomography. *Am J Ophthalmol.* 2003 Apr;135(4):513-20.

[63] Gupta PK, Asrani S, Freedman SF, et al. Differentiating glaucomatous from non-glaucomatous optic nerve cupping by optical coherence tomography. *Open Neurol J.* 2011 Jan 26;5:1-7.

[64] Leung CK, Cheung CY, Weinreb RN, et al Evaluation of retinal nerve fiber layer progression in glaucoma: a comparison between the fast and the regular retinal nerve fiber layer scans. *Ophthalmology.* 2011 Apr;118(4):763-7

[65] Batta P, Engel HM, Shrivastava A, et al. Effect of partial posterior vitreous detachment on retinal nerve fiber layer thickness as measured by optical coherence tomography. *Arch Ophthalmol.* 2010 Jun;128(6):692-7.

[66] Ophir A, Martinez MR, Mosqueda P, Trevino A. Vitreous traction and epiretinal membranes in diabetic macular oedema using spectral-domain optical coherence tomography. *Eye (Lond).* 2010 Oct;24(10):1545-53.

[67] Mirza RG, Johnson MW, Jampol LM. Optical coherence tomography use in evaluation of the vitreoretinal interface: a review. *Surv Ophthalmol.* 2007 Jul-Aug;52(4):397-421.

[68] De Boer JF, Cense B, B. Park H, et al. Improved signal-to-noise ratio in spectral-do*main compared with time-domain optical coherence tomography. *Optics Letters.* November 1, 2003 / Vol. 28, 21.

[69] Knight OJ, Chang RT, Feuer WJ, Budenz DL. Comparison of retinal nerve fiber layer measurements using time domain and spectral domain optical coherent tomography. *Ophthalmology.* 2009 Jul;116(7):1271-7.

[70] Sung KR, Kim DY, Park SB, Kook MS. Comparison of retinal nerve fiber layer thickness measured by Cirrus HD and Stratus optical coherence tomography. *Ophthalmology.* 2009 Jul;116(7):1264-70.

[71] Vieira P, Manivannan A, Lim CS, Sharp P, Forrester JV. Tomographic reconstruction of the retina using a confocal scanning laser ophthalmoscope. *Physiol Meas.* 1999 Feb;20(1):1-19.

[72] Kalaboukhova L, Vanja Fridhammar V, Lindblom B. Glaucoma follow-up by the Heidelberg Retina Tomograph. *Graefe's Archive for Clinical and Experimental Ophthalmology* Volume 244, Number 6, 654-662.

[73] Kilintzis V, Pappas T, Chouvarda I, et al. Novel Heidelberg retina tomograph-based morphological parameters derived from optic disc cupping surface processing. *Invest Ophthalmol Vis Sci.* 2011 Feb 16;52(2):947-51.

[74] Balasubramanian M, Bowd C, Weinreb RN, Zangwill LM. Agreement between the Heidelberg Retina Tomograph (HRT) stereometric parameters estimated using HRT-I and HRT-II. *Optom Vis Sci.* 2011 Jan;88(1):140-9.

[75] Vizzeri G, Weinreb RN, Martinez de la Casa JM, Alencar LM, Bowd C, Balasubramanian M, Medeiros FA, Sample P, Zangwill LM. Clinicians agreement in establishing glaucomatous progression using the Heidelberg retina tomograph. *Ophthalmology.* 2009 Jan;116(1):14-24.

[76] Weinreb RN, Bowd C, Zangwill LM. Glaucoma detection using scanning laser polarimetry with variable corneal polarization compensation. *Arch Ophthalmol.* 2003 Feb;121(2):218-24.

[77] Bagga H, Greenfield MD, William DS, Feuer J, Quantitative assessment of atypical birefringence images using scanning laser polarimetry with variable corneal compensation *American Journal of Ophthalmology* Volume 139, Issue 3, March 2005, 437-446.

[78] Kim HG, Heo H, Park SW. Comparison of scanning laser polarimetry and optical coherence tomography in preperimetric glaucoma. *Optom Vis Sci.* 2011 Jan; 88(1):124-9.

[79] Pablo LE, Ferreras A, Schlottmann PG. Retinal nerve fibre layer evaluation in ocular hypertensive eyes using optical coherence tomography and scanning laser polarimetry in the diagnosis of early glaucomatous defects. *Br J Ophthalmol.* 2011 Jan;95(1):51-5.

[80] Aptel F, Sayous R, Fortoul V, Beccat S, Denis P. Structure-function relationships using spectral-domain optical coherence tomography: comparison with scanning laser polarimetry. *Am J Ophthalmol.* 2010 Dec;150(6):825-33.

[81] López-Peña MJ, Ferreras A, Polo V, Larrosa JM, Pablo LE, Honrubia FM. Relationship between standard automated perimetry and retinal nerve fiber layer parameters measured with laser polarimetry. *Arch Soc Esp Oftalmol.* 2010 Jan;85(1):22-31.

3

End Stage Glaucoma

Tharwat H. Mokbel

Mansoura University Mansoura,
Egypt

1. Introduction

Glaucoma is the second leading cause of blindness in the general population. The definition of end-stage glaucoma may be based on a very constricted visual field, or a markedly severed visual acuity (Gillies& Brooks et al., 2000). Many factors have been postulated to put the patient at a high risk. Achieving an individually fashioned target IOP is supposed to minimize the risk of glaucoma progression (Nouri-Mahdavi & Hoffman et al., 2004). Medical regimens may induce significant short and long term IOP fluctuations. Surgery should be considered in end stage glaucoma. Trabeculectomy has been reported to be associated with less diurnal IOP fluctuation compared to maximum medical therapy. Wipe-out phenomenon is a rare complication and may be considered as a blast from the past. Meanwhile, Trabeculectomy has many surgical difficulties. Emphasis on guidelines for a successful trabeculectomy without toil is presented, besides the new modalities to achieve a favorable outcome.

2. What is end stage glaucoma?

There is no universally accepted definition of end-stage glaucoma. It may be based on a very constricted visual field, less than 10 or a visual acuity of 20/200 or worse that is attributable to glaucoma (Gillies & Brooks et al., 2000).

2.1 Importance

Glaucoma is the second leading cause of irreversible blindness in the general population, and the leading cause of blindness in black patients. Besides, patients with end-stage glaucoma have a high risk of further disease progression. Although peripheral vision is seriously affected, these patients may maintain good central vision sufficient enough to perform simple daily tasks.

2.2 Diagnostic challenge

End stage glaucoma carries a diagnostic challenge. Visual field examination is either unreliable or impossible. Only when a central island of vision remains, visual field tests of the central degrees should be chosen. Small changes in the visual field may be deleterious to central vision but it can be difficult to differentiate them from inter-test fluctuation. Small neuroretinal rim changes may correspond to significant changes in the visual acuity. On the other hand, OCT may be useful in the detection of glaucomatous progression. In advanced or progressive glaucoma, imaging can be justified every 3-4 months to look for change (Bartz-Schmidt & Thumann G et al., 1999).

2.3 Risk factors for progression

Many factors have been proved to increase the risk of glaucoma progression in end stage glaucoma, The most important are elevated intraocular pressure (IOP), IOP fluctuations, male gender, less formal education, severity of disease, pseudoexfoliation syndrome, worsening visual fields during follow up, optic disc hemorrhage, advanced stage of disease, migraine, patient's expected longevity, and the possibility of systemic diseases e.g hypertension, diabetes, and myopia (Law & Nguyen et al., 2007).

3. Target IOP in end stage glaucoma

Target IOP is the IOP that minimizes the risk of glaucoma progression with minimum impact on the quality of life. Although the concept of a target IOP is debated, it is recommended that every patient should have an individualized target IOP and re-estimated according to the follow up. Target IOP may be a percent reduction from a baseline IOP or may be an absolute IOP reduction. It is generally assumed that aiming to achieve a target IOP of at least a 20% reduction from the initial pressure at which damage occurred is a useful starting point. For moderate and advanced damage, a 30 and 40% decrease of IOP from baseline, respectively, is proposed. In each individual, the efficacy of any treatment lowering the IOP less than 15% should be questioned. The range of IOP fluctuations should also be considered and when in doubt a diurnal curve is indicated. Besides, the greater the pre-existing glaucoma damage, the lower the target IOP should be. It is clinically relevant that in eyes with severe pre-existing damage, any further damage may be functionally important. Thus, IOP should be set low in end-stage glaucoma. Target pressures seem to drop to lower and lower levels each decade. Even a more lower target IOP may be needed if other risk factors are present specially diabetes mellitus and hypertension. Severe pre-existing damage in the fellow eye is another possible risk factor, as well as a positive family history of visual handicap caused by primary open-angle glaucoma (POAG). A further 3% IOP lowering for each risk factor or for each decade of life expectancy is advised. Periodical re-evaluation and adjustments are necessary if the visual field continues to worsen at a rate that is clinically significant, it may be necessary to aim for a lower target IOP after other causes have been excluded (Miglior & Bertuzzi , 2010)..

3.1 Medical versus interventional strategy

The target IOP may not be achieved despite maximum medical therapy. Even if end stage glaucoma could be controlled medically, the lack of adherence and persistence with medication regimens may induce significant short and long term IOP fluctuations. These fluctuations have a deleterious effect on the visual outcomes. Medication may be inappropriate in some clinical situations. Extremely high IOP may be unlikely to be sufficiently reduced by medications. In this case medical treatment may be initiated briefly in order to operate at lower IOP.Some patients may have secondary conditions that interfere with the ability to administer medication such as dementia, mental illness, or arthritis.Economic problems are also challenges for patients in many locations. This may limit or effectively exclude access to medical treatment for glaucoma. Limited access to medical resources may be based on other factors such as distance from medical care and limited availability of practitioners and medications.On the other hand, glaucoma procedures are associated with more tight IOP control and minimal IOP fluctuations. There is a growing evidence that glaucoma procedures are more helpful in prevention of visual field loss when further IOP reduction is needed despite maximum medical therapy. There are no clearly defined and accepted rules to decide when surgery is the appropriate therapeutic choice, but there are principles that seem to guide this decision. Several assumptions underlie the recommendation of surgery for the treatment of glaucoma. Among these are the observation that surgical IOP lowering stops or slows progressive glaucoma damage. Even more, greater IOP lowering can be achieved with surgery than with medication in many patients, while surgery has greater risk than medical treatment of glaucoma. Intra-operative risks such as suprachoroidal haemorrhage, and post-operative risks such as hypotony and bleb related infection can result in rapid and profound visual loss.For example, trabeculectomy has been reported to be associated with less diurnal IOP fluctuation compared with maximum medical therapy in patients with end stage glaucoma . On the contrary, if the central fixation has already been lost, glaucoma procedures add no more beneficial effect and it is suggested to consider withholding surgery.

4. Surgical intervention in end stage glaucoma

4.1 Surgical options of end stage glaucoma

The surgical options for end stage glaucoma are generally the same as those of earlier stages of glaucoma. Many trabeculectomy modalities are suitable for end stage glaucoma. While trabeculectomy is the treatment of choice in primary open angle glaucoma, consider lens removal (combined surgery) in patients with end-stage chronic angle closure glaucoma. This offers the best chance to deepen the anterior chamber and widen the angle. Trabeculectomy with antimetabolites reduces IOP more compared with trabeculectomy alone. Ologen collagen matrix is a new promising modality that carries a superior advantage over conventional trabeculectomies and antimetabolites. Glaucoma drainage implants are indicated after glaucoma filtration surgery failure, on the other hand cycloablation in the form of cyclophotocoagulation or cyclocryotherapy are indicated for eyes with poor vision.

4.2 Preoperative preparation

A proper preoperative preparation is essential for a successful glaucoma surgery outcome. Adequate management of blood pressure, coagulation profile by the physician is crucial .Preoperative Visual field is important for medical and medico-legal reasons. Topical corticosteroids such as fluoromethelone may be used to calm down any claimed inflammation. Glaucoma lowering agents should be stopped several days in advance.

4.3 Anaesthetic precautions

Ophthalmic anaesthesia planning is of great help in end stage glaucoma surgery. General anaethesia is considered for one-eyed patients as possible. Certain precautions are mandatory during local anesthesia particularly reduction of the volume, addition of hyaluronidase and avoidance of orbital compression. Facial block is important to produce enough facial akinesia. Subtenon or peribulbar anaethesia do worth consideration particularly for myopia.

4.4 Difficulties of surgical intervention in end stage glaucoma

It has been well noticed that procedures in end stage glaucoma carries more surgical difficulties. This is because of the possibility of previous operations (glaucoma or cataract) and the long term use of topical glaucoma drugs. These co-morbidities have negative effects on the conjunctiva, and on the outcome of a new operation.

5. Conventional trabeculectomy in end stage glaucoma

Trabeculectomy should be fashioned properly and with extreme caution in end stage glaucoma to achieve the best favorable outcomes. Fornix-based flaps are preferred for better exposure of the sclera and less chance of a posterior scar formation. A corneal traction suture is suggested to avoid formation of a superior rectus haematoma.An anterior segment infusion system through the paracentesis is helpful in stabilizing the IOP during surgery, decrease the risk of serious complications, and enable more accurate suturing of the scleral flap. Bleb is fashioned under the upper lid to minimize discomfort and bleb-related complications, such as leak or infection. The scleral flap must be sufficiently large and of adequate thickness to provide resistance to aqueous outflow, especially if antimetabolites are used. Besides, the side incisions are left incomplete (1–2 mm from limbus) to encourage posterior flow and achieve a diffuse bleb. Scleral flap sutures can be pre-placed while the eye is still firm. Adjustment of sutures of the scleral flap should be based on intraoperative evaluation of flow.

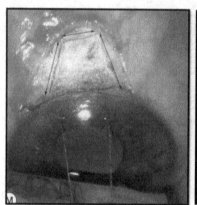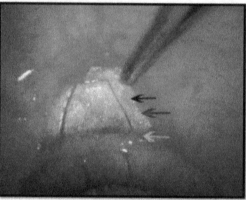

Fig. 1. (RT) Fornix-based flaps for better exposure of the sclera and less chances of a posterior scar. A corneal traction suture avoids the formation of a superior rectus haematoma, (LT) The scleral flap must be sufficiently large and of adequate thickness to provide resistance to aqueous outflow. (Fellman, 2009)

Many modalities of scleral flap sutures are of great help. Among those are fixed interrupted sutures that can be lasered later, releasable sutures that can be pulled out postoperatively and adjustable sutures that can be loosened transconjunctivally. Meticulous conjunctival closure is a priority to avoid hazardous postoperative bleb leakage and hypotony. Careful postoperative IOP measurement is indicated to detect early IOP spikes which could result in optic nerve damage. Bleb leakage and signs of inflammation should always be examined.

6. Trabeculectomy with antimetabolites

Tissue healing can be modulated with antimetabolites to improve outcomes of trabeculectomy. Antimetabolites are not very often used for the first trabeculectomies, but are mandatory after previous trabeculectomy or cataract surgery and for combined cataract-trabeculectomy surgery. Also they are indicated with trabeculectomy failure in the other eye and for dark skin and young patients. Antimetabolites are applied with a low dose, short duration, and on the largest possible area. While preoperative subconjunctival mitomycin-C (MMC) has less cytotoxic effect on the ciliary body compared with intraoperative episcleral application, both preoperative and intraoperative applications of MMC are effective in controlling IOP with a safer course and less postoperative complications in preoperative subconjunctival injection. Argon laser trabeculoplasty as an adjuvant therapy before or after trabeculectomy is an issue of controverse. Black and white patients with advanced glaucoma respond differently. Blacks with end stage glaucoma benefit more from a regimen that begins with laser surgery, and whites benefit more from one that begins with trabeculectomy.

7. Glaucoma filtering surgery with amniotic membrane transplantation

7.1 Principle
Antimetabolites may influence the integrity of the conjunctival barrier, resulting in a thin-walled avascular bleb (Hutchinson & Grossniklaus et al., 1997). The end result is often poor epithelialization and increased susceptibility to leakage and hypotony or infection, sometimes months after surgery (Parrish & Minckler, 1996). On the other hand, amniotic membrane exhibits a number of characteristics that might be of benefit in glaucoma surgery, that is good epithelization, good integration with the surrounding tissue, a low healing response, suppression of TGF-B activity and poor immunogenicity (Willoch & Nicolaissen, 2003). These features of amniotic membrane make it an attractive tissue for use in glaucoma surgery. It has been used in filtration surgery as an adjunct to reduce scarring, for repair of leaking blebs and as a cover for valve implant (Fujishima & Shimazaki et al., 1998).

7.2 Operative technique

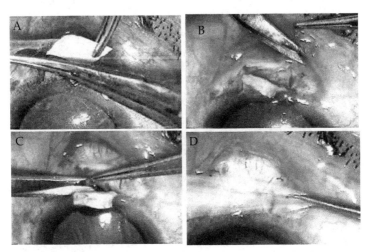

Fig. 2. (A) Peeling of aminiotic membrane from Nitro celluose paper, (B) Amniotic membrane graft is placed under the scleral flap and suturing of the graft to the sclera, (C) Trabeculectomy measuring 2X3 mm is done (D) Second graft over the scleral flap (Mokbel & El-hefny et al., 2005)

Fornix based conjunctival flap, care was taken to ensure haemostasis during the whole surgical procedure. Scleral flap was done measuring 4x5 mm. Previously prepared amniotic membrane which is preserved in Dulbeccos Modified Eagles Media (DME) at -80°C and was known to be free from HIV, HCV, HBV and syphilis was used Fig. 2(A). Amniotic membrane graft measuring 3x8 mm with its epithelial side up was placed between the scleral flap and deep sclera and attached to the scleral with four 10-0 nylon sutures at the corners Fig. 2(B). The amniotic membrane was then retracted and trabeculectomy measuring 2x3 mm was done Fig. 2(C). The scleral flap was then closed by two 10/0 nylon sutures. A second graft of amniotic membrane measuring 1.5x1.5 cm was placed over the sclera and attached near the limbus by two 10-0 nylon sutures and posteriorly by other two sutures Fig. 2(D). The conjunctiva was then closed using two 8/0 virgin sutures at the corners. Postoperatively each patient recieved a subconjunctival injection of Dexamethazone and garamycin followed by topical application of 5 times daily tobramycin & Dexamethazone drops for 4 weeks. All antiglaucoma medications were stopped (Mokbel & El-hefny et al., 2005).

8. Ologen collagen matrix

Ologen is porcine extracellular matrix made of atelocollagen cross-linked with glycosaminoglycan. Ologen is a biodegradable scaffolding matrix that induces a regenerative wound healing process without the need for antifibrotic agents. It is well known that episcleral fibrosis and sub-conjunctival scarring are the major causes of failure in glaucoma filtering surgery. Ologen collagen matrix can creat the sub-conjunctival bleb and modulate the wound healing for the surgery. Ologen collagen matrix is a 3-D scaffold porous structure that can guide fibroblast to grow randomly, instead of linear alignment. This can reduce sub-conjuctival and trabdoor scars. Thus, Ologen collagen matrix carries the

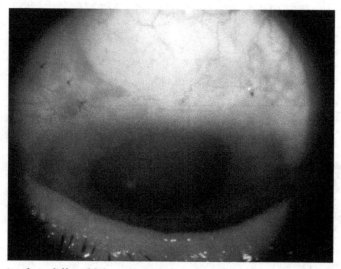

Fig. 3. Ologen implant,diffuse bleb and a well formed anterior chamber (photo of the author)

advantage of lowering IOP more safely and efficiently than standard trabeculectomy with MMC, with the merit of less possibility of bleb leaks and endophthalmitis compared with antimetabolites (Sarkisian, 2010).

The collagen matrix helps to limit hypotony through a tamponading effect over the scleral flap. On the other hand Ologen collagen matrix carry the disadvantage of increased cost, besides the difficulty of laser suture lysis.

8.1 Technique

According to the surgeon preference, limbal - or a fornix-based conjunctival flap are accepted. A loose stitch sclera flap is done in order to encourage aqueous flow for the filtering surgery. Ologen collagen matrix disc is implanted over the scleral flap. No suture is required to secure the implant, and as soon as it touches the sclera, it absorbs aqueous and molds to cover the scleral tissue. Collagen matrix therefore need not be presoaked or prepared in any way. After the collagen matrix's placement, the surgeon closes the conjunctiva in his or her usual meticulous fashion to ensure that the wound is watertight.

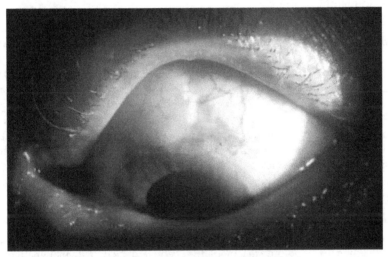

Fig. 4. Ologen implant, next day after surgery (photo of the author)

Ologen currently comes in two sizes for glaucoma filtering surgery: 6 X 2 mm and 12 X 1 mm. The numbers 6 and 12 stands for the diameter of the round implant, and the numbers 2 and 1 refer to its thickness. Ologen is biodegradable in 90 to 180 days. Ologen has been approved by the FDA in August 2009 (Sarkisian, 2010).

9. Aqueous shunting procedures with glaucoma drainage devices

Glaucoma drainage devices (GGDs) are indicated when trabeculectomy is unlikely to be successful. Besides, GDDs should be considered for socioeconomic or logistical issues relating to safety, follow-up care, etc. GDDs that do not have mechanisms to restrict aqueous flow require a suture ligature or internal stent or other flow restricting mechanism because the restriction of flow of aqueous humor from the eye is important in the prevention of postoperative hypotony. There are several type of devices; however, they can be divided into two categories:anterior drainage devices and posterior drainage devices. Most posterior drainage devices are composed of a silicone or Silastic tube that is placed into the eye (through the limbus or pars plana) and through which aqueous humor passes into the episcleral-subconjunctival space near the globe's equator. In this area there is an episcleral plate that is designed to maintain an aqueous reservoir. There are three design features which distinguish different implants; the presence of a valve or mechanism to restrict the flow of aqueous humor from the eye, the surface area and configuration of the episcleral plate, and the the material used.Drainage devices without a built in flow restriction mechanism, such as the Molteno, Baerveldt, and Schocket band implants, may be inserted in a one-stage procedure, where the flow of aqueous is restricted by a suture ligature around the tube or an internal stent. On the other hand krupin Valve implant and Ahmed Glaucoma Valve implant have pressure-sensitive valves or mechanisms which restrict the flow of aqueous from the eye (Mokbel, 2005).

10. Cyclodestruction

Cyclodestructive procedures aim to decrease aqueous humor secretion by damaging the ciliary processes, thereby reducing intraocular pressure (IOP). Modalities for cyclodestruction include cyclocryotherapy, and cyclophotocoagulation, using the Nd:YAG or diode laser. Endoscopic, non-contact and contact modes of cyclophotocoagulation are available, with the contact diode mode most widely used, laser diode cyclophotocoagulation is the procedure of choice for end stage glaucoma when trabeculectomy and drainage implants have a high probability for failure or have high risk of surgical complications. Less intense laser therapy on a repeated basis rather than a single high dose treatment is suggested to minimize complications of treatment. The effectiveness of treatment should be assessed after 3-4 weeks, at which time re-treatment may be considered.

11. Risk of losing vision

The patient should be informed about the relative risk of losing vision from a surgical procedure in end-stage glaucoma eyes. Visually devastating complications include chronic hypotony (leading to hypotony maculopathy), retinal detachment, malignant glaucoma, corneal decompensation, endophthalmitis, and phthisis bulbi. A detailed clearly written patient consent is important.It should entail all the potential hazards from suggested surgical procedure.

11.1 Wipe-out phenomenon
The wipe-out phenomenon is unexplained vision loss following glaucoma surgery. Wipe-out phenomenon data comes from older retrospective reports using older surgical techniques. Newer data does not report the occurrence of the wipe-out phenomenon.

12. Conclusion

In end stage glaucoma there is a higher incidence of visual loss than early glaucoma. So, frequent patient monitoring and quick decision making should be done.The target IOP in end stage glaucoma is lower than in early stage. Surgery should be considered in end stage glaucoma. Wipe-out phenomenon is a rare complication and may be considered as a blast from the past.

13. References

Bartz-Schmidt K. U., Thumann G., Jonescu-Cuypers C. P., et al. (1999) Quantitative morphologic and functional evaluation of the optic nerve head in chronic open-angle glaucoma. *Surv Ophthalmol* 44; 1, pp.541-553.

Fellman R. (2009). Trabeculectomy, In: *Glaucoma volume two surgical management*, Shaarawy T. & Sherwood M. & Hitchings R. and Crowston J. pp.(111-150), Saunders, 978-0-7020-2978-3,China.

Fujishima H., Shimazaki J., Shinozaki N., Tsubota K. (1998) Trabeculectomy with the use of amniotic membrane for uncontrollabe glaucoma. Ophthalmic Surg. 29; pp.928-943.

Gillies W. E., Brooks A. M., Strang N. T. (2000). Management and prognosis of end stage glaucoma. *Clin Experiment Ophthalmol*, 28, PP.(405-408).

Hutchinson A. K., Grossniklaus H. E., Brown R. H., McManus P. E. and Bradley G. K. (1997) Clinicopathologic features of excised mitomycin filtering bleb. Arch Ophthalmol 112, pp. 74-79.

Law S. K., Nguyen A. M., Coleman A. L., et al. (2007) Severe loss of central vision in patients with advanced glaucoma undergoing trabeculectomy. *Arch Ophthalmol,* 125, pp.1044-1050.

Miglior S. and Bertuzzi F. (2010). IOP: Target Pressures, In: *Pearls of Glaucoma Management,* Giaconi, J. & Law, S. & Coleman A. and Caprioli J. pp.(99-104), Springer-Verlag Berlin Heidelberg, 978-3-540-68238-7, New York.

Mokbel T., (2005) Long term clinical experience with Ahmed valve in refractory glaucoma. *Bull. Ophthalmol. Soc . Egypt, 98(3); pp 479-484.*

Mokbel T., El-hefny E., El-bendary A. (2005) Glaucoma filtering surgery with amniotic membrane transplantation. *Bull. Ophthalmol. Soc. Egypt, 98(3); pp 419-423.*

Nouri-Mahdavi K., Hoffman D., Coleman A. L., et al. (2004) Predictive factors for glaucomatous visual field progression in the Advanced Glaucoma Intervention Study. *Ophthalmology* 111; pp1627-1635.

Palmberg, P. (2005).outcome measures for Studies of glaucoma surgery, In: Glaucoma urgery Open Angle Glaucoma, Weinreb,R and Crowston,J.pp(1-7), Kugler, ISBN 90 6299 203 X, Netherlands.

Parrish R. K. II and Minckler D. (1996) "Late endophthalmitis" filtering surgery time bomb? Ophthalmology. 103, pp. 1167-1168.

Sarkisian, S. (2010). A Replacement for Antimetabolites? Ologen is a new product that modulates wound healing in glaucoma surgery. *Glaucoma Today.*winter2010,pp.22-24 .

Topouzis, F. (2010). Procedural Treatments:Surgery in End-Stage Glaucoma, In: *Pearls of Glaucoma Management,* Giaconi J & Law S. & Coleman A. and Caprioli J. pp.(323-330), Springer-Verlag Berlin Heidelberg, ISNB 978-3-540-68238-7, New York.

Willoch C. M., Nicolaissen B. (2003). Amnion sheilded trabeculectomy. Acta Ophthalmologica
       Scand. pp.658-659.

4

Update on Modulating Wound Healing in Trabeculectomy

Hosam Sheha

Ocular Surface Center & Tissue Tech Inc., Miami, Florida
United States

1. Introduction

Trabeculectomy is the most commonly used surgical procedure for managing medically uncontrolled glaucoma. It reduces intraocular pressure (IOP) by creating an artificial drainage pathway of the aqueous humor from the anterior chamber to the subconjunctival space, forming a filtering bleb. Aqueous humor in the subconjunctival space may then exit by multiple pathways including transconjunctival filtration and absorption through the episcleral veins (Fig. 1).

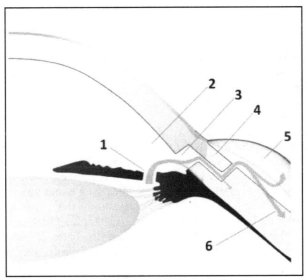

Fig. 1. Aqueous pathway after trabeculectomy through peripheral iridectomy (1) to the anterior chamber (2), the internal ostium (3), the route under the scleral flap (4), and the edge of the scleral flap to be absorbed via the bleb wall (5), and the episcleral venous plexus (6)

The success of trabeculectomy has been limited by postoperative fibrosis at the surgery site, leading to bleb failure months or years after surgery. High risk factors that lead to the failure in trabeculectomy include previous ocular surgery, specific types of glaucoma e.g. secondary

glaucoma such as neovascular, uveitic, post-traumatic, and lens-induced glaucoma, and to a lesser extent, young age and black race (Sturmer et al, 1993; Broadway and Chang, 2001).
Several surgical and pharmacologic techniques have been introduced to enhance the success in eyes with poor surgical prognoses. Until now, no effective and safe agent has been identified that can inhibit fibrosis, without complications, in the glaucoma filtering wound created by trabeculectomy. Although antimetabolites have revolutionized glaucoma surgery, the use of these agents is still associated with substantial risk (Chen, 1983). The common clinical practice of using mitomycin C (MMC) in trabeculectomy as an anti-fibrotic and anti-metabolic agent has achieved only limited success in cases with high-risk glaucoma while raising notable sight-threatening complications such as hypotony, bleb leaks, and infection (Lama and Fechtner, 2003).
To circumvent complications caused by MMC, there is a great need to improve the outcome of trabeculectomy by identifying a physiological modulator that may suppress pathological fibrosis without compromising the normal reparative wound healing process.
Our recent clinical research suggests that amniotic membrane (AM) could be a physiological modulator of wound healing that prevents scar formation in the subconjunctival space. We have demonstrated that AM not only prevents scar formation via its anti-inflammatory and anti-scarring actions but also serves as a spacer integrated into the intra-bleb structure to avert early over-filtration complications associated with trabeculectomy, and to stabilize the patency of the filtering fistula for prolonged maintenance of the bleb function (Sheha et al, 2008). This chapter reviews recent advances in the use of amniotic membrane as a biological modulator of wound healing that suppresses pathological fibrosis in trabeculectomy.

2. Wound healing process following trabeculectomy

Wound healing is triggered by activating the body's innate immunity and is characterized by inflammation in the acute phase, granulation tissue formation in the intermediate phase, and scarring in the chronic phase. This wound healing process is mediated by a number of cell types and is orchestrated by complex arrays of growth factors, cytokines, chemokines, and non-protein mediators. Trabeculectomy differs from most surgical procedures in that inhibition of wound healing is desirable to achieve surgical success (Dvorak, 1986).
Experimental and human studies have outlined a sequence of events that occurs in early bleb failure (Summarized in Fig. 2) (Skuta and Parrish, 1987). After surgical trauma, plasma proteins, including fibrinogen, fibronectin, and plasminogen, form a gel-like fibrin-fibronectin matrix, into which inflammatory cells (including monocytes and macrophages), new capillaries, and fibroblasts migrate. Macrophages from monocytes appear in about 12 hours, reaching peak numbers around day 3. These macrophages activate an inflammatory response, including the activation of lymphocytes and fibroblasts. T-cells appear on day 5, and after reaching a peak in numbers by the end of two weeks, they are activated into specific T-cells, which release various cytokines to control the activity and proliferation of fibroblasts. The fibrin-fibronectin matrix is eventually degraded by inflammatory cells, and fibroblasts subsequently synthesize fibronectin, interstitial collagens, and glycosaminoglycans to form fibrovascular granulation tissue (Desjardins et al, 1986; Grierson et al, 1988; Reichel et al, 1998; Miller et al, 1989; Chang et al, 2000).
The proliferated fibroblasts gradually begin to differentiate; this process is suspected to be mediated by various factors: transforming growth factor (TGF)-beta (Wipff et al, 2007), connective-tissue growth factor (CTGF) (Sherwood, 2006), Rho-associated serine-threonine

kinase (ROCK1) (Meyer-ter-Vehn et al, 2006), and the matrix-metalloproteinases (MMPs) (Chintala et al, 2005). Unlike undifferentiated fibroblasts, the newly-differentiated myofibroblasts transform the secreted extracellular matrix into an actin-based component which creates stronger scar tissue (Desmouliere et al, 1993). Blood vessels retract over time and fibroblasts largely disappear as the tissue is remodeled to form a dense collagenous subconjunctival scar.

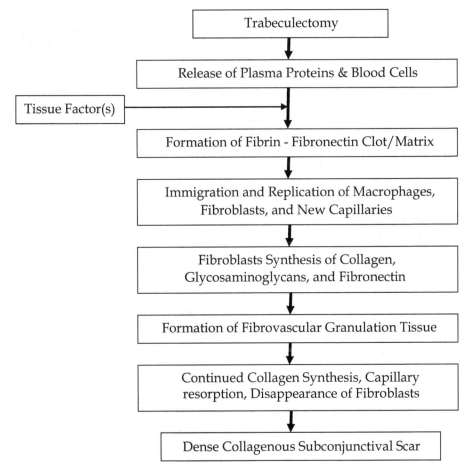

Fig. 2. Events of wound healing in trabeculectomy failure

3. Risk factors and potential causes of trabeculectomy failure

3.1 External factors
External factors at the episceral-conjunctival interface are responsible for most cases of trabeculectomy failure. Fibroblast proliferation, synthesis of the extracellular matrix, and subsequent development of subconjunctival fibrosis play prominent roles in external failure. Chemotactic factors for fibroblasts include lymphokines, complement, native collagens of

types I to V, fibronectin, some proteolytic digestion fragments of collagen and fibronectin, and platelet-derived growth factor (Ross et al, 1986).

Intense preoperative and postoperative inflammation induces a cellular response that accelerates wound healing. The presence of blood beneath the conjunctiva may also increase the probability of bleb failure. As noted above, serum derivatives including fibronectin and platelet-derived growth factor may stimulate fibroblast migration and proliferation. In addition, macrophages, which may be activated by blood, appear to play a key role in inducing the fibroproliferative response in wound repair (Leibovich and Ross, 1975). Extrapolation of these observations to trabeculectomy wound healing is consistent with the clinical impression that the presence of blood increases the likelihood of postoperative fibrosis.

3.2 Intraocular factors

In the absence of scar formation, an inadequate opening into the anterior chamber due to scleral remnants or Descemet's membrane in the fistula may lead to primary failure. Blockage of the filtration site by prolapsed iris, vitreous, or ciliary body may also lead to early postoperative failure (Maumenee, 1960). Many of these potential causes of bleb failure can be avoided by careful surgical technique. A spacer during surgery can enhance the likelihood of a patent fistula.

4. Measures to improve the trabeculectomy outcome

Trabeculectomy success relies on the continued patency of the fistula and the continued ability of the filtering bleb created out of the conjunctiva to absorb aqueous humor. Thus, the success of the procedure lies not only on the surgical technique but also the intraoperative and postoperative measures to minimize scar formation.

Preoperative inflammation should be treated with anti-inflammatory agents, usually corticosteroids. Miotics, which break down the blood-aqueous barrier, should be discontinued at least two weeks before trabeculectomy. Treatment of postoperative inflammation is also important. Cycloplegic agents help restore the blood-aqueous barrier and may reduce the release of plasma proteins, which may contribute to the postoperative healing response.

With respect to surgical technique, tissue trauma should be minimized by avoiding unnecessary manipulation of the conjunctiva, Tenon and iris. Hemostasis should be performed to decrease bleeding. Removal of the inner sclerectomy block should establish a patent channel without remnants of Descemet's membrane. A basal iridectomy prevents postoperative iris incarceration at the filtering site.

Although a fornix-based conjunctival flap might prevent scarring of the posterior conjunctiva and Tenon's capsule, randomized studies of limbus versus fornix-based conjunctival flaps in primary trabeculectomies failed to document significant differences in surgical success between the two techniques (Shuster et al, 1984; Traverso et al, 1987). The effect of the excision of Tenon's capsule on trabeculectomy success is also controversial.

5. Pharmacologic modulation of wound healing

Unlike most surgical procedures, success of glaucoma filtering surgery is achieved through the inhibition of wound healing. The use of pharmacologic agents is based on suppression of proliferation of cells, mainly fibroblasts, which would limit the healing at the site of the fistulizing surgery and consequently limit postoperative scarring.

5.1 Corticosteroids

As stated above, the initial steps in wound healing are inflammation and coagulation, leading to a cascade of biological events including cellular, hormonal, and growth factor release. These events finally lead to scar tissue formation (Skuta and Parrish, 1987). Corticosteroids regulate wound healing through the inhibition of macrophage functions, such as phagocytosis and the release of enzymes like collagenase, plasminogen activator, and growth factors, and thus suppress inflammation. Specific anti-inflammatory effects include suppression of fibrin deposition, capillary permeability, migration of leukocytes and macrophages, and phagocytic activity (Starita et al, 1985). Corticosteroids also inhibit vascular permeability and fibroblast proliferation (Lama and Fechtner, 2003). Tissue culture studies of human Tenon capsule fibroblasts have shown that corticosteroids inhibit cell attachment and proliferation (Nguyen and Lee, 1992).

Postoperative topical corticosteroids have been reported to significantly increase the success of trabeculectomy (Araujo 1995). Sub-Tenon injection of triamcinolone acetonide (TA) appears to be a more effective mean of high-dose corticosteroid delivery and may increase the success rate of trabeculectomy (Hosseini 2007). Tham and associates reported that the use of TA (1.2 mg) injection into filtration blebs at the conclusion of trabeculectomy was associated with good intraocular pressure (IOP) control for 3 months (Tham 2006). However, Yuki et al reported no significant differences between the success rates of trabeculectomy with or without intraoperative sub-Tenon injection of 20 mg TA within the 12-month follow-up period (Yuki, 2009).

Besides intra- and post-operative administration, some studies have highlighted the beneficial effect of preoperative use of corticosteroids and non steroidal anti-inflammatory agents in improving the success rate of filtration surgery. Baudouin demonstrated that fluorometholone drops one month before filtering surgery has effectively reduced inflammation, as indicated by the expression of human leukocyte antigen (HLA)-DR after impression cytological analysis (Baudouin 2002). Breusegem compared preoperative topical anti-inflammatory medications to placebo before trabeculectomy. Significantly fewer postoperative needling procedures were needed in the steroid-treated group (5%) than in the placebo group (41%). Furthermore, none of the patients in the steroid group required topical IOP-lowering medication to maintain a subtarget IOP, compared with 24% of patients in the placebo group. However, there was no significant overall difference in absolute IOP values or in relative IOP reduction between two groups at any point (Breusegem 2010). Despite the aforementioned advantages, topical steroids pose a risk for steroid-induced IOP elevation and cataract.

5.2 Antimetabolites

Anti-mitotic agents such as MMC and 5-fluorouracil (5-FU) help suppress post-surgical scarring by causing widespread non-selective cell death and apoptosis. The intraoperative application of MMC in trabeculectomy was introduced by Chen (Chen, 1983), while Heuer was the first to report the use 5-FU postoperatively as subconjunctival injections (Heuer et al, 1984).

While 5-FU can be used both for intraoperative application and postoperative injection (Parrish et al, 2001), the use of MMC as a postoperative injection is not as widely accepted as

5-FU (Apostolov and Siarov, 1996). The concentration of 5-FU used intraoperatively is 50 mg/mL applied for up to 5 minutes. The concentration of MMC used intraoperatively ranges from 0.1-0.5 mg/mL applied for 2-5 minutes, depending on the risk of failure. The antifibrotic agent can be applied to the scleral bed before or after the scleral flap is made, using cellulose sponges. The antifibrotic-soaked sponges should be applied to the area where aqueous flow is desired and should not be placed too close to the limbus or in contact with the wound edges. After all the sponges have been removed, the site is irrigated with copious amounts of saline solution to remove residual antifibrotic agents.

Although anti-mitotic agents improved the success rate of trabeculectomy (Chen et al, 1990;Kitazawa et al, 1991), there is an increased risk of early postoperative complications such as hypotony, bleb rupture, and infectious endophthalmitis (Shields et al, 1993; Greenfield and Parrish, 1996; Singh et al, 2000; WuDunn et al, 2002; Palanca-Capistrano et al, 2009). Another common late complication is bleb leakage, which may cause other serious complications such as infection, hypotony related maculopathy, and corneal endothelial decompensation (Greenfield et al, 1996; Nuyts et al, 1994). Thus, understanding, mechanisms of wound healing following MMC treatment is important to reduce bleb-related complications of leakage.

As a mechanism of MMC action, it is commonly accepted that inhibiting fibroblast proliferation leads to decreased conjunctival adhesion and maintaining the bleb (Lama and Fechtner, 2003). In terms of the pharmacokinetics of MMC, the t1/2 in blood doses of 30, 20, and 10 (mg/body) is 50, 43, and 10 minutes, respectively (Fujita, 1982). This suggests that the half-life of MMC is very short. Because we use MMC at a dosage of less than 1% on the sclera for several minutes in trabeculectomy, its effective lifespan seems to be less than several hours. As stated above, fibroblasts appear and are activated at 12 hours after surgery by macrophages and various cytokines that are released from T-cells. Therefore, it seems unreasonable that MMC directly suppresses fibroblasts' proliferation.

It is more likely that MMC initially suppresses the proliferation of mast cells, including chymase-positive cells which may promote inflammatory response. As a result of this, fibroblast proliferation is then restrained (Okada et al, 2009). In fact, topical instillation of an anti-mast-cell agent, tranilast, was useful for filtering bleb formation and IOP

reduction (Chihara et al, 2002). Therefore, suppression of mast cells might be related to formation of the filtering bleb. In addition, chymase inhibition might play a role in maintaining filtering blebs for an extended period of time. It has been reported that a chymase inhibitor prevents adhesion for up to three months in an abdomen adhesion model (Okamoto et al, 2004), so bleb formation may be maintained for a long period if MMC inhibits chymase function after tissue injury. Further investigation is needed to verify that chymase inhibitors are appropriate for glaucoma surgeries.

5.3 Anti-vascular endothelial growth factor (VEGF) antibodies

Pathologic angiogenesis is frequently associated with massive inflammation and migration of fibroblasts. It was shown that cultured conjunctival fibroblasts could be stimulated to produce VEGF by pro inflammatory cytokines (sano-Kato et al, 2005), and Tenon's capsule fibroblasts were inhibited by angiogenesis inhibitors (Wong et al, 1994). Based on these findings, it is imaginable that a selective inhibition of growth factors such as VEGF could be an approach to prevent or treat extensive wound healing. To further elucidate the direct effect of anti-VEGF agents on fibroblasts, Guerriero et al. illustrated in vitro effects of bevacizumab on human corneal and conjunctival fibroblast cell lines. Their research concluded that when corneal stromal fibroblasts are exposed to bevacizumab, loss of cell-to-cell adhesions and morphological changes are seen. They further stated that these changes are dose-dependent (Guerriero et al. 2006).

Currently, two therapeutic anti-VEGF antibodies exist; bevacizumab and ranibizumab. The use of subconjunctival bevacizumab 1mg in 0.04ml to treat a failing filtering bleb in addition to a needling procedure has been described in one patient (Kahook et al, 2006b). This patient showed an immediate decrease in IOP and was symptomatically improved as well. Bevacizumab has also been used in neovascular glaucoma (Kahook et al, 2006a; Michels et al, 2005). Kapetansky et al. studied the utility of subconjunctival bevacizumab injections administered proximal to blebs after trabeculectomy at the earliest sign of vascularization (Kapetansky et al, 2007). They noted that nearly two thirds of the blebs had an observable reduction in vascularity while decreasing IOP from a mean of 17.8 to 14mmHg 1 month after injection. Improved results were noted when the injections were given earlier in the postoperative phase. Coote et al presented a case of subconjunctival injection of bevacizumab that resulted in a dramatic reduction of bleb vascularity for 6 weeks. In their case, even 6 months after injection, a healthy bleb with minimal scar tissue was seen (Coote et al., 2008).

Ranibizumab is a fully humanized monoclonal antibody-fragment and therefore has a low molecular weight, which results in good tissue penetration. The antibody deactivates all isoforms of VEGF-A. Although intraocular injection of the drug showed no toxic side effects in an animal model (Manzano et al, 2006), the disadvantage of this form of application in trabeculectomy is the short half life of the drug. Although ranibizumab has a longer intravitreal half-life (6 days), this form of application does not cover the main peak of scarring reaction that is occurring around 2-3 weeks after surgery (Choi et al, 2010). For example, Purcell et al. noted decreased IOP and bleb vascularization after bleb needle revision using ranibizumab. But, this effect was short-lived, as increased vascularization was noted after 1 month of follow-up (Purcell, et al. 2008).

Further studies are needed to better understand how anti-VEGF agents might benefit patients undergoing glaucoma filtration surgery. There are ongoing safety studies to better analyze the importance of route of administration – intracameral, sub-Tenon and intravitreal – and to determine whether unknown side effects co-exist. It is important to delineate duration of action when anti-VEGF agents are injected in the intra or sub-Tenon's space and how this might influence efficacy.

6. Amniotic membrane as a modulator of trabeculectomy wound healing

6.1 Fetal strategy of wound healing

The amniotic membrane shares the same cell origin as the fetus. The majority of the studies testify the clinical efficacy of amniotic membrane transplantation (AMT) in gearing adult wound healing toward regeneration with minimal inflammation and scarring, suggesting that amniotic membrane (AM), like the fetal tissue, carries similar features that may not only facilitate regeneration but also inhibit scar formation (Mast et al, 1992; Adzick and Lorenz, 1994)

A number of mechanisms have been put forth to explain the AM's biological actions in modulating adult wound healing toward the fetal direction with anti-inflammation, anti-scarring and anti-angiogenesis. (Tseng et al, 2004).

It remains unclear whether such therapeutic actions are directly or indirectly linked to modulate healing and differentiation. AM has been shown to down-regulate transforming growth factor-β signaling in cultured normal conjunctival fibroblasts (Tseng et al., 1999; Lee et al., 2000) and to inhibit the cellular migration triggered by vascular endothelial growth factor (VEGF) (Shey et al., 2011). Furthermore, AM can exert potent anti-inflammatory effects by facilitating macrophage apoptosis (Li et al, 2006).

6.2 Preliminary studies

Several investigators have explored the clinical efficacy of deploying AM as an adjunctive therapy to improve the surgical outcome of various glaucoma procedures, including trabeculectomy (Sheha et al, 2010). They have shown that transplantation of a single (Fujishima et al, 1998; Lu and Mai, 2003; Yue et al, 2003; Drolsum et al, 2006) or folded (Bruno et al, 2006; Eliezer et al, 2006) sheet of AM under the scleral flap (Fujishima et al, 1998; Yue et al, 2003; Drolsum et al, 2006; Bruno et al, 2006), and/or under the conjunctiva (Yue et al, 2003; Drolsum et al, 2006; Bruno et al, 2006; Eliezer et al, 2006), with additional MMC (Fujishima et al, 1998; Drolsum et al, 2006; Bruno et al, 2006), reduces IOP in eyes with refractory glaucoma. Experimental rabbit studies demonstrated that the AM, inserted under the scleral flap, achieves the same reduction of subconjunctival fibroblasts and macrophages around the trabeculectomy sites as that achieved by MMC (Demir et al, 2002; Wang et al, 2005), as well as reduces the number of fibroblasts at trabeculectomy sites when inserted under the scleral flap even without MMC (Zhong et al, 2000; Barton et al, 2001).

6.3 Potential advantages of AM

We have conducted the first prospective randomized trial to demonstrate the clinical efficacy of transplanting a single layer of cryopreserved AM under and around the scleral flap (Fig. 3), in conjunction with application of MMC in refractory glaucoma. In this study of 37 eyes, 18 received 0.2 mg/ml MMC under the flap for 2 min while 19 received additional implantation of cryopreserved AM under and around the scleral flap (Sheha et al, 2008).

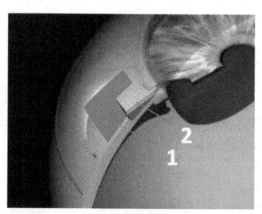

Fig. 3. AMT in trabeculectomy. AM (1) inserted under and around the scleral flap (2)

In the control MMC only group, IOP continuously rose between 3 and 12 months postoperatively. The incidence of encapsulated blebs, which are caused by collagen-producing fibroblasts (Ophir, 1992), was greater in the control group (38.9% vs. 5.3%) at 12 months postoperatively. This indicates that the effect of MMC was not sufficient to suppress scar formation, potentially due to its short half-life.

At 12 months postoperatively, the group with AM transplantation achieved significantly higher rates of complete (IOP ≤ 21 mmHg without medications) and qualified success (IOP ≤ 21 mmHg with or without additional medications). Furthermore, the resultant blebs were diffuse and translucent, but still retained normal vascularity (Fig. 4A). This bleb morphology was notably different from a MMC-induced ischemic bleb, which is prone to develop late complications such as bleb leak and infection (Fig. 4B). There were significantly fewer early postoperative complications such as shallow anterior chamber and choroidal effusion. These beneficial effects may be attributed to the fact that AM inserted under the scleral flap effectively halts rapid drainage of aqueous humor from the trabeculectomy site to reduce immediate hypotony from overfiltration and reduces scarring in the filtration site in the long run.

Hence, it is plausible that AM implanted in subconjunctival and subscleral spaces might reduce the adverse side effects intrinsically associated with MMC and with over-filtration, making AM a unique natural biological modulator that may exert a similar anti-scarring action to MMC while eliminating the potential sight-threatening complications known to MMC.

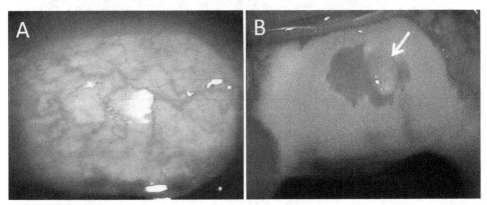

Fig. 4. Comparison between functioning bleb with normal vascularity after AMT (A) and ischemic leaking bleb after MMC (B); arrow indicates the bleb leak revealed by fluorescein staining (B)

The aforementioned favorable results could be attributed to a synergistic beneficial effect of MMC and AM on controlling fibrosis at the trabeculectomy site. It remains unclear whether the AM can substitute MMC completely in trabeculectomy. Furthermore, the mechanism through which the AM exerts its effects as well as its fate in the subscleral space over time remains largely unknown. The AM may not only prevent scar formation via its known anti-inflammatory and anti-scarring actions but may also serve as a spacer integrated into the internal bleb structure to stabilize the patency of the filtering fistula and maintain a functioning bleb.

Currently we are studying the fate of AM and internal bleb morphology. Although histological studies showed that human AM dissolves at 1 month postoperatively in rabbits (Wang et al, 2005), we do not know whether similar AM dissolution also occurred in human patients. We have gathered preliminary data supporting the feasibility of using anterior segment optic coherence tomography (OCT) to detect the presence of AM and the evidence of host cell integration into the AM after being transplanted in the subconjunctival space to cover the glaucoma shunt tube. Our results showed that implanted AM maintained its thickness over a period of 12 months (Anand et al, 2011).

6.4 Evidence of AM anti-angiogenic action

Pathologic angiogenesis that is frequently associated with uncontrolled inflammation may lead to fibrosis. While reducing fibrosis in subconjunctival and subscleral spaces as shown above, AM was found to deliver anti-angiogenic actions to resolve rubeosis iridis that is known to occur in neovascular glaucoma. In our study, there were 7 eyes with neovascular glaucoma in each group, which was accompanied by circumcorneal congestion, neovascularization at the angle and the iris in the form of rubeosis iridis (Fig. 5A), and hyphema (Fig. 6A). Interestingly, 2 weeks following implantation of AM, we observed rapid resolution of the circumcorneal congestion and dramatic regression of the anterior chamber neovascularization (Fig. 5B) and hyphema (Fig. 6B). The effect was persistent through 12 months of follow-up.

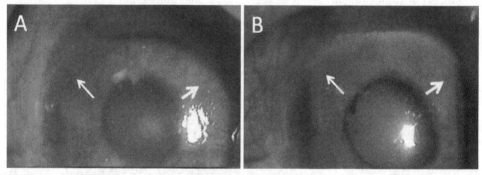

Fig. 5. Resolution of rubeosis iridis (arrows) in neovascular glaucoma

Hence, our study was the first showing AM's anti-angiogenic clinical efficacy. Because such an action was not associated with reduction of the normal vascularity of the bleb (Fig.4A), we speculate that AM's anti-angiogenic action is preferentially directed toward abnormal neovascularization. This novel therapeutic action against neovascularization may add an extra benefit in the management of high-risk neovascular glaucoma.

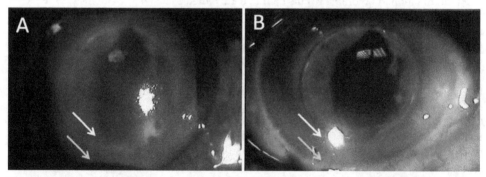

Fig. 6. Rapid resolution of rubeosis iridis (white arrow) and hyphema (green arrow) in neovascular glaucoma

7. Future research

Our preliminary studies designate that the implantation of AM to lower IOP in trabeculectomy represents a significant advance in treating glaucoma by eliminating complications associated with MMC and over-filtration. Further understanding of the fate of AM via imaging studies will not only confirm its anti-inflammatory and anti-scarring effects but will also teach us how intrableb wound healing can be modulated by the AM regarding integration into the surrounding operated tissue. Such knowledge will further strengthen our belief that AM can be a natural biological matrix derived from the fetus that may modulate adult wound healing toward regeneration through the reduction of inflammation, scarring, and unwanted new blood vessel formation. Further proof of the anti-angiogenic action of AM in reverting neovascularization in cases of neovascular glaucoma will generate a direct impact on using AM to treat ocular diseases where angiogenesis threatens vision. We expect that such a treatment will be more effective than the conventional approach based on an antibody blockade against VEGF, because AM not only suppresses angiogenesis mediated by VEGF and other growth factors, but also curtails inflammation and scarring. This innovative concept can then be applied to other parts of the body where pathological fibrosis or angiogenesis is considered detrimental and undesirable.

8. Financial disclosure and acknowledgement

The clinical research mentioned in this article was supported in part by grant #EY019785 from the National Eye Institute via TissueTech, Inc., which owns US patents on the method of preparation and clinical uses of human amniotic membrane. The content is solely the responsibility of the author and does not necessarily represent the official views of the National Eye Institute or the National Institutes of Health. The author thanks Lingyi Liang, MD, PhD and Shunsuke R. Sakurai for assistance in editing the text.

9. References

Adzick NS, Lorenz HP. (1994). Cells, matrix, growth factors, and the surgeon. The biology of scarless fetal wound repair. *Ann Surg*, Vol.220, pp.10-18.

Anand A, Sheha H, Teng C, Liebmann JM, Ritch R, Tello C. (2011). Use of Amniotic Membrane Graft in Glaucoma Shunt Surgery. *Ophthalmic Surg Lasers Imaging*.

Apostolov VI, Siarov NP. (1996). Subconjunctival injection of low-dose Mitomycin-C for treatment of failing human trabeculectomies. *Int Ophthalmol*, Vol.20, No.1-3, pp.101-105.

Araujo SV, Spaeth GL, Roth SM, Starita RJ. A ten-year follow-up on a prospective, randomized trial of postoperative corticosteroids after trabeculectomy. Ophthalmology 1995; 102:1753–1759.

Barton K, Budenz D, Khaw PT, Tseng SCG. (2001). Glaucoma filtration surgery using amniotic membrane transplantation. *Invest Ophthalmol Vis Sci*, Vol.42, pp.1762-1768.

Baudouin C, Nordmann JP, Denis P, et al. Efficacy of indomethacin 0.1% and fluorometholone 0.1% on conjunctival inflammation following chronic application of antiglaucomatous drugs. Graefes Arch Clin Exp Ophthalmol 2002;240:929–35.

Breusegem C, Spielberg L, Van Ginderdeuren R, Vandewalle E, Renier C, Van de Veire S, Fieuws S, Zeyen T, Stalmans I. Preoperative Nonsteroidal Anti-inflammatory Drug or Steroid and Outcomes after Trabeculectomy. Ophthalmology 2010;117:1324–1330

Broadway DC, Chang LP. (2001). Trabeculectomy, risk factors for failure and the preoperative state of the conjunctiva. *J Glaucoma*, Vol.10, No.3, pp.237-249.

Bruno CA, Eisengart JA, Radenbaugh PA, Moroi SE. (2006). Subconjunctival placement of human amniotic membrane during high risk glaucoma filtration surgery. *Ophthalmic Surg Lasers Imaging*, Vol.37, No.3, pp.190-197.

Chang L, Crowston JG, Cordeiro MF, Akbar AN, Khaw PT. (2000). The role of the immune system in conjunctival wound healing after glaucoma surgery. *Surv Ophthalmol*, Vol.45, No.1, pp.49-68.

Chen CW, Huang HT, Bair JS, Lee CC. (1990). Trabeculectomy with simultaneous topical application of mitomycin-C in refractory glaucoma. *J Ocul Pharmacol*, Vol.6, No.3, pp.175-182.

Chen C. (1983). Enhanced intraocular pressure controlling effectiveness of trabeculectomy by local application of mitomycin C. *Trans Asia Pac Acad Ophthalmol*, Vol.9, pp.172-177.

Chihara E, Dong J, Ochiai H, Hamada S. (2002). Effects of tranilast on filtering blebs: a pilot study. *J Glaucoma*, Vol.11, No.2, pp.127-133.

Chintala SK, Wang N, Diskin S, Mattox C, Kagemann L, Fini ME, Schuman JS. (2005). Matrix metalloproteinase gelatinase B (MMP-9) is associated with leaking glaucoma filtering blebs. *Exp Eye Res*, Vol.81, No.4, pp.429-436.

Choi JY, Choi J, Kim YD. (2010). Subconjunctival bevacizumab as an adjunct to trabeculectomy in eyes with refractory glaucoma: a case series. *Korean J Ophthalmol*, Vol.24, No.1, pp.47-52.

Coote MA, Ruddle JB, Qin Q, Crowston JG (2008). Vascular changes after intra-bleb injection of bevacizumab. *J Glaucoma* Vol.17, No., pp.517-518.

Demir T, Turgut B, Akyol N, Ozercan I, Ulas F, Celiker U. (2002). Effects of amniotic membrane transplantation and mitomycin C on wound healing in experimental glaucoma surgery. *Ophthalmologica*, Vol.216, No.6, pp.438-442.

Desjardins DC, Parrish RK, Folberg R, Nevarez J, Heuer DK, Gressel MG. (1986). Wound healing after filtering surgery in owl monkeys. *Arch Ophthalmol*, Vol.104, No.12, pp.1835-1839.

Desmouliere A, Geinoz A, Gabbiani F, Gabbiani G. (1993). Transforming growth factor-beta 1 induces alpha-smooth muscle actin expression in granulation tissue myofibroblasts and in quiescent and growing cultured fibroblasts. *J Cell Biol*, Vol.122, No.1, pp.103-111.

Drolsum L, Willoch C, Nicolaissen B. (2006). Use of amniotic membrane as an adjuvant in refractory glaucoma. *Acta Ophthalmol Scand*, Vol.84, No.6, pp.786-789.

Dvorak HF. (1986). Tumors: wounds that do not heal. Similarities between tumor stroma generation and wound healing. *N Engl J Med*, Vol.315, No.26, pp.1650-1659.

Eliezer RN, Kasahara N, Caixeta-Umbelino C, Pinheiro RK, Mandia C, Jr., Malta RF. (2006). Use of amniotic membrane in trabeculectomy for the treatment of glaucoma: a pilot study. *Arq Bras Oftalmol*, Vol.69, No.3, pp.309-312.

Fujishima H, Shimazaki J, Shinozaki N, Tsubota K. (1998). Trabeculectomy with the use of amniotic membrane for uncontrolled glaucoma. *Ophthalmic Surg Lasers,* Vol.29, pp.428-431.

Fujita H. (1982). [Pharmacokinetics of mitomycin C and its derivative (KW-2083)]. *Gan To Kagaku Ryoho,* Vol.9, No.8, pp.1362-1373.

Greenfield DS, Parrish RK. (1996). Bleb rupture following filtering surgery with mitomycin-C: clinicopathologic correlations. Ophthalmic Surg Lasers, Vol.27, No.10, pp.876-877.

Greenfield DS, Suner IJ, Miller MP, Kangas TA, Palmberg PF, Flynn HW, Jr. (1996). Endophthalmitis after filtering surgery with mitomycin. *Arch Ophthalmol,* Vol.114, No.8, pp.943-949.

Guerriero E, Yu JU, Kahook MY. (2006) Morphologic evaluation of bevacizumab (Avastin) treated corneal stromal fibroblasts. *Invest Ophthalmol Vis Sci, Vol*47, E-Abstract 1642.

Grierson I, Joseph J, Miller M, Day JE. (1988). Wound repair: the fibroblast and the inhibition of scar formation. *Eye (Lond),* Vol.2 (Pt 2), pp.135-148.

Heuer DK, Parrish RK, Gressel MG, Hodapp E, Palmberg PF, Anderson DR. (1984). 5-fluorouracil and glaucoma filtering surgery. II. A pilot study. *Ophthalmology,* Vol.91, No.4, pp.384-394.

Hosseini H, Mehryar M, Farvardin M. Focus on triamcinolone acetonide as an adjunct to glaucoma filtration surgery. Med Hypotheses 2007;68:401– 403

Kahook MY, Schuman JS, Noecker RJ. (2006a). Intravitreal bevacizumab in a patient with neovascular glaucoma. *Ophthalmic Surg Lasers Imaging,* Vol.37, No.2, pp.144-146.

Kahook MY, Schuman JS, Noecker RJ. (2006b). Needle bleb revision of encapsulated filtering bleb with bevacizumab. Ophthalmic Surg Lasers Imaging, Vol.37, No.2, pp.148-150.

Kapetansky FM, Pappa KS, Krasnow MA, et al (2007). Subconjunctival injection(s) of bevacizumab for failing filtering blebs. *Invest Ophthalmol Vis Sci* 2007 [E-Abstract 837

Kitazawa Y, Kawase K, Matsushita H, Minobe M. (1991). Trabeculectomy with mitomycin. A comparative study with fluorouracil. *Arch Ophthalmol,* Vol.109, No.12, pp.1693-1698.

Lama PJ, Fechtner RD. (2003). Antifibrotics and wound healing in glaucoma surgery. *Surv Ophthalmol,* Vol.48, No.3, pp.314-346.

Lee S-B, Li D-Q, Tan DTH, Meller D, Tseng SCG. (2000). Suppression of TGF-b signaling in both normal conjunctival fibroblasts and pterygial body fibroblasts by amniotic membrane. *Curr Eye Res,* Vol.20, pp.325-334.

Leibovich SJ, Ross R. (1975). The role of the macrophage in wound repair. A study with hydrocortisone and antimacrophage serum. *Am J Pathol,* Vol.78, No.1, pp.71-100.

Li W, He H, Kawakita T, Espana EM, Tseng SCG. (2006). Amniotic membrane induces apoptosis of interferon-gamma activited macrophages in vitro. *Exp Eye Res,* Vol.82, No.2, pp.282-292.

Lu H, Mai D. (2003). [Trabeculectomy combined amniotic membrane transplantation for refractory glaucoma]. *Yan Ke Xue Bao,* Vol.19, No.2, pp.89-91.

Manzano RP, Peyman GA, Khan P, Kivilcim M. (2006). Testing intravitreal toxicity of bevacizumab (Avastin). *Retina,* Vol.26, No.3, pp.257-261.

Mast BA, Diegelmann RF, Krummel TM, Cohen IK. (1992). Scarless wound healing in mammalian fetus. *Surgery,* Vol.174, pp.441-451.

Maumenee AE. (1960). External filtering operations for glaucoma: the mechanism of function and failure. *Trans Am Ophthalmol Soc,* Vol.58, pp.319-328.

Meyer-ter-Vehn T, Sieprath S, Katzenberger B, Gebhardt S, Grehn F, Schlunck G. (2006). Contractility as a prerequisite for TGF-beta-induced myofibroblast transdifferentiation in human tenon fibroblasts. *Invest Ophthalmol Vis Sci,* Vol.47, No.11, pp.4895-4904.

Michels S, Rosenfeld PJ, Puliafito CA, Marcus EN, Venkatraman AS. (2005). Systemic bevacizumab (Avastin) therapy for neovascular age-related macular degeneration twelve-week results of an uncontrolled open-label clinical study. *Ophthalmology,* Vol.112, No.6, pp.1035-1047.

Miller MH, Grierson I, Unger WI, Hitchings RA. (1989). Wound healing in an animal model of glaucoma fistulizing surgery in the rabbit. Ophthalmic Surg, Vol.20, No.5, pp.350-357.

Nguyen KD, Lee DA. Effect of steroids and nonsteroidal anti-inflammatory agents on human ocular fibroblast. Invest Ophthalmol Vis Sci 1992;33:2693-2701

Nuyts RM, Felten PC, Pels E, Langerhorst CT, Geijssen HC, Grossniklaus HE, Greve EL. (1994). Histopathologic effects of mitomycin C after trabeculectomy in human glaucomatous eyes with persistent hypotony. *Am J Ophthalmol,* Vol.118, No.2, pp.225-237.

Okada K, Sugiyama T, Takai S, Jin D, Ishida O, Fukmoto M, Oku H, Miyazaki M, Ikeda T. (2009). Effects of mitomycin C on the expression of chymase and mast cells in the conjunctival scar of a monkey trabeculectomy model. *Mol Vis,* Vol.15, pp.2029-2036.

Okamoto Y, Takai S, Miyazaki M. (2004). Significance of chymase inhibition for prevention of adhesion formation. *Eur J Pharmacol,* Vol.484, No.2-3, pp.357-359.

Ophir A. (1992). Encapsulated filtering bleb. A selective review--new deductions. *Eye,* Vol.6 (Pt 4), pp.348-352.

Palanca-Capistrano AM, Hall J, Cantor LB, Morgan L, Hoop J, WuDunn D. (2009). Long-term outcomes of intraoperative 5-fluorouracil versus intraoperative mitomycin C in primary trabeculectomy surgery. *Ophthalmology,* Vol.116, No.2, pp.185-190.

Parrish RK, Schiffman JC, Feuer WJ, Heuer DK. (2001). Prognosis and risk factors for early postoperative wound leaks after trabeculectomy with and without 5-fluorouracil. *Am J Ophthalmol,* Vol.132, No.5, pp.633-640.

Purcell JM, Teng CC, Tello C, et al (2008). Effect of needle bleb revision with ranibizumab as a primary intervention in a failing bleb following trabeculectomy. *Invest Ophthalmol Vis Sci* 2008. [E-Abstract 4165]

Reichel MB, Cordeiro MF, Alexander RA, Cree IA, Bhattacharya SS, Khaw PT. (1998). New model of conjunctival scarring in the mouse eye. *Br J Ophthalmol,* Vol.82, No.9, pp.1072-1077.

Ross R, Rainee EW, Bowen-Pope DF. (1986). The biology of platelet-derived growth factor. Cell, Vol.46, pp.155-169.

Sano-Kato N, Fukagawa K, Okada N, Kawakita T, Takano Y, Dogru M, Tsubota K, Fujishima H. (2005). TGF-beta1, IL-1beta, and Th2 cytokines stimulate vascular endothelial growth factor production from conjunctival fibroblasts. *Exp Eye Res,* Vol.80, No.4, pp.555-560.

Sheha H, Liang L, Tseng SCG (2010). Amniotic Membrane Grafts for Glaucoma Surgery. In: Paul N.Schacknow, John R.Samples, editors. *The Glaucoma Book;* A Practical, Evidence-Based Approach to Patient Care.New York:Springer. p. 861-869.

Sheha H, Kheirkhah A, Taha H. (2008). Amniotic membrane transplantation in trabeculectomy with mitomycin C for refractory glaucoma. *J Glaucoma,* Vol.17, No.4, pp.303-307.

Sherwood MB. (2006). A sequential, multiple-treatment, targeted approach to reduce wound healing and failure of glaucoma filtration surgery in a rabbit model (an American Ophthalmological Society thesis). *Trans Am Ophthalmol Soc,* Vol.104, pp.478-492.

Shey E, He H, Sakurai S, Tseng SC. (2011) Inhibition of Angiogenesis by HC{middle dot}HA, a Complex of Hyaluronan and the Heavy Chain of Inter-{alpha}-Inhibitor, Purified from Human Amniotic Membrane. Invest Ophthalmol Vis Sci. [Epub ahead of print]

Shields MB, Scroggs MW, Sloop CM, Simmons RB. (1993). Clinical and histopathologic observations concerning hypotony after trabeculectomy *with* adjunctive mitomycin C. *Am J Ophthalmol,* Vol.116, pp.673-683.

Shuster JN, Krupin T, Kolker AE, Becker B. (1984). Limbus- v fornix-based conjunctival flap in trabeculectomy. A long-term randomized study. Arch Ophthalmol, Vol.102, No.3, pp.361-362.

Singh K, Mehta K, Shaikh NM, Tsai JC, Moster MR, Budenz DL, Greenfield DS, Chen PP, Cohen JS, Baerveldt GS, Shaikh S. (2000). Trabeculectomy with intraoperative mitomycin C versus 5-fluorouracil. Prospective randomized clinical trial. *Ophthalmology,* Vol.107, No.12, pp.2305-2309.

Skuta GL, Parrish RK. (1987). Wound healing in glaucoma filtering surgery. *Surv Ophthalmol,* Vol.32, No.3, pp.149-170.

Starita RJ, Fellman RL, Spaeth GL, Poryzees EM, Greenidge KC, Traverso CE. (1985). Short- and long-term effects of postoperative corticosteroids on trabeculectomy. *Ophthalmology,* Vol.92, No.7, pp.938-946.

Sturmer J, Broadway DC, Hitchings RA. (1993). Young patient trabeculectomy. Assessment of risk factors for failure. *Ophthalmology,* Vol.100, No.6, pp.928-939.

Tham CC, Li FC, Leung DY. Intrableb triamcinolone acetonide injection after bleb-forming filtration surgery (trabeculectomy, phacotrabeculectomy, and trabeculectomy revision by needling): a pilot study. Eye 2006;20:1484–1486.

Traverso CE, Tomey KF, Antonios S. (1987). Limbal- vs fornix-based conjunctival trabeculectomy flaps. *Am J Ophthalmol,* Vol.104, No.1, pp.28-32.

Tseng SCG, Espana EM, Kawakita T, Di Pascuale MA, Wei Z-G, He H, Liu TS, Cho TH, Gao YY, Yeh LK, Liu C-Y. (2004). How does amniotic membrane work? *The Ocular Surface,* Vol.2, No.3, pp.177-187.

Tseng SCG, Li D-Q, Ma X. (1999). Suppression of Transforming Growth Factor isoforms, TGF-b receptor II, and myofibroblast differentiation in cultured human corneal and limbal fibroblasts by amniotic membrane matrix. *J Cell Physiol,* Vol.179, pp.325-335.

Wang L, Liu X, Zhang P, Lin J. (2005). [An experimental trial of glaucoma filtering surgery with amniotic membrane]. *Yan Ke Xue Bao,* Vol.21, No.2, pp.126-131.

Wipff PJ, Rifkin DB, Meister JJ, Hinz B. (2007). Myofibroblast contraction activates latent TGF-beta1 from the extracellular matrix. *J Cell Biol,* Vol.179, No.6, pp.1311-1323.

Wong J, Wang N, Miller JW, Schuman JS. (1994). Modulation of human fibroblast activity by selected angiogenesis inhibitors. *Exp Eye Res,* Vol.58, No.4, pp.439-451.

WuDunn D, Cantor LB, Palanca-Capistrano AM, Hoop J, Alvi NP, Finley C, Lakhani V, Burnstein A, Knotts SL. (2002). A prospective randomized trial comparing intraoperative 5-fluorouracil vs mitomycin C in primary trabeculectomy. *Am J Ophthalmol,* Vol.134, No.4, pp.521-528.

Yue J, Hu CQ, Lei XM, Qin GH, Zhang Y. (2003). Trabeculectomy with amniotic membrane transplantation and combining suture lysis of scleral flap in complicated glaucoma. *Zhonghua Yan Ke Za Zhi,* Vol.39, No.8, *pp.476-480.*

Yuki K, Shiba D, Kimura I, Ohtakey Y, Tsubota K. Trabeculectomy With or Without Intraoperative Sub-Tenon Injection of Triamcinolone Acetonide in Treating Secondary Glaucoma Am J Ophthalmol 2009;147:1055–1060

Zhong Y, Zhou Y, Wang K. (2000). Effect of amniotic membrane on filtering bleb after trabeculectomy in rabbit eyes. *Yan Ke Xue Bao,* Vol.16, No.2, pp.73-6, 83.

5

Novel Glaucoma Surgical Devices

Parul Ichhpujani[1] and Marlene R. Moster[2]
[1]Glaucoma Facility, Department of Ophthalmology,
Government Medical College and Hospital, Chandigarh,
[2]Anne and William Goldberg Glaucoma Service,
Wills Eye Institute, Philadelphia, PA,
[1]India
[2]USA

1. Introduction

An ideal glaucoma procedure is the one that is easy to perform, reproducible, with a low incidence of early postoperative hypotony, and long-term adequate IOP control. Furthermore, it should be minimally cataractogenic, allow rapid visual recovery and have the potential to be combined with phacoemulsification without one procedure potentially affecting the outcome of the other. Unfortunately, the quest for an ideal glaucoma procedure is on. The Landmarks in the course of surgical innovations for glaucoma management highlight the fact that we have come a long way.

Landmarks in the history of surgical innovations for glaucoma

- 1857 – Albrecht von Graefe: Surgical iridectomy "to reduce aqueous production" in glaucoma. Iridectomy helped many cases of angle closure, but not by the mechanism proposed.
- 1859 – Coccius: Iridectomy with iris inclusion
- 1876 – Argyll-Robertson: Scleral trephination
- 1878 – Louis De Wecker: Anterior sclerectomy
- 1903 – Bader and Lagrange: Iridosclerectomy
- 1905 – Heine: Cyclodialysis
- 1906 – Soren Holth: Iridenclesis
- 1909 – Elliot: Corneoscleral trephination
- 1924 – Preziozi: Electrocautery to create a full thickness fistula between the anterior chamber and the subconjunctival space.
- 1936 – Otto Barkan: Goniotomy for chronic glaucoma in adults.
- 1956 – Meyer-Schwickerath: Laser iridotomy with a xenon arc photocoagulator.
- 1958 – Harold Scheie: Modified Preziozi's procedure. Entered the eye with a knife and then used cautery to extend the scleral wound.
- 1968 – Cairns: Trabeculectomy. Removed a rectangular section of trabecular meshwork and deep cornea. He aimed to remove a block of the canal of Schlemm to get aqueous to flow freely into its cut ends.

- 1968 – Anthony Molteno: Glaucoma drainage device that directly shunted aqueous from the anterior chamber into a episcleral reservoir.
- 1976 – Theodore Krupin: First valved glaucoma drainage tube, at first without a reservoir.
- 1979 – James B. Wise and Stanton L. Witter: Argon laser "trabeculoplasty."
- 1982 – Robert Ritch: Iridoplasty for acute angle closure crisis unresponsive to medication.
- 1983 – Chen Wu Chen: Mitomycin C as an adjunctive in trabeculectomy.
- 1984 – 5-Fluorouracil was first reported in an animal model and in a pilot study in glaucoma filtering surgery.
- 2002 - ExPRESS miniature glaucoma shunt
- 2003 - Reay Brown and Mary Lynch: EYEPASS glaucoma shunt
- 2004 - George Baerveldt and Don Minckler: FDA approved, Trabectome microelectrocautery device
- 2004 - Richard Hill and Mory Ghareb: Trabecular micro-bypass stent, iStent. Undergoing FDA review
- 2005 – Deep light Gold shunt
- 2009 - Bruce Shields: Aquashunt
- 2009 - Transcend CyPass glaucoma implant

2. Trabeculectomy

Despite several available options, trabeculectomy — arguably is the most-performed glaucoma surgery till today. Although improved techniques and the adjunctive use of antimetabolites has enhanced long-term success as measured by intraocular pressure (IOP) control, trabeculectomy has a sizeable risk profile to glaucoma patients, over both the short and long term.

Blebitis, bleb related endophthalmitis, hypotony, overfiltration, bleb leaks, bleb fibrosis and encapsulation, bleb overhang, corneal endothelial cell loss, dellen, and aqueous misdirection are among the many risks associated post trabeculectomy. (Borisuth et al, 1999)

3. Drainage devices

Glaucoma drainage devices (GDD) were initially developed for use in complex glaucoma patients, many of whom had failed medical, laser, and prior surgical treatments. (Molteno, 1969; Krupin et al., 1976; Lloyd et al., 1994 & Coleman et al., 1995) Typically, these devices consist of a tube placed into the anterior chamber to allow for aqueous humor to flow posteriorly into an encapsulated filtration area typically 10–12 mm posterior to the limbus, into a reservoir sutured to the sclera.

Though complications associated with anterior bleb formation were avoided, GDD resulted in a high risk of hypotony and overfiltration, sometimes leading to suprachoroidal hemorrhage. As a result several measures for flow restriction and regulation were adopted, but despite all efforts complication profile of GDD is significant. Overfiltration, fibrosis, tube exposure, tube occlusion, tube retraction and diplopia to list a few potential complications. (Kupin et al., 1995; Ticho and Ophir, 1993 & Gedde et al., 2007)

Since neither trabeculectomy nor GDDs are without their fair share of complications, the quest for the development and advancement of glaucoma surgery to provide alternative means of shunting aqueous humor out of the anterior chamber is on.

Surgical procedures augmenting either conventional outflow pathway or uveoscleral outflow pathway have been developed. For conventional outflow enhancement, goniosurgical procedures (Epstein et al., 1985) and surgeries involving schlemm canal (both ab interno and ab externo) have recently emerged as successful surgical options.

Surgical approaches to augment suprachoroidal outflow have also been explored with cyclodialysis, suprachoroidal implants, seton devices, and most recently, an ab externo gold shunt placed in the suprachoroidal space. (Pinnas and Boniuk, 1969; Krejci, 1972; Ozdamar et al., 2003; Jordan et al., 2006)

Type	Glaucoma surgery
Non penetrating	Viscocanalostomy Deep sclerectomy Canaloplasty
Minimally penetrating	Ex-PRESS glaucoma filtration device Trabecular micro-bypass iStent Trabectome microelectrocautery Gold microshunt (GMS) device Eyepass implant
Penetrating	Trabeculectomy

Table 1. Types of glaucoma surgeries

This chapter, addresses the available knowledge for the novel drainage devices; devices which attempt to assist with flow regulation such as the Ex-PRESS mini-glaucoma shunt (Alcon Laboratories, Inc., Fort Worth, TX) (Wamsley et al., 2004), Schlemm's canal surgical procedures, including nonpenetrating canaloplasty surgery (Lewis et al., 2007), the Glaukos trabecular micro-bypass iStent (Nichamin, 2009) the Trabectome microelectrocautery device (Nguyen, 2008) and the suprachoroidal outflow gold microshunt device (GMS) (Melamed et al., 2009) (Table 1).Published data is limited as many of these devices are currently in investigation and undergoing clinical trials.

4. Minimally penetrating procedures

4.1 Ex-PRESS glaucoma filtration device
Ophthalmic surgery has evolved over the last several decades into sophisticated microsurgery involving continually smaller incisions. The Ex-PRESS shunt is on the forefront of this evolution toward smaller incision glaucoma filtration surgery. Since there is an added cost to using the Ex-PRESS rather than trabeculectomy, its place in the surgical management of glaucoma has not been clear so far.

Device

Ex-PRESS stands for "excessive pressure regulating shunt system".

The Ex-PRESS implant is a miniature unvalved glaucoma implant. It was originally developed by Optonol, Ltd. (Neve Ilan, Israel), as an alternative procedure to trabeculectomy and to the other types of glaucoma filtering surgery for patients with open angle glaucoma (Nyska et al., 2003). Now, it is available as EX-PRESS Glaucoma Filtration Device (Alcon Laboratories, Inc., Fort Worth, TX).

The device is approximately 3 mm long, stainless steel tube (outer diameter 400 μm (27 gauge)) with a beveled, sharpened, rounded tip, a disc-like flange (<1 mm²) at the device proximal end, and a spur-like projection that prevents its extrusion. (Nyska et al., 2003; Geffen et al., 2010) The external flange and inner spur are angled to conform to the anatomy of the sclera, and the distance between them corresponds to the scleral thickness at the site of implantation.

The EX-PRESS® Glaucoma Filtration Device is preloaded on a specially designed disposable introducer, the EX-PRESS® Delivery System (EDS). The EDS is an inserter designed to maintain the correct orientation of the EX-PRESS® Glaucoma Filtration Device throughout the implantation procedure. The commercially available versions are: R-50, P-50 and P-200. (Table 2; Figure 1)

Characteristic	Ex PRESS R50	Ex PRESS P50	Ex PRESS P200
External body device	Round	Round	Round
Device length	2.96	2.64	2.64
Internal lumen size	50	50	200
Tip shape	Pointed	Pointed	Pointed
Backplate shape	Uniform	Vertical split	Vertical split
Preincision needle gauge	27G	25G	25G

Table 2. Comparative characteristics of the available models of Ex- PRESS implant

Indications

- Open Angle Glaucoma refractory to medical and laser treatment
- Open Angle Glaucoma with a failed filtration procedure
- Combined glaucoma and cataract procedure (Ex-PRESS may have the advantage of faster visual recovery compared with trabeculectomy)
- Aphakic glaucoma (As no iridectomy is required with the Ex-PRESS implantation, there is less risk of vitreous moving forward through a new iridectomy)
- Sturge-Weber syndrome and other situations as high hyperopia and nanophthalmos (Since chances of choroidal effusions following trabeculectomy are high in these subset of patients; Ex-PRESS implantation may offer a safer alternative because of its lower rate of prolonged postoperative hypotony)

Contraindications

The implantation of the EX-PRESS® Glaucoma Filtration Device is contraindicated if one or more of the following conditions exist:

- Presence of ocular disease such as uveitis, ocular infection, severe dry eye or severe blepharitis.
- Pre-existing ocular or systemic pathology that, in the opinion of the surgeon, is likely to cause postoperative complications following implantation of the device.
- Patient diagnosed with angle closure glaucoma.

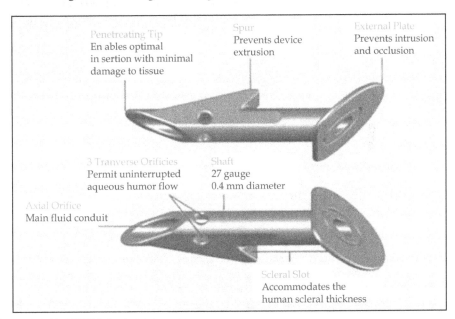

Fig. 1. R 50 Ex-PRESS device

Surgical procedure

Originally, the device was designed to be inserted at the limbus directly under the conjunctiva with formation of a subconjunctival bleb which served as a flow modulator. Poor conjunctival covering of the device, conjunctival erosions over the external flange and conjunctival scarring with subsequent decreased aqueous humour filtration, were some of the complications that were encountered because of direct subconjunctival implantation. (Kaplan Messa et al., 2002; Gandolfi et al., 2002; Traverso et al., 2005; Wamsley et al., 2004; Stewart et al., 2005; Rivier et al., 2007; Tavolato et al., 2006; Garg et al., 2005) Conjunctivoplasty or tube removal had to be performed to avoid secondary infection.

To overcome these complications, Dahan and Carmichael suggested implanting the device under a limbus based 50% deep scleral flap extending into clear cornea. (Dahan and Carmichael, 2005) This operation is similar to standard trabeculectomy without the need of an iridectomy or scleral removal.

This implant may also be used in deep sclerectomy to simplify the difficult dissection of Schlemm's canal and Trabeculo-Descemet's membrane.

4.2 Placement of device under a scleral flap

To place the Ex-PRESS filtration device, a conjunctival peritomy, limbal or fornix-based, is first created as in conventional trabeculectomy. Gentle cautery is applied to the sclera prior to creation of a scleral flap. The dimensions of the scleral flap may need to be slightly larger than the trabeculectomy flap and it should be initiated more posteriorly in order to ensure full coverage of the shunt plate.

Scleral spur is identified by a white, glistening band of fibers that crosses the bed of this section. The blue zone is a transition zone to the clear cornea. The surgeon should make sure that they implant the EX-PRESS device in the anterior chamber, just at the level of the scleral spur, but not too far posteriorly. It is important for the device to enter the eye exactly at the anterior aspect of the scleral spur and for it to remain at the iris plane so that it does not point downward towards the iris.

Once the scleral spur has been visualized, the anterior chamber should be filled with viscoelastic or air in the area of anticipated shunt entry. Rather than an ostium created by a punch, trephine, or scissors, a 25- or 27-gauge needle or a 400 µm wide blade is used to enter the anterior chamber at the level of the scleral spur, parallel to the iris, and the Ex-PRESS device is injected into this needle tract.

Complications

The Ex-PRESS device relies on nonphysiologic subconjunctival flow as its mechanism of IOP lowering. As a result, all of the issues that limit trabeculectomy and the complication profile associated with blebs accompany the Ex-PRESS shunt too, but to a much lesser extent.

Recently, external blockade of the tube has been reported as a possible device-related complication of Ex-PRESS implants, which can be visualized on a systematic gonioscopic examination. (Bagnis et al., 2011) It should be considered whenever IOP increases and a flat bleb is observed. Neodymium: Yttrium Argon Garnet (Nd:YAG) laser at the tip of the device is a viable therapeutic option to treat the external occlusion of Ex-PRESS devices, regardless the nature of the obstruction. Obstruction may also occur inside the lumen of the device where it may not be visualized by gonioscopy, at the point where the diameter constricts to 50 mm. Since this constriction point is close to the opening into the anterior chamber, Nd:YAG laser works in this scenario as well (Netland, 2011).

Corneal dislocation of the Ex-PRESS implant may occur and when associated with ocular hypertension, needs surgical treatment. (Vetrugno et al., 2011) Before considering a trabeculectomy, it could be valuable to attempt an implant reposition. Reopening of the conjunctiva and the scleral flap, excision of the corneal tissue covering the flange, and stitching the implant to the sclera with polyprolene suture has been tried with success.

The Magnetic Resonance Imaging (MRI) systems in clinical use today operate with magnetic fields ranging from 0.2 to 3.0 Tesla. To ascertain MRI compatibility, the Ex-PRESS glaucoma drainage device (316L stainless steel) has been examined for magnetic field interactions under standard 1.5, 3.0, and 4.7 T MRI scanning protocols. (Seibold et al., 2011) During induced torque testing, no displacement was noted under 1.5 and 3.0 T conditions, although a significant amount of displacement occurred in the 4.7 T environment. Increasing amounts of angular deflection were demonstrated at all three field strengths. So, it should be remembered that Ex-PRESS moves in the presence of high magnetic fields.

4.3 Scientific evidence so far

Ex-PRESS versus trabeculectomy

Maris et al in a retrospective comparative case series analysed data of 49 eyes with the Ex-PRESS and 47 eyes with a standard trabeculectomy. (Maris et al., 2007) The authors noted that although the mean IOP was significantly higher in the early postoperative period in the Ex-PRESS group compared with the trabeculectomy group, the reduction of IOP was similar in both groups after 3 months. The number of postoperative glaucoma medications in both groups was not significantly different. Kaplan-Meier survival curve analysis showed no significant difference in success between the two groups (P = 0.594). The success rate at an average of 11 months was 90% for the Ex-PRESS shunt compared with 92% for trabeculectomies at last follow up. Early postoperative hypotony and choroidal effusion were significantly more frequent after trabeculectomy than after Ex-PRESS implants under a scleral flap (P < 0.001). There was no difference between a limbal based or a fornix based approach with either procedure (trabeculectomy vs. Ex-PRESS shunt). After 3 months, the percentage decrease in IOP was similar for the groups, Ex-PRESS group (39.9 to 46.6%) and the trabeculectomy group (28.6 to 45.4%). For IOP control during the postoperative period, a significantly greater number of laser suture lysis procedures were performed in the Ex-PRESS group compared with the control group. The authors concluded that the Ex-PRESS implant under a scleral flap had similar IOP-lowering efficacy with a lower rate of early hypotony compared with trabeculectomy.

Ex-PRESS in previously operated eyes

Moster and co workers reported intermediate-term results of the Ex-PRESS implant (R-50 and T-50), under a scleral flap in previously operated eyes (cataract or failed glaucoma surgeries). (Lankaranian et al., 2010) To compare the outcome between patients who had previous trabeculectomy or cataract surgery the definition of success was IOP of 5-15mmHg. One hundred eyes of 100 patients were studied. The mean follow-up period was 27 ± 13.2 months (range: 12-66). Success was defined as complete if IOP was 5-21 mmHg without medication or surgical intervention, and qualified if IOP was within the same range with glaucoma medication. Success was complete in 60 (60%) and qualified in 24 (24%) eyes. The mean preoperative IOP of 27.7 ± 9.2 mm Hg (range, 14-52 mmHg) with 2.73 ± 1.1 drugs declined to 14.02 ± 5.1 mm Hg with 0.72 ± 1.06 drugs at the last follow up (P < 0.0001). The causes of failure were uncontrolled IOP (11%), bleb needling (4%), and persistent hypotony (1%). Bleb needling may induce an erratic wound healing response in some cases and lead to failure. The probability of success in the patients with previous cataract surgery and trabeculectomy at 3 years was 60.6% and 50.9%, respectively. Figure 2 shows Ex-PRESS implant in a case with previously failed trabeculectomy.

Ates and coworkers studied 15 eyes with postpenetrating keratoplasty glaucoma unresponsive to medical antiglaucomatous therapy in which Ex-PRESS mini glaucoma shunt implantation was done. (Ates et al., 2010)

IOP decreased from 41.46 mm Hg to 12.06 mm Hg over a mean follow-up of 12.2 months (P<0.001).

IOP was below 21 mm Hg in 14 of 15 eyes (93.3%) with or without antiglaucomatous drugs. Complete success (IOP<21 mm Hg without medication) rate was 86.6%. Average number of antiglaucomatous drug usage decreased from 3.20 (range: 2 to 4) preoperatively to 0.26 postoperatively (range: 0 to 3) (P<0.001). In 93.3% of the cases, the decrease in IOP was 30%

or above postoperatively. After Ex-PRESS implantation, clear grafts remained clear while edematous grafts became clearer due to IOP decrease. Neither biomicroscopy nor pachymetry showed worsening of preoperatively opaque grafts.

Similarly, Vetrugno and colleagues also reported good results in vitrectomized patients who required glaucoma surgery for persistent ocular hypertension (Vetrugno et al., 2010).

Ex-PRESS with deep sclerectomy

Bissig and colleagues did a prospective, nonrandomized trial to study Deep Sclerectomy with the Ex-PRESS X-200 implant in 26 eyes. (Bissig et al., 2010) A posterior deep sclerectomy was dissected without opening the Schlemm's canal and an Ex-PRESS X-200 device was inserted under the scleral flap into the anterior chamber to drain aqueous humour into the intrascleral space. Eighty-five percent of patients achieved an IOP < 18 mmHg with or without medication and 69% without medication. Post-operative complications were hyphaema (15%), wound leak (15%), encysted blebs (54%) and bleb fibrosis in 8% of patients.

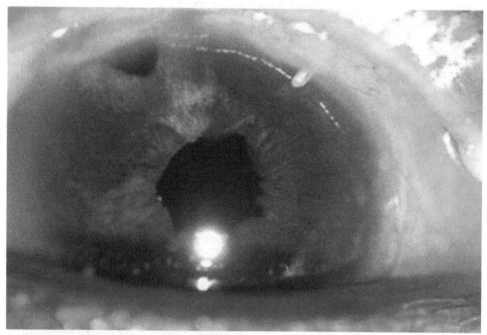

Fig. 2. Ex-PRESS in a previously failed glaucoma surgery

Gindroz and coworkers conducted a prospective study reporting on modified deep sclerectomy using the Ex-PRESS LR-50 in combined cataract and glaucoma surgery in 24 eyes. (Gindroz et al., 2011) Preoperative data had, IOP: 18.1±5.3 mmHg, best-corrected visual acuity (BCVA): 0.6±0.3, and number of medications: 2.3±1.1. The IOP decreased by 25.4% at 24 months and by 27.0% at 48 months. At 24 months, 19 patients (86.3%) achieved a BCVA of 0.5 or better, and at 48 months the mean BCVA was 0.7±0.3. At the last visit, the mean number of medications reduced to 0.6±0.8 (P<0.05). The complete and qualified success rates were 45.6% and 85.2%. No conjunctival erosions over the Ex-PRESS LR-50 were noted.

Ex-PRESS with phacoemulsification

Kanner and co workers implanted Ex-PRESS device under a scleral flap either as a single procedure in 231 eyes of 200 patients or combined with cataract surgery in 114 eyes of 100 patients, for a total of 345 eyes in 300 patients who received the implant. (Kanner et al., 2009) They found that the Ex-PRESS implant under a scleral flap could lower IOP alone or in combination with cataract surgery. The most common device-related complication was blockage of the lumen of the implant, which was effectively treated with Nd:YAG laser treatment of the tube tip in the anterior chamber.

4.4 Place in surgical armamentarium

The advantages of this device as an adjunct to filtration surgery may be a lowered incidence of early postoperative hypotony and elimination of the need for a surgical iridectomy. The device is easily placed either temporally or nasally in an eye with prior scarring, as long as there are 2 to 3 clock hours of mobile conjunctiva available. There is often enough conjunctivae available between the side port vitrectomy scars to form a posterior bleb following a pars plana vitrectomy. Ex-PRESS requires less healthy tissue than for placement of a traditional drainage implant.

Since the resulting blebs are usually low and diffuse, there is little risk of developing delle or bleb dysethesias, even when the surgery is located off to one side.

In eyes with prior failed trabeculectomies, Ex-PRESS can help to reestablish the aqueous flow without having to repeat the original procedure. The Ex-PRESS fits easily in the middle ground between a repeat trabeculectomy and a larger glaucoma drainage device like a Baerveldt, Molteno, or an Ahmed tube shunt.

Additionally, because of the technical familiarity of trabeculectomy, the learning curve for the incorporation of this device into filtering surgery is not a steep one, and it has shown to be effective when combined with phacoemulsification.

Initial doubts about the Ex-PRESS filtration device are decreasing with recent advances offering possibly a wider spectrum of indications while diminishing the potential complications.

5. Trabecular bypass devices

The site of abnormal outflow resistance within the meshwork is probably the juxtacanalicular tissue adjacent to Schlemm's canal, a layer of the meshwork approximately 10 μm thick. Removal or bypassing this thin layer of tissue should decrease the elevated IOP, without the need for creating a hole in the sclera and a filtration bleb.

Recent work has focused on using small tubes to bypass the meshwork, creating a direct route from the anterior chamber into Schlemms' canal. (Razeghinejad and Spaeth, 2011)

5.1 Trabecular micro-bypass iStent

Device

The iStent® trabecular micro-bypass stent (Glaukos Corp, Laguna Hills, California) is the first ab-interno micro bypass stent. It is a heparin-coated with Duraflo (Edwards Lifesciences, Irvine, CA), nonferromagnetic, surgical grade titanium (Ti6Al4V ELI) stent less than one mm in length and approximately 0.3 mm in height, with a snorkel length of 0.25 mm and a nominal snorkel bore diameter of 120 μm. It is about 1/5000 of the size of the Baerveldt implant. (Samuelson et al., 2011) The iStent® is inserted through a small temporal clear corneal incision, bypassing the trabecular meshwork, and placed in Schlemm's canal at the lower nasal quadrant. The dimensions of the stent are customized for a natural fit and retention within the 270µ canal space, with three retention arches to ensure secure placement.

Indications

- Mild-to-moderate primary open angle glaucoma
- Pigmentary glaucoma
- Pseudoexfoliative glaucoma, stand alone or in combination with cataract surgery.

Contraindications

- Presence of ocular disease such as uveitis, ocular infection
- Patients diagnosed with angle closure glaucoma

Surgical technique

The iStent® is preloaded in a single-use, light release force, sterile applicator (Figure 3) with a secure, rotatable grip to facilitate manipulation and placement into Schlemm's canal. Separate orientations of the stent are available for the right and left eye. iStent® implantation can be performed under topical anesthesia. Prior to implanting the iStent®, the angle anatomy and targeted stent site must be in clear view. The Swan-Jacob gonioprism is used to inspect the angle to ensure a good view at the nasal implant location. The iStent® is implanted through the same small, temporal, clear corneal incision used for phacoemulsification or a 1.5 mm incision when the stent is implanted as a stand-alone procedure. iStent in inserted in trabecular meshwork with *"Penetrate, lift and slide"* insertion technique.

For best possible angle visualization; iStent® insertion should be performed from the temporal side with the microscope magnified 12X and tilted towards the surgeon. The patient's head is tilted away from the surgeon.

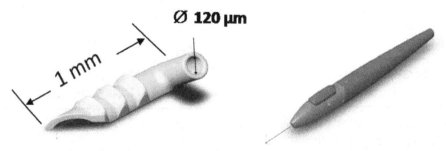

Fig. 3. Snorkel shaped iStent; iStent Applicator

Implantation is performed in the nasal position (3 to 4 o'clock for the right eye; 8 to 9 o'clock for the left eye) with the tip of the implant directed inferiorly. The tip of the stent should approach the trabecular meshwork at 15° angle to facilitate penetration of the tissue (Figure 4). Excessive resistance indicates that the approach is too perpendicular to the trabeculum. Once the stent is covered with meshwork it is released by pressing the applicator button. Only the proximal end of the stent remains visible in the anterior chamber. The iStent® is seated into position by gently tapping the side of the snorkel with the applicator tip. A small reflux of blood from the Schlemm's canal reflects correct positioning of the stent. Extraction of the viscoelastic material and hydration of the corneal incision conclude the procedure.

Proper stent placement is confirmed by flushing the anterior chamber of any refluxed blood, performing a high-magnification examination to confirm that the base of the implant is parallel with the circumferential axis of the Schlemm canal, and gently nudging the snorkel to confirm that the snorkel axis is parallel with the iris plane and that the base is well seated and fully through the trabecular meshwork.

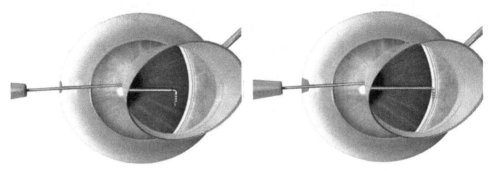

Fig. 4. Technique of iStent implantation

Complications

The stent is small (1 mm) and hence it may sometimes be difficult to verify exact placement of the implant via gonioscopy, particularly in cases of corneal edema, peripheral anterior synechiae, or an uncooperative or anxious patient. In such cases there is a possibility of accidentally misplacing the iStent. Ichhpujani and coworkers carried out an in vitro study, in which they used a human cadaver eye, unsuitable for transplantation, as a model to visualize the position of the stent. (Ichhpujani et al., 2010) They reported that in cases where gonioscopy is not successful, UBM can aid in localization of the iStent, in both the anterior and posterior chambers, provided the probe is moved to provide a favorable signal, whereas AS-OCT is limited to detection of stents in the anterior chamber alone and B-scan is of no value.

A theoretical problem with bypass of the meshwork is blood reflux from Schlemm's canal into the anterior chamber via the tube, creating a microhyphema. Any activity that raises episcleral venous pressure higher than IOP, such as prolonged bending with the head down or vigorous Valsalva maneuver, would be most likely to cause this problem. Since such maneuvers also increase IOP by increasing the choroidal blood volume, this would counter the elevated episcleral venous pressure. This may explain why microhyphemas have not been reported till date with an iStent.

5.2 Scientific evidence so far

US iStent Study group assessed the safety and efficacy of the iStent in combination with cataract surgery in subjects with mild to moderate open-angle glaucoma. (Samuelson et al., 2011) A total of 240 eyes with mild to moderate open-angle glaucoma with IOP ≤ 24 mmHg controlled on 1 to 3 medications were randomized to undergo cataract surgery with iStent implantation (treatment group) or cataract surgery only (control). The primary efficacy measure was unmedicated IOP≤ 21 mmHg at 1 year. The study met the primary outcome, with 72% of treatment eyes versus 50% of control eyes achieving the criterion ($P< 0.001$). At 1 year, IOP in both treatment groups was statistically significantly lower from baseline values. Sixty-six percent of treatment eyes versus 48% of control eyes achieved ≥20% IOP reduction without medication ($P<$ 0.003). The overall incidence of adverse events was similar between groups with no unanticipated adverse device effects.

The ocular hypotensive efficacy seen with the stent in this study was found to be consistent with the trabecular bypass mechanism of action and results described in literature. (Fea, 2010; Spiegel et al., 2008 & 2009)

Compared with cataract surgery alone, implantation of the iStent concomitant with cataract extraction significantly increases trabecular outflow facility, reduces IOP and the number of medications. (Fernandez- Barrientos et al., 2010)

A study in cultured human anterior segments has shown that a single stent created the largest change in IOP, resulting in a mean of 12.4 ± 4.2 mm Hg, corresponding to an 84% increase in facility of outflow. Interestingly, IOP seemed to reach a baseline level of approximately 12 mm Hg, even with multiple stents. (Bahler et al., 2004)

The probable explanation is that only one is enough to bypass the barrier of the Schlemm's canal and the lumen of the iStent is large enough to drain the aqueous as if the Schlemm's wall is well functioning.

5.3 Place in the surgical armamentarium

The iStent is believed to reestablish natural trabecular outflow, and it leaves the conjunctiva untouched, and avoids the lifelong risk of complications associated with filtering blebs. Thus, iStent implantation in patients with mild to moderate open-angle glaucoma undergoing cataract surgery represents a novel therapeutic approach that provides clinically significant reductions in IOP and medication use.

5.4 Trabectome electrocautery device

Device

The Trabectome surgical device was cleared by the US Food and Drug Administration in January 2004 for the treatment of adult and juvenile open-angle glaucoma. The concept is similar in principle to *ab interno* trabeculotomy, the key difference being that a microelectrocautery device is used to ablate a strip of the trabecular meshwork and inner wall of Schlemm's canal, thus allowing direct access of aqueous to the collector channels. This theoretically bypasses the main site of resistance to aqueous outflow and reestablishes the natural drainage passageway out of the eye.

The Trabectome consists of a disposable footpedal activated handpiece and a console to adjust infusion, aspiration and electrosurgical energy. The handpiece consists of a 19-gauge infusion sleeve, a 25-gauge aspiration port, and a bipolar electrocautery unit 150 µm away from an insulated footplate (Figure 5). The footplate is 800 µm in length from the heel to the tip, has a maximum width of 230 µm, and maximum thickness of 110 µm.

Indications

Trabectome may be an excellent surgical option for patients who require postoperative IOPs in the mid-to-high teens. It can be combined with cataract surgery.

- Early to moderate Primary open-angle glaucoma
- Pigmentary and pseudoexfoliative glaucoma.
- Patients with elevated IOP despite previous glaucoma surgery (trabeculectomy or a drainage tube)

Contraindications

Angle closure with or without peripheral anterior synechiae is the only contraindication. Trabecular meshowork without pigment may pose difficulty for proper gonioscopic identification of structures.

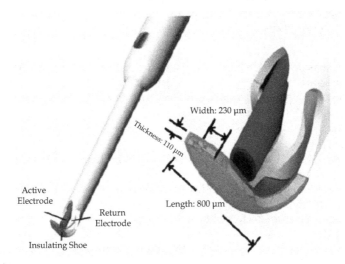

Fig. 5. Trabectome hand piece

Surgical procedure

Surgery is carried out with a temporal approach through a clear corneal incision of 1.6-1.8 mm to accommodate the electrocautery unit. Alternatively, when combined with clear cornea coaxial phacoemulsification, the main incision may be used for the Trabectome handpiece. Ophthalmic visco-devices are used to inflate and stabilize the anterior chamber and a gonioprism is used for direct visualization of the angle. Once the instrument has been inserted into Schlemm's canal, the foot pedal is depressed to begin electrocautery. The surgeon's hand simultaneously moves in one direction to ablate the tissue until the tip of the handpiece has reached the limit of visibility. The handpiece may then be turned to achieve ablation in the opposite direction again, to the limits of view. Total arc length amenable to treatment through a single incision is 60-90°. Tissue debris released during electrocautery can obscure the view hence aspiration and continuous irrigation are carried out. A clear corneal suture is applied and intracameral air is injected at the conclusion of Trabectome ablation to prevent postoperative hyphema.

When combined Trabectome and cataract surgery are done then the ab interno trabeculotomy is completed before starting the phacoemulsification. This order of operation prevents the formation of phacoemulsification-related corneal edema that could impair visualization of the angle structures.

Too low power settings and rapid movement of the handpiece should be avoided as it may lead to inadvertent tear of the trabecular meshwork and cause tissue from the inner wall of Schlemm's canal to accumulate in the gap of the footplate. In addition, the surgeon should make sure that the eye does not rotate during the treatment, as this indicates excessive pressure on the posterior wall of Schlemm's canal.

Many surgeons advocate the use of pilocarpine 1% 1 to 2 hours prior to Trabectome-only surgery to improve surgical visualization of the angle and to protect the crystalline lens in phakic patients. Postoperatively, pilocarpine can enhance aqueous outflow and prevent the development of peripheral anterior synechiae. The tapering of glaucoma medications is generally undertaken approximately 1 month after surgery.

The procedure has a learning curve, especially for surgeons not familiar with operating temporally or with various patient head positions.

Complications

Transient hyphemas are the typical complication, clearing within a few days. Other complications are rare in this procedure, but can include iridodialysis, cyclodialysis, and IOP spike. Sustained hyphema, wound leak, infection, choroidal effusion, and hemorrhage are not typically seen after this procedure.

5.5 Scientific evidence so far

Minckler et al reported a retrospective case series of 1127 Trabectome surgeries, with 738 Trabectome-only and 366 Trabectome-cataract surgeries. (Minckler et al., 2008) Overall, IOP reduced to 39% at 24 months (n=50), and with Trabectome only cases (n=46) the reduction was 40%. Surgery combined with cataract removal (n=45) showed an 18% decrease in IOP at 12 months. Medications were decreased by at least half in each cohort.

Francis et al for the Trabectome study group reported the short-term results of combined phacoemulsification and trabeculotomy by the internal approach with a follow-up to 21 months. (Francis et al., 2008) This prospective interventional case series comprised of 304 consecutive eyes with open-angle glaucoma and cataract having combined phacoemulsification and trabeculotomy with a Trabectome. The mean IOP was 20.0 mm Hg ±6.3 (SD) preoperatively, 14.8±3.5 mm Hg at 6 months, and 15.5±2.9 mm Hg at 1 year. There was a corresponding drop in glaucoma medications from 2.65±1.13 at baseline to 1.76±1.25 at 6 months and 1.44±1.29 at 1 year. Subsequent secondary glaucoma procedures were performed in 9 patients. The only frequent complication, blood reflux in 239 patients (78.4%), resolved within a few days.

Previous laser trabeculoplasty does not appear to significantly impact IOP, but may increase the need for glaucoma medication in patients undergoing Trabectome surgery (Vold and Dustin, 2010).

5.6 Place in surgical armamentarium

Early clinical experience with this technology has shown that patient selection, surgical technique, and postoperative medical management affect patients' outcomes. Though it is efficacious in IOP lowering, we still do not know what is the maximal amount of IOP lowering that can be attained, and whether this relates to other factors such as episcleral venous pressure.

5.7 Canaloplasty

Canaloplasty is an *ab externo* procedure which entails 360° intubation of Schlemm's canal, along with suture-assisted distension of the canal in order to restore physiologic outflow via the conventional pathway without the formation of a fistula or bleb (Khaimi, 2009). The iTrack 250 flexible microcatheter (iScience Interventional, Menlo Park, CA) for canaloplasty received FDA approval in 2008.

Device

The iScience device has a 45-mm working length flexible polymer microcatheter of 200-mm shaft diameter with a rounded 250-mm tip diameter (Figure 6).The catheter consists of a central support wire designed to provide a backbone for guidance during advancement and to add resistance to potential kinking of the microcatheter. The optical fibers in the microcatheter allow for transmission of a red blinking light from a laser-based micro-illumination system to the tip to assist in visualization and localization of the tip during passage. The microcatheter possesses a true lumen for the delivery of substances such as viscoelastic to expand the canal during passage or retraction. The proximal end of the device connects to the nonsterile laser-based micro-illumination light source on a mayo stand from one arm, with another arm connected to a sterile screw-mechanism syringe designed to assist in controlled injection of viscoelastic into Schlemm's canal.

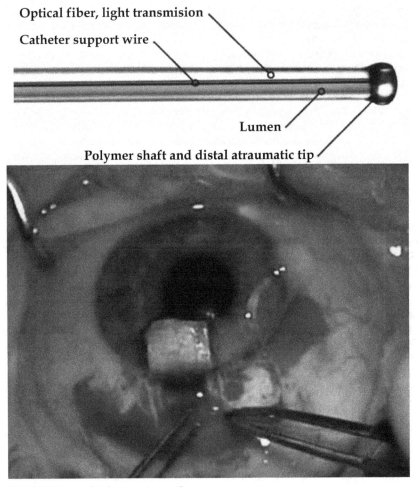

Fig. 6. iTrack250A canaloplasty microcatheter

Indications

• Mild-to-moderate open angle glaucoma
• Pigmentary glaucoma (Ichhpujani et al., 2011)
• Pseudoexfoliative glaucoma

Contraindications

• Scarring from prior trabeculectomy
• Patients with obvious scarring in Schlemm's canal due to prior medication use, laser, surgery or corneoscleral trauma at the limbus
• Anomalies in the anterior chamber angle

Surgical procedure

The chosen surgical site is the superior sclera and hence a traction suture is needed for maintaining a downgaze position. For a corneal traction a careful site selection is required so as to ensure the suture is placed several clock hours away from the intended surgical site.

A fornix based conjunctival peritomy is done leaving an anterior skirt of conjunctiva attached to the limbus with blunt dissection carried out posteriorly. Light wet field cautery is applied to the sclera, being careful to avoid aqueous and ciliary veins. A superficial parabolic scleral flap of approximately 5 mm anterior–posterior length by 5 mm width and one-third scleral thickness is fashioned with the help of a crescent knife, forward into clear cornea. A deep inner scleral flap is then created approximately 1 mm inside from the edge of the superficial scleral flap. An approximately 100 mm thick layer of sclera should be left covering the choroid at the base of the deep dissection. Once the white limbus-parallel fibers of the scleral spur are visible at the deep dissection, fibers of the outer wall of Schlemm's canal should be visible by lifting of the deep flap with a toothed forceps. A paracentesis incision should be made in the clear cornea to lower the IOP to prevent outward bulging of Descemet's membrane and the inner wall of Schlemm's canal, reducing the likelihood of penetration into the anterior chamber during the ensuing delicate dissection. The deep flap is now advanced forward approximately another 1 mm to expose Descemet's membrane. Mermoud forceps can be used to delicately strip the inner wall of Schlemm's canal away. The corneal stroma should be separated from Descemet's window with surgical sponges such as Merocel. Once the window has been fashioned, the underside of the deep flap is scored with a sharp tip blade at the very anterior aspect and cut off with Vannas scissors. Each cut end of Schlemm's canal is then intubated with a 150-mm outer bore viscocanalostomy cannula, and a miniscule amount of high viscosity sodium hyaluronate is injected into each end to dilate the ostia and facilitate entrance of the iScience device into the canal.

With the help of nontoothed forceps, the microcatheter is introduced into one of the cut ends of Schlemm's canal and advanced 360° until the tip emerges from the other cut end of the canal. In a minority of patients successful catheterisation through the entirety of the canal fails. At times the microcatheter may pass into the suprachoroidal space posterior to Schlemm's canal. In such cases, the catheter should be immediately retracted and passage attempted in the opposite direction. Once the microcatheter has been passed 360° and the tip has emerged, a 10–0 Prolene suture with the needles cut off is tied around the shaft of the device near the tip with the two loose ends tied to the loop. The device is then withdrawn slowly from the opposite direction with controlled injection of viscoelastic every 2-3 clock hours, taking care not to cause Descemet's detachment.

Once the catheter has been removed, the 10–0 Prolene is cut from the tip, leaving two single 10–0 Prolene sutures in the canal with two loose ends emerging from each cut end of

Schlemm's canal. Each suture is tied to itself in a slipknot fashion with some back and forth movement in the canal, known as "flossing, " to ensure that the suture sits anteriorly in Schlemm's canal. Suture tension is then assessed by pulling the suture knot posteriorly, until it is only barely able to reach the scleral spur. Suture tension is felt to play an important role in canaloplasty, where a greater suture tension results in more distension of Schlemm's canal with resultant greater IOP reduction and increased flow. The superficial scleral flap is then placed back into position and sutured in a watertight fashion with interrupted 10–0 nylon sutures. Conjunctiva is also closed in a water tight fashion with 10-0 vicryl sutures.

Complications

In trabeculectomy the natural anterior chamber fluid outflow is by-passed via an artificial fistula. Unlike trabeculectomy, canaloplasty attempts to re-establish the physiological anterior chamber fluid draining system by means of dilation of Schlemm's canal and its collector channels. If the anterior chamber pressure temporarily lowers the level of the venous capillary pressure, it is consistent with a patent piping system when a reverse flow with blood reflux into the anterior chamber can be observed as long as a minimal physiological pressure gradient from the anterior chamber in the direction of channel Schlemm's canal has been restored. Thus, an anterior chamber haemorrhage shows the desired consistency of the draining system and hence it should logically be expected after each successful procedure where hypotony in the postoperative period occurs. (Koch et al., 2010)

The surgery is technically challenging and hence there is a learning curve. Microhyphema (7.9%), early and late IOP elevations (7.9% and 2.4%, respectively), wound hemorrhage (2.4%), suture extrusion (1.6%), Descemet membrane detachment (DMD) (1.6%), and hypotony (0.8%) have been reported. (Grieshaber et al., 2010; Palmiero et al., 2010) Trabeculo-Descemet window fibrosis may occur in postoperative course.

5.8 Scientific evidence so far

Lewis and coworkers reported 3-year results of the safety and efficacy of canaloplasty either as a standalone procedure or in combination with cataract surgery in adult open angle glaucoma subjects. (Lewis et al., 2011) Three years postoperatively, all study eyes (n = 157) had a mean IOP of 15.2 mm Hg ± 3.5 (SD) and mean glaucoma medication use of 0.8 ± 0.9 compared with a baseline IOP of 23.8 ± 5.0 mm Hg on 1.8 ± 0.9 medications. Eyes with combined cataract-canaloplasty surgery had a mean IOP of 13.6 ± 3.6 mm Hg on 0.3 ± 0.5 medications compared with a baseline IOP of 23.5 ± 5.2 mm Hg on 1.5 ± 1.0 medications. Intraocular pressure and number of medication, in all eyes were significantly decreased from baseline at every time point (P<0.001). Late postoperative complications included cataract (12.7%), transient IOP elevation (6.4%), and partial suture extrusion through the trabecular meshwork (0.6%).

Koerber reported a comparative case series of 30 eyes of 15 adult patients with bilateral primary open-angle glaucoma who underwent canaloplasty in one eye and viscocanalostomy in the contralateral eye. (Koerber, 2011) With a follow-up period of 18 months, both the canaloplasty and viscocanalostomy groups showed statistically significant reductions in mean IOP (P<0.01) and number of supplemental medications (P<0.01) as compared with preoperative values. In the canaloplasty cohort, eyes had a mean IOP of 14.5±2.6 mm Hg on 0.3±0.5 medications at 18 months postoperatively as compared with preoperative levels of 26.5±2.7 mm Hg on 2.1±1.0 medications. In the viscocanalostomy cohort, eyes had a mean IOP of 16.1±3.9 mm Hg on 0.4±0.5 medications at 18 months as compared with preoperative levels of 24.3±2.8 mm Hg on 1.9±0.8 medications (P=0.02). No patient in either cohort experienced significant complications. The author concluded that canaloplasty showed slightly better efficacy to viscocanalostomy in the reduction of IOP (P=0.02).

Grieshaber and coworkers have shown that Canaloplasty produced a sustained long-term reduction of IOP in 60 eyes of black Africans with POAG independent of preoperative IOP. (Grieshaber et al., 2010)

5.9 Place in surgical armamentarium

The analogy of cardiac surgery is most appropriate to educate patients. In some patients, cardiac surgeons can stent or dilate the obstructed vessel with a less invasive angioplasty, while in others with more serious disease, surgeons may have to open the chest and perform a more complex procedure." For glaucoma patients, this means transitioning from canaloplasty to trabeculectomy.

6. Deeplight gold micro shunt

Device

The GMS (SOLX Ltd, Boston, Massachusetts) is a nonvalved flat-plate drainage device made from 24-K medical-grade (99.95%) gold. The device is composed of two leaflets fused together vertically concealing nine channels within the body that connect the anterior openings to the posterior ones (Figure 7). Two different models of the device exist, the GMS (XGS-5) and the GMS Plus (XGS-10), both measuring 5.2 mm long, 2.4 mm wide anteriorly and 3.2 mm wide posteriorly, but differing in weight and channel size. The XGS-5 model weighs 6.2 mg and is 60mm in thickness with the channels measuring 25mm in width and 44mm in height while the XGS-10 model weighs 9.2 mg and the channels measure 25mm in width by 68mm in height. Aqueous humor from the anterior chamber exiting through the uveoscleral pathway to the suprachoroidal space is enhanced by this device by allowing fluid to travel both through the channels in the shunt and also around the body of the shunt. (Melamed et al., 2009)

Indications

The suprachoroidal space appears to be an excellent pathway option for those patients who have had failed trabeculectomy or Schlemm's canal procedures.

Contraindications

- Recent angle closure glaucoma episode
- Uveitic glaucoma, iridocorneal endothelial syndrome, traumatic glaucoma, or neovascular glaucoma
- Other significant ocular disease, except cataract
- Active ocular infection
- Expected ocular surgery in next 12 months
- No suitable quadrant for implant

Surgical procedure

After a 4 mm fornix-based conjunctival peritomy, an approximately 3.5 mm scleral incision is created 2 mm posterior to the limbus or slightly further posteriorly in high myopes (can be inserted in any quadrant but easier in superotemporal quadrant). The dissection is carried out to near full thickness depth, where the choroid is visible through a thin layer of sclera. A scleral pocket at 95% depth is then created by tunneling anteriorly towards the scleral spur. At this point, a vertical incision is made into the choroidal space and a small amount of suprachoroidal anesthesia and viscoelastic are administered with a blunt cannula. Via a sideport incision viscoelastic is filled in the anterior chamber at the anticipated site of entry of the gold shunt. Alternatively, an AC maintainer can be used and an entry is made into the anterior chamber at the level of the scleral spur through the previously constructed scleral tunnel.

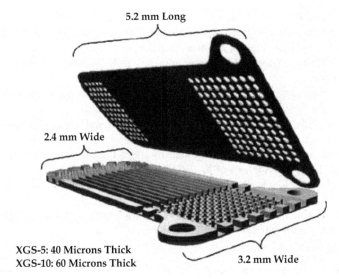

Fig. 7. Gold microshunt

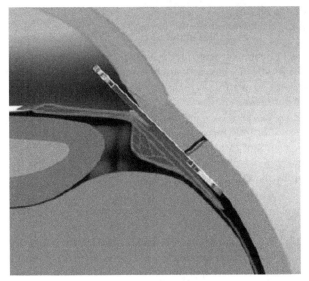

Fig. 8. Cross-section of eye showing correct GMS position

The shunt is placed through the scleral incision, ensuring the head of the device is in the anterior chamber (Figure 8). Positioning of the shunt is achieved posteriorly in the suprachoroidal space using a sharp 27-gauge needle against the shunt to gently encourage it into the suprachoroidal pocket expanded previously by viscoelastic while grasping the wound with a toothed forceps. A "Push then pull" approach works well while inserting the shunt through scleral incision in the anterior chamber.

Alternatively, an instrument such as a Sinskey hook can be utilized on the lateral positioning holes. All of the shunt openings on the posterior aspect should be concealed under the posterior scleral lip of the wound. The anterior aspect of the wound can also be manipulated through the anterior chamber to aid in positioning of the shunt. Intraoperative gonioscopy can help to confirm the proper and intended positioning of the gold shunt in the anterior chamber.

The overlying scleral wound is tightly sutured with 4–5 interrupted 10-0 nylon sutures to ensure watertight closure, as subconjunctival reservoir is not the intended mode of filtration in this surgical procedure. Finally, a 10-0 vicryl horizontal mattress suture is placed to reappose conjunctiva. The crescent-shaped anterior aspect of the shunt consists of a positioning hole, which can be used to adjust shunt positioning with an instrument such as a Sinskey hook. The posterior aspect of the shunt likewise possesses two lateral wings for shunt manipulation. Flow is directed through and around the shunt via the natural pressure gradient from the anterior chamber to the suprachoroidal space.

Placement of GMS in anterior chamber allows future access with 790nm Ti: sapphire laser and goniolens to selectively open specific windows.

Complications

Mild hyphema, hypotony, choroidal effusion, haemorrhage or detachment and shunt migration have been noted in few cases, in decreasing order of their occurrence.

6.1 Surgical evidence so far

Melamed and colleagues reported results of implantation of the GMS in 38 patients with uncontrolled glaucoma in a prospective 2-center study. (Melamed et al., 2009) The mean follow-up time was 11.7 months. The IOP decreased a mean (SD) of 9 mmHg from 27.6 (4.7) to 18.2 (4.6) mmHg (P <0.001). Surgical success was achieved in 30 patients (79%) (IOP >5 and <22 mm Hg, with or without antiglaucoma medication). Eight patients had mild to moderate transient hyphema.

Mastropasqua and co workers used in vivo confocal microscopy to show that successful GMS implantation significantly increased conjunctival microcysts density and surface at the site of the device insertion. (Mastropasqua et al., 2010) These findings suggest that the enhancement of the aqueous filtration across the sclera may be one of the possible outflow pathways exploited by the shunt.

6.2 Place in surgical armamentarium

The European Agency for the Evaluation of Medicinal Products (EMEA) gave this shunt CE approval in October 2005. It is undergoing Phase III trials in USA. The results till date appear promising. One of the advantages with gold micro-shunt is that in addition to working as an implantable microscopic shunt, the level of IOP control can be titrated by the laser. Additional micro channels can be opened with the laser in the clinicians' office.

6.3 EYEPASS Bi-Directional glaucoma implant

Device

The Eyepass Bi-Directional glaucoma implant (GMP Vision Solutions, Inc.) consists of a dual 6.0 mm long silicone tube bonded at 1 end for less than 1.0 mm, creating a Y-shape (Figure 9). (Dietlein et al., 2008) The inner diameter of the silicone tube is 125 µm and the outer diameter is 250 µm, making the tube narrow enough to fit the lumen of the Schlemm canal. The implant is sterilized by gamma radiation and is a single-use device that should be stored at a temperature between 15°C and 30°C.

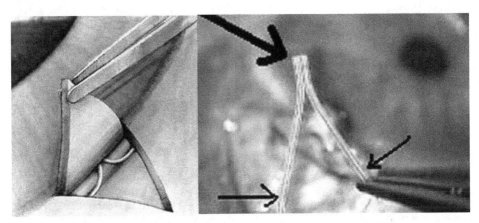

Fig. 9. Eyepass bidirectional implant

Surgical procedure

It can be used as a standalone procedure or in combination with cataract surgery. After a fornix-based superomedial conjunctival dissection and a mild wet field cautery, a two-third thickness triangular scleral flap with a 4 mm basis is dissected. Before the Schlemm canal is unroofed, clear corneal cataract surgery is performed. This is followed by the Schlemm canal unroofing by dissecting a second scleral flap or by opening the canal with small Vannas scissors. Before the Eyepass device is implanted in both lumina of the Schlemm canal, the openings on both sides of the canal are dilated by gentle injection of an OVD such as sodium hyaluronate 1.0% [Healon] through a viscocanalostomy cannula. Thereafter, the arms of the "Y" are inserted into the lumina of the Schlemm canal without exerting pressure in the direction of the anterior chamber. After both ends are buried in the Schlemm canal, the bonded end is inserted into the anterior chamber via a paracentesis almost 1.0 mm from the trabecular meshwork, toward the center of the anterior chamber and under the scleral flap. The implant does not need to be secured by sutures. The scleral flap is sutured to a watertight fit using interrupted 10-0 nylon sutures. The conjunctiva is closed with 8-0 polyglactin (Vicryl) sutures at the limbus.

Complications

The implant actually acts as a wick underneath the scleral flap, encouraging transscleral filtration in the early days after surgery; hence early postoperative hypotony may occur. Intraoperative perforation of the trabecular meshwork may also occur. Since this procedure entails conjunctival dissection, it may compromise other future ab-externo glaucoma surgery.

6.4 Surgical evidence so far

Dietlein et al conducted a small study to evaluate the safety and pressure-reducing efficacy of the Y-shaped Eyepass glaucoma implant in 12 glaucoma and cataract patients and found that combined cataract surgery with Eyepass shunt implantation was safe and appeared to be beneficial in glaucomatous eyes with cataract not requiring a low target IOP. (Dietlein et al., 2008) Perforation of the trabecular meshwork during Eyepass implantation occurred in 2 eyes requiring explantation and conversion to trabeculectomy. In the remaining 10 eyes, the mean maximum IOP was 30.4 mm Hg preoperatively, 12.0 mm 1 day postoperatively, 17.2 mm Hg at 4 weeks, and 18.3 mm at the end of the preliminary follow-up.

In case of trabecular meshwork perforation while inserting an arm of Eyepass, whether opening just 1 arm of the canal could achieve sufficient degree of surgical success is yet to be ascertained. Over the long term, the transscleral filtration seems to play a minor role in the IOP reducing effect of the Eyepass implant because of scarring and no antimetabolite induced favourable wound modulation. Role of antimetabolites to improve transscleral filtration is questionable at present.

6.5 Place in surgical armamentarium

The implant is currently undergoing Phase III trials.

7. Cypass micro stent

Device

Cypass (Transcend) is made from a biocompatible material (polyimide) and features a unique delivery system. The CyPass is a micro-implantable device, 6 mm in length, with a small lumen of 300 im (Figure 10). It allows for an *ab interno* surgical approach, which spares the conjunctiva, does not penetrate the sclera and leaves the trabecular meshwork intact.

Surgical procedure

It is implanted in the suprachoroidal space through a clear corneal incision, which coincides with the phacoemulsification incision in combined procedures. A special inserter is used to make the distal end of the device penetrate into the suprachoroidal space, while the proximal collar remains in the anterior chamber. Three rings on the collar keep the device in place, preventing movement.

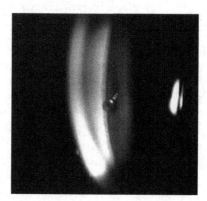

Fig. 10. Cypass microstent

7.1 Scientific evidence so far

Early clinical results, with the Cypass being placed in combination with cataract surgery (study by Transcend; unpublished data), showed promising results, with a 42% IOP decrease and a 60% decrease in medication use at six months.

Ongoing clinical trials

Combination cypass and cataract surgery trial (COMPASS): Transcend's 480 patient domestic pivotal clinical trial, combines the Cypass and cataract surgery. Enrollment began in the second half of 2009 and the company hopes to complete it by the end of 2011 or in early 2012.

Cypass clinical evaluation trial (CYCLE): This is a European prospective, non-randomized multi-center trial that includes "all-comers" with a goal to assess the Cypass in a broad variety of glaucoma patients.

DUETTE: This is another European trial. Evaluating two different versions of the Cypass in a prospective and randomized study.

Place in surgical aramamentarium

Cypass has been found to have few and minor complications compared with filtering procedures. In addition, it is a repeatable procedure, which leaves an intact superior conjunctiva, allowing filtering procedures to be performed at a later stage in case of failure. Preliminary findings need to be confirmed in prospective trials with larger series, evaluating long-term results.

8. Conclusion

The current gold standard, trabeculectectomy, has done well for many medically refractory glaucoma patients in the past 40 years. Despite its efficacy in lowering IOP, relatively easy learning curve, it is fraught with not only short time but lifetime potential sight threatening issues. Glaucomatologists and bioengineers are leaving no stone unturned to find a better alternative which addresses the flaws of trabeculectomy. Ex-PRESS glaucoma filtration implant, Trabectome electrocautery device, iStent, Canaloplasty, Gold microshunt and Eyepass bidirectional valve are few milestones along the path of finding an ideal glaucoma device. Although for most devices, the studies are ongoing and the verdict on long term safety and efficacy is awaited, the future definitely seems promising. One size does not fit all in glaucoma. Much remains to be resolved about all these new innovative procedures in glaucoma. It is not wise to abandon time-tested trabeculectomy but it's time to be more selective in choosing surgical procedures.

9. References

Ates, H, Palamar, M, Yagci, A, Egrilmez, S. (2010) Evaluation of Ex-PRESS mini glaucoma shunt implantation in refractory postpenetrating keratoplasty glaucoma. *J Glaucoma.*; 19:556-60.

Bagnis, A, Papadia, M, Scotto, R, Traverso, CE. (2011) Obstruction of the Ex-PRESS Miniature Glaucoma Device: Nd: YAG Laser as a Therapeutic Option. *J Glaucoma.* 2011 Mar 21. (Epub ahead of print).

Bahler, CK, Smedley, GT, Zhou, J, Johnson, DH (2004). Trabecular bypass stents decrease intraocular pressure in cultured human anterior segments. *Am J Ophthalmol.*; 138:988–94.

Bissig, A, Feusier, M, Mermoud, A, Roy, S. (2010) Deep sclerectomy with the Ex-PRESS X-200 implant for the surgical treatment of glaucoma. *Int Ophthalmol.*; 30:661-8.

Borisuth, NS, Phillips, B, Krupin T. (1999). The risk profile of glaucoma filtration surgery. *Curr Opin Ophthalmol*, 10, 2:112–116.

Coleman, AL, Hill, R, Wilson, MR, et al (1995). Initial clinical experience with the Ahmed glaucoma valve implant. *Am J Ophthalmol*, 120:23–31.

Dahan, E, Carmichael, TR. (2005) Implantation of a miniature glaucoma device under a scleral flap. *J Glaucoma*; 14:98-102.

Dietlein, TS, Jordan, JF, Schild, A, et al. (2008) Combined cataract-glaucoma surgery using the intracanalicular Eyepass glaucoma implant: first clinical results of a prospective pilot study. *J Cataract Refract Surg.*; 34:247-52.

Epstein, DL, Melamed, S, Puliatio, CA, Steinert, RF. (1985). Neodymium: YAG laser trabeculopuncture in open-angle glaucoma. *Ophthalmology*, 92:931–937.

Fea, AM (2010). Phacoemulsification versus phacoemulsification with micro-bypass stent implantation in primary open-angle glaucoma: randomized double-masked clinical trial. *J Cataract Refract Surg.*, 36:407-12.

Fernández-Barrientos, Y, García-Feijoó, J, Martínez-de-la-Casa JM, Pablo LE, Fernández-Pérez C, García Sánchez J. (2010). Fluorophotometric study of the effect of the glaukos trabecular microbypass stent on aqueous humor dynamics. *Invest Ophthalmol Vis Sci.*, 51:3327-32.

Francis, BA, See, RF, Rao, NA, et al (2006). Ab interno trabeculectomy: development of a novel device (Trabectome) and surgery for open-angle glaucoma. *J Glaucoma*.15:68-73.

Francis, BA, Minckler, D, Dustin, L, Kawji, S, Yeh, J, Sit, A, Mosaed S, Johnstone M; (2008) Trabectome Study Group. Combined cataract extraction and trabeculotomy by the internal approach for coexisting cataract and open-angle glaucoma: initial results. *J Cataract Refract Surg.*; 34:1096-103.

Gandolfi S, Traverso CF, Bron A, Sellem E, Kaplan-Messas A, Belkin M. (2002) Short-term results of a miniature drainage implant for glaucoma in combined surgery with phacoemulsification. *Acta Ophthalmol Scand Suppl*; 236:66.

Garg, SJ, Kanitkar, K, Weichel, E, Fischer, D. Trauma-induced extrusion of an Ex-PRESS glaucoma shunt presenting as an intraocular foreign body. *Arch Ophthalmol* 2005; 123:1270-2.

Gedde, SJ, Schiffman, JC, Feuer, WJ, Herndon, LW, Brandt, JD, Budenz DL (2007). Treatment outcomes in the tube versus trabeculectomy study after one year of follow-up. *Am J Ophthalmol*, 143:9–22.

Geffen, N, Trope, GE, Alasbali, T, et al (2010). Is the EX-PRESS glaucoma device magnetic resonance imaging safe? *J Glaucoma*, 19:116-118.

Gindroz, F, Roy, S, Mermoud, A, Schnyder, CC (2011).Combined Ex-PRESS LR-50/IOL implantation in modified deep sclerectomy plus phacoemulsification for glaucoma associated with cataract. *Eur J Ophthalmol.*, 21:12-9.

Grieshaber, MC, Pienaar, A, Olivier, J, Stegmann, R. (2010) Canaloplasty for primary open-angle glaucoma: long-term outcome. *Br J Ophthalmol.*, 94:1478-82.

Ichhpujani, P, Katz, LJ, Gille, R, Affel, E (2010). Imaging modalities for localization of an iStent (®). *Ophthalmic Surg Lasers Imaging*, 41:660-3.

Ichhpujani, P, Barahimi, B, Shields, CL, Eagle, RC Jr, Katz LJ (2011). Canaloplasty for pigmentary glaucoma with coexisting conjunctival lymphoma. *Ophthalmic Surg Lasers Imaging.* Feb 10; 42 Online:e10-1. doi: 10.3928/15428877-20110203-01.

Jordan, JF, Engels, BF, Dinslage, S, et al (2006). A novel approach to suprachoroidal drainage for the surgical treatment of intractable glaucoma. *J Glaucoma*, 15:200–205.

Kaplan-Messas, A, Traverso, CF, Sellem, E, Zbigniew, Z, Belkin, M. (2002) The Ex-PRESS™ miniature glaucoma implant in combined surgery with cataract extraction: prospective study. *Invest Ophthalmol Vis Sci*; 43:3348A

Kanner, EM, Netland, PA, Sarkisian, SR, et al (2009). Ex-PRESS miniature glaucoma device implanted under a sclera flap alone or combined with phacoemulsification cataract surgery. *J Glaucoma*.; 18:488–491.

Koch, JM, Heiligenhaus, A, Heinz, C. (2010) Canaloplasty and Transient Anterior Chamber Haemorrhage: a Prognostic Factor? *Klin Monbl Augenheilkd*. Nov 16. [Epub ahead of print]

Koerber, NJ (2011). Canaloplasty in One Eye Compared With Viscocanalostomy in the Contralateral Eye in Patients With Bilateral Open-angle Glaucoma. *J Glaucoma*. Jan 26. [Epub ahead of print]

Khaimi, MA. (2009) Canaloplasty using iTrack 250 Microcatheter with Suture Tensioning on Schlemm's Canal. *Middle East Afr J Ophthalmol*.; 16:127-9.

Krejci, L. (1972) Cyclodialysis with hydroxyethyl methacrylate capillary strip. *Ophthalmologica*; 164:113–121.

Krupin, T, Podos, SM, Becker, B, Newkirk, JB. (1976). Valve implants in filtering surgery. *Am J Ophthalmol*, 81:232–235.

Kupin, TH, Juzych, MS, Shin, DH, Khatana, AK, Olivier, MM (1995).Adjunctive mitomycin C in primary trabeculectomy in phakic eyes. *Am J Ophthalmol*, 119:30–39.

Lankaranian, D, Razeghinejad, MR, Prasad, A, et al (2010). Intermediate-term results of the Ex-PRESS miniature glaucoma implant under a scleral flap in previously operated eyes. *Clin Experiment Ophthalmol*. Dec 22. doi: 10.1111/j.1442-9071.2010.02481.x. [Epub ahead of print].

Lewis, RA, von Wolff, K, Tetz, M, et al (2007). Canaloplasty: circumferential viscodilation and tensioning of Schlemm's canal using a flexible microcatheter for the treatment of open-angle glaucoma in adults: interim clinical study analysis. *J Cataract Refract Surg*; 33:1217–1226.

Lewis, RA, von Wolff, K, Tetz, M, et al. (2011) Canaloplasty: Three-year results of circumferential viscodilation and tensioning of Schlemm canal using a microcatheter to treat open-angle glaucoma. *J Cataract Refract Surg*.; 37:682-90.

Lloyd, MA, Baerveldt, G, Heuer, DK, et al. (1994). Initial clinical experience with the Baerveldt implant in complicated glaucomas. *Ophthalmology*, 101:640–650.

Maris, PJ, Jr, Ishida, K, Netland, PA. (2007) Comparison of trabeculectomy with Ex-PRESS miniature glaucoma device implanted under scleral flap. *J Glaucoma* 16: 14 – 19.

Mastropasqua, L, Agnifili, L, Ciancaglini, M, et al (2010). In vivo analysis of conjunctiva in gold micro shunt implantation for glaucoma. *Br J Ophthalmol*.; 94:1592-6.

Melamed, S, Ben Simon, GJ, Goldenfeld, M, Simon, G (2009).Efficacy and safety of gold micro shunt implantation to the supraciliary space in patients with glaucoma: a pilot study. *Arch Ophthalmol*; 127:264-9.

Minckler, DS, Mosaed, S, Dustin, L, Francis, BA. (2008) Trabectome (trabeculectomy-internal approach): additional experience and extended follow-up. *Trans Am Ophthalmol Soc*.106:1-12.

Molteno, ACB. (1969) New implant for drainage in glaucoma: clinical trial. *Br J Ophthalmol*, 53:606-615.

Netland, PA. Obstruction (Also Known as Occlusion or Blockage) of the Ex-PRESS Miniature Glaucoma Device. *J Glaucoma*. Mar 21. [Epub ahead of print]

Nichamin, LD. (2009) Glaukos iStent Trabecular Micro-Bypass. *Middle East Afr J Ophthalmol*., 16 (3):138-40.

Nguyen, QH. Trabectome: a novel approach to angle surgery in the treatment of glaucoma. *Int Ophthalmol Clin.* Fall; 48:65-72.

Nyska, A, Glovinsky Y, Belkin M, Epstein Y. (2003) Biocompatibility of the Ex-PRESS miniature glaucoma drainage implant. *J Glaucoma*; 12:275-80.

Ozdamar, A, Aras, C, Karacorlu, M (2003). Suprachoroidal seton implantation in refractory glaucoma: a novel surgical technique. *J Glaucoma*; 12:354–359.

Palmiero, PM, Aktas, Z, Lee, O, Tello, C, Sbeity, Z (2010). Bilateral Descemet membrane detachment after canaloplasty. *J Cataract Refract Surg.*; 36:508-11.

Pinnas, G, Boniuk, M. (1969) Cyclodialysis with teflon tube implants. *Am J Ophthalmol*; 68:879–883.

Razeghinejad, MR, Spaeth, GL. (2011). A history of the surgical management of glaucoma. *Optom Vis Sci.*, 88:E39-47.

Rivier, D, Roy, S, Mermoud, A. (2007). Ex-PRESS R-50 miniature glaucoma implant insertion under the conjunctiva combined with cataract extraction. *J Cataract Refract Surg*, 33:1946-52.

Samuelson, TW, Katz, LJ, Wells, JM, Duh, YJ, Giamporcaro JE (2010); US iStent Study Group. Randomized evaluation of the trabecular micro-bypass stent with phacoemulsification in patients with glaucoma and cataract. *Ophthalmology.*; 118:459-67.

Seibold, LK, Rorrer, RA, Kahook, MY. (2011). MRI of the Ex-PRESS stainless steel glaucoma drainage device. *Br J Ophthalmol.*, 95:251-4.

Spiegel, D, Wetzel, W, Neuhann, T, et al. (2009).Coexistent primary open-angle glaucoma and cataract: interim analysis of a trabecular micro-bypass stent and concurrent cataract surgery. *Eur J Ophthalmol.*, 19:393-9.

Spiegel, D, García-Feijoó, J, García-Sánchez, J, Lamielle, H. (2008). Coexistent primary open-angle glaucoma and cataract: preliminary analysis of treatment by cataract surgery and the iStent trabecular micro-bypass stent. *Adv Ther.*; 25:453-64.

Stewart, RM, Diamond, JG, Ashmore, ED, Ayyala, RS. (2005). Complications following Ex-PRESS glaucoma shunt implantation. *Am J Ophthalmol*, 140:340-1.

Tavolato, M, Babighian, S, Galan, A (2006). Spontaneous extrusion of a stainless steel glaucoma drainage implant (Ex-PRESS). *Eur J Ophthalmol*; 16:753-5.

Ticho, U, Ophir, A. (1993). Late complications after glaucoma filtering surgery with adjunctive 5-fluorouracil. *Am J Ophthalmol*, 115:506–510.

Traverso, CE, De Feo, F, Messas-Kaplan, A, Denis, P, Levartovsky, S, Sellem, E, et al. (2005) Long term effect on IOP of a stainless steel glaucoma drainage implant (Ex-PRESS) in combined surgery with phacoemulsification. *Br J Ophthalmol*; 89:425-9.

Wamsley, S, Moster, MR, Rai, S, Alvim, HS, Fontanarosa, J. (2004) Results of the use of the Ex-PRESS miniature glaucoma implant in technically challenging, advanced glaucoma cases: a clinical pilot study. *Am J Ophthalmol*; 138:1049-51.

Wamsley, S, Moster, MR, Rai, S, Alvim, H, Fontanarosa, J, Steinmann, WC. (2004). Optonol Ex-PRESS miniature tube shunt in advanced glaucoma. *Invest Ophthalmol Vis Sci*; 45:994A.

Vetrugno, M, Ferreri, P, Sborgia, C (2010). Ex-PRESS miniature glaucoma device in vitrectomized eyes. *Eur J Ophthalmol.*; 20:945-7.

Vetrugno, M, Ferreri, P, Cardascia, N, Sborgia, C. (2011)Surgical reposition of a dislocated Ex-PRESS miniature device. *Eur J Ophthalmol.*; 21:212-4.

Vold, SD, Dustin, L. Impact of laser trabeculoplasty on trabectome ((r)) outcomes. *Ophthalmic Surg Lasers Imaging.* 2010; 41:443-51.

6

Cyclodestructive Procedures

Sima Sayyahmelli and Rakhshandeh Alipanahi

From the Glaucoma Division, Tabriz Medical Sciences University, Tabriz,
Iran

1. Introduction

Several method used when an initial filtering procedure is not adequate to control the refractory glaucoma and when resumption of medical therapy,revision of original surgery, repeat filtering surgery at a new site, or aqueous shunt implantation is not successful; finally all cyclodestructive procedures reduce aqueous secretion by destroying part of the secretory ciliary epithelium portion of the ciliary body including cyclocryotherapy, contact and non-contact trans-scleral thermal lasers such as continuous-wave with the 1064-nm Nd:YAG, argon, and portable 810-nm semiconductor Diode laser.[1-4] Cryotherapy, the original technique, is increasingly being supplanted by laser photocoagulation, originally with the 1064-nm Nd:YAG laser and lately with the portable 810-nm semiconductor Diode laser.[2-3] An endoscopic laser delivery system has been advocated for use with cataract surgery or in pediatric, pseudophakic, or aphakic eyes. Use of the argon laser aimed at the ciliary processes through a goniolens is possible in a small percentage of patients. Transcleral diod laser cyclophotocoagulation (CPC) reducing aqueous secretion by destroying, is generally considered to be better tolerated and perhaps more effective than cyclocryotherapy, and it has a lower incidence of complications such as postoperative pain, inflammation, phthisis bulbi and retinal detachment, possibly because of better absorption of this wave length by the pigmented tissues of the ciliary body. Diode laser cyclophotocoagulation (CPC) is often the choice treatment of lOP-lowering in painful blind eyes or in eyes unlikely to respond to other modes of therapy. Interventions methods such as retrobulbar alcohol injection, retrobulbar chlorpromazine injection, or enucleation are rarely performed now because of improved CPC techniques. Treatment of glaucoma in the pediatric population is frequently challenging and may require multiple surgical interventions. In the past it was used mainly in uncontrolled end-stage secondary glaucoma with minimal visual potential mainly to control pain. However it is now apparent that it can also be used in eyes with reasonably good vision which may be retained provided control of IOP is adequate. This section studies the indications, success rate and long term efficacy and complications of the cyclodestructive procedures in refractory glaucoma. Laser cycloablation is generally considered to be better tolerated and perhaps more effective than cyclocryotherapy.[3,4] The most commonly used technique for cyclodestructive surgery is the transscleral approach, in which the destructive element must pass through conjunctiva, sclera, and ciliary musculature, before reaching and destroying the ciliary processes. These procedures have the advantages of being noninvasive and relatively quick and easy because of variable success in adults (34-92%) and significant postoperative pain and complications including phthisis and retinal detachment, transscleral neodymium:YAG (Nd:YAG) and Diode lasers are replacing cyclocryotherapy as the preferred form of cyclodestruction in these eyes.[5-7] The cyclophotocoagulation has a lower incidence of complications such as pain, postoperative inflammation and phthisis bulbi, possibly because of better absorption of this wave length by the pigmented tissues of the ciliary body.[7-9] Several methods of Diode laser photocyclocoagulation have been reported to lower IOP and reduce pain in the eyes of refractory glaucoma Diode cyclophotocoagulation and sequential tube shunt following primary tube shunt failure in childhood glaucoma showed similar efficacy and complication rates. Ten to fifty percent of patients with primary congenital glaucoma fail goniotomy surgery and require further surgical intervention, Childhood glaucoma associated with systemic or ocular anomalies and secondary glaucoma such as that associated with congenital aphakia or pseudophakia have a worse surgical prognosis compared to primary congenital glaucoma. Trabeculectomy surgery with adjunctive mitomycin has a lower chance of successful control of children less than two years of age and in children who have had congenital cataract surgery. Additionally, compared to adults, the adjunctive use of anti-fibrotic agents with trabeculectomy in children may be associated with greater risk of late bleb-related infections. When a tube shunt fails to adequately control the intraocular pressure, limited treatment options remain. These options include a sequential tube shunt in another quadrant of the eye revision or replacement of the existing tube shunt, or a cyclodestructive procedure (usually transscleral or endoscopic Diode cyclophotocoagulation or cyclocryotherapy). Both tube shunts and transscleral Diode cyclophotocoagulation have been examined for treatment of refractory pediatric glaucoma. Compare the results of Contact Diod Laser Cyclophotocoagulation Versus Cyclocryotherapy in Refractory Glaucoma.[10-15]

Ciliary ablation is indicated to lower IOP in eyes that have glaucoma resistant to conventional medical and surgical therapies (refractory glaucoma, neovascular glaucoma, congenital glaucoma, secondary glaucoma, Post-surgical glaucoma, poor visual potential or that are poor candidates for incisional surgery(because of the small risk of sympathetic ophthalmia), painful blind eyes or in eyes unlikely to respond to other modes of therapy were treated with transscleral Diode laser Cyclophotocoagulation (CPC).

Ciliary ablation is relatively contraindicated in eyes with good vision because of the risk of loss of visual acuity.

Preoperative evaluation is the same as for incisional glaucoma surgery.

2. Methods and considerations

All patients signed an informed consent for the Ciliary body ablation procedures, after an explanation of the risks and benefits. Cyclophotocoagulation was performed under local anaesthesia (A sub-Tenon or peri bulbar) with the Laser settings arc 1.5-2 sec and 1500-2000 mW with semiconductor Diode laser system (810 nm laser wavelength) with a spherical polished tip oriented by a handpiece, "G-Probe.". Figures 1 and 2. Duration was set at 2000 ms (2 seconds), and the initial power setting was 1750 MW. After the edge of the probe is aligned with the limbus, approximately 17-19 applications are placed 270° around the limbus, with a power of 1.5-2 Wand a duration of approximately 2 seconds The power was increased in 250 MW increments to a maximum of 2000 MW until an audible 'popping' sound is heard, and then the power was reduced by 250 MW to just below that level. Approximately 2-40 burns arc (typically five per quadrant for 270 degrees of treatment) placed 1.2 mm posteriorly to the limbus over 180 °but avoiding the posterior ciliary nerves at 3 and 9 o'clock. In all cases, the probe tips were carefully examined. The Diode laser handpiece attachment from one manufacturer is shown in figure 2. A strong topical steroid is prescribed hourly on the day of treatment and then q.i.d. for 2 weeks. Oral non-steroidal anti-inIlammatory agents are prescribed for 2 days. Figure 1 showed cyclodestructive procedures to relieve pain. Figure 2 showed Semiconductor Diode laser. Figure 3 showed "G probe" handpiece for contact Diode TCP.

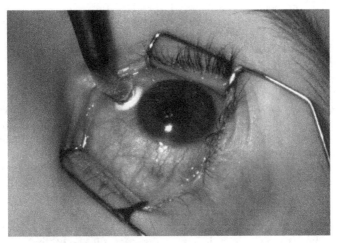

Fig. 1. Cyclodestructive procedures to relieve pain

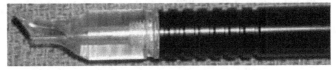

Fig. 2. Semiconductor Diode laser (IRIS Oculight SLx, Iris Medical Inc) for Diode contact TCP

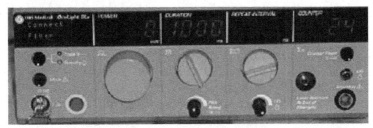

Fig. 3. Showed "G probe" handpiece for contact Diode TCP

Frequently more than one treatment session is required for adequate pressure control. The outcome of cycloDiode therapy was determined in terms of:

1. Success rate: defined as the percentage of eyes achieving and IOP between 5 and 21mm Hg with or without topical medication with cessation of oral carbonic anhydrase inhibitor use in all eyes after cycloDiode therapy at their final follow-up visit.

2. Response rate: defined as the percentage of patients achieving >30% drop from baseline IOP with cessation of oral carbonic anhydrase inhibitor use. This included eyes that developed hypotony (IOP<5mm Hg).
3. Failure rate: defined as percentage of patients who developed hypotony (IOP<5mm Hg) or phthisis, or those whose IOP drop was <30% from baseline.

The success rate is dependent on the type of glaucoma, frequently more than one treatment session is required for adequate pressure control and the procedure has to be repeated. Pain relief is generally good. After surgery intra ocular pressure and mean number of antiglaucoma medications would be dropped.

Criteria for success included intraocular pressure (IOP) of 21 mmHg or less with no devastating complications or need for further glaucoma surgery.

Pain following these procedures may be substantial, and patients should be provided with adequate analgesics, including narcotics, during the immediate postoperative period.

Cyclophotocoagulation may be associated with vision loss, prolonged hypotony, pain, inflammation, cystoid macular edema, hemorrhage, and even phthisis bulbi. Sympathetic ophthalmia is a rare but serious complication. Mildpostoperative pain and anterior segment innammation are common. Serious complications are rare and include conjunctival burns, prolonged uveitis, hyphema, chronic hypotony, phthisis bulbi, scleral thinning, corneal decompensation and retinal or choroidal detachment. However, since the aim of the procedure is usually to relieve pain. Vision-threatening complications do not have the same significance as those following conventional filtering procedures.

Transscleral Diode laser cycloablation is a recognized therapeutic approach to refractory glaucoma that involves photocoagulation of the pars plicata of the ciliary body with consequent reduction of aqueous secretion.[7,11] Diode laser cyclophotocoagulation appeared to be an effective and safe primary surgical treatment of medically uncontrolled chronic angle closure glaucoma, with intraocular pressure lowering effect persisting for up to two years.[16]

TSCPC has a significant ocular hypotensive effect on glaucoma refractory to both tube shunt and medical therapy.[17]

An unqualified success after cycloablation would be the attainment of a target IOP without the need for further medication, coupled with preservation of visual function. CycloDiode therapy appears to be effective in lowering IOP, in both the short and long term. Endoscopic cyclophotocoagulation (ECP) was introduced as an alternative to trans-scleral cyclophotocoagulation for treating refractory glaucomas in order to minimise complications such as phthisis and hypotony by providing direct visualisation of the ciliary processes. Glaucoma following penetrating keratoplasty, which has an incidence ranging from 10–52%, often proves refractory to medical treatment.[1-3] We introduce a case of refractory post-PKP glaucoma in order to demonstrate the efficacy of ECP in treating post-PKP glaucoma and to describe its potential delayed effect in achieving intraocular pressure control Diode Laser Transscleral Cyclophotocoagulation as Primary Surgical Treatment for Medically Uncontrolled Chronic Angle Closure Glaucoma Long-Term Clinical Outcomes.[17] Endoscopic cyclophotocoagulation (ECP) was introduced as an alternative to trans-scleral cyclophotocoagulation for treating refractory glaucomas in order to minimise complications such as phthisis and hypotony by providing direct visualisation of the ciliary processes. Glaucoma following penetrating keratoplasty, which has an incidence ranging from 10–52%, often proves refractory to medical treatment.[1-3] We introduce a case of refractory post-PKP glaucoma in order to demonstrate the efficacy of ECP in treating post-PKP glaucoma and to describe its potential delayed effect in achieving intraocular pressure control Diode Laser Transscleral Cyclophotocoagulation as Primary Surgical Treatment for Medically Uncontrolled Chronic Angle Closure Glaucoma Long-Term Clinical Outcomes Diode Laser Transscleral Cyclophotocoagulation for Refractory Glaucoma.[18]

Contact Diode laser transscleral cyclophotocoagulation is useful in eyes with refractory glaucoma in which the risks of outflow surgery are deemed unacceptable, Diode laser transscleral cyclophotocoagulation (DCPC) is one of the most widely used methods of ciliary body ablation, with reported success rates ranging from 40% to 80% cyclodestructive procedures are generally reserved for eyes with glaucoma refractory to other forms of medical or surgical intervention. In the past 10 years, cyclocryotherapy has been replaced by other techniques, especially laser cyclophotocoagulation with Nd:YAG or Diode laser systems,[5-10] that achieve good results with a lower complication rate.[19-24] Diode laser transscleral cyclophotocoagulation is effective in lowering the intraocular pressure in chronic angle-closure glaucoma and its effect lasts for at least 1 year.[20] Transscleral Diode laser cyclophotocoagulation is an effective and safe method for the treatment of advanced, refractory glaucoma. However, repeated treatments are often necessary. Success of treatment depends on the age of patients, previous surgery, and the type of glaucoma.[21] Types of glaucoma that are often difficult to treat include neovascular glaucoma, posttraumatic glaucoma, glaucoma associated with aphakia severe congenital/developmental glaucoma, postretinal surgery glaucoma, glaucoma associated with penetrating keratoplasties, and glaucoma in eyes with scarred conjunctiva from surgery or disease processes.[22] Delgado et al. (2003) reported that use of noncontact transscleral neodymium:yttrium-aluminum-garnet cyclophotocoagulation for NVG in 115 eyes, while providing long-term IOP reduction, was associated with complications that included inflammation, visual loss, and hypotony, and that repeat treatments may be necessary to main good control of IOP.[27] Table 1showed demographics and treatment results of Transscleral diode laser cyclophotocoagulation at the different studies.

	No. of eyes (%)	Age (yrs) (range)	Follow-up (mos)	Successfully treated eyes (%)	Reference number
A. Mistlberger et al	93	9–92	12	74.2%	19
Mr J P Diamond et al	263	4–99	17	89%	15
Ness et al	32	22-92	17.1	28.6	17
Bloom et al	34		34.1	34.1	9
Sood and Beck	9	1-15	12	66.7%	13
Jimmy et al	14	48- 76	12	92.3%	16
T. Schlote et al.	93	9–92	12	74.2%	21
F. A. Hauber and W. J. Scherer	47	38–100	12	94.4%)	24
Ataullah, Biswas, Artes, et al	53	6–90	23.1	84%	25
Iliev, Gerber	131	69-84	30.1	69.5%	26

Table 1. Demographics and treatment results of Transscleral diode laser cyclophotocoagulation at the different studies

Previous studies have demonstrated this, with ocular hypotensive responses.[7-9] Our study showed that in 50.6 % of patients the IOP was below 21 mmHg.

Complications of transscleral Diode CPC include conjunctival surface burns that may occur if tissue debris becomes coagulated on the tip and chars. We inspected all tips for this and found no debris. In addition, increased perilimbal conjunctival pigmentation may occur. One of patients had hypotony and phthisis after treatment 21 months after treatment. The risks of hypotony and phthisis are directly proportional to the dosage of laser energy delivered in a treatment session,[7] although, a clear relationship between treatment energy and IOP response, which is essential to accurate prediction of desirable effect, remains to be demonstrated. The published literature suggests that this type of treatment is usually reserved for eyes with end stage disease and poor visual potential. In conclusion, this study showed an increase of visual acuity after transscleral Diode laser cyclophotocoagulation therapy. Diode laser cyclophotocoagulation produces very characteristic injury to pars plicata, which frequently extends into pars plana, but with only mild persisting inflammation. Ciliary processes are, however, frequently spared within the treatment zone and may account for early or late treatment failure.[22-24]

Histopathological studies of enucleation specimens following laser cyclophotocoagulation (Diode and Nd:YAG laser) and cyclocryotherapy have been performed in humans [25-29] and animals.[12, 30-35] We have previously reported histopathology of two cases of clinical failure following Diode laser cyclophotocoagulation.[36] This study examines histological outcomes in nine cases in humans, and correlates this with the clinical c course in each eye.[28] Repeated use of the G-probe in transscleral cyclophotocoagulation, with ethylene oxide sterilization in between, resulted in an average decrease of 3% in laser energy delivered per repeated cycle of use up to the fourth cycle. No signs of physical damage were found.[25-28]

Laser G-probes remain functional after repeated use and ethylene oxide resterilization for up to four cycles. No visible physical damage to the probes was identified. It is safe and cost-effective to reuse G-probe for transscleral cyclophotocoagulation with ethylene oxide sterilization, provided the surgeon stays alert for signs of probe damage. This alertness should be retained regardless of whether new or old G-probes are used.[29-30] We noticed microscopic contamination of the G-probe by the tear film fluid in all the probes examined by us. The review of literature indicates that repeated use of the G-probe is not uncommon. The types of techniques used for making it suitable for repeated use indicate that it is not universally recognized that the lumen of the G-probe can accumulate fluid during the procedure, which makes it potentially hazardous when used for other patients.

Treatment with cyclophotocoagulation in patients with refractory glaucoma leads to increase in acuity and lower intraocular pressure. In our opinion the G-probe should not be reused as inadequately reprocessed G-probe can lead to risk of nosocomial infections, serious iatrogenic complications, and medico-legal problems.[30] Underlying diagnosis of neovascular glaucoma is a significant risk factor for hypotony post TCP. Hypotony was defined as IOP <5 at the end of 1-year follow-up period. Factors, such as underlying diagnosis, total energy used, age, earlier operations, and retreatment rates, which may influence the development of hypotony were analyzed using univariate analysis.[31-32]

CycloDiode therapy is highly effective but there is a significant risk of hypotony, which may be reduced by applying lower energy in cases of very high pretreatment IOP and in neovascular glaucoma.The dose-response association remains unpredictable, although a linear relation was found for neovascular glaucoma. Cyclophotocoagulation is necessary in some intractable cases but should be avoided whenever possible because of its potential adverse effects on the lens and the retina. retrobulbar alcohol injection, retrobulbar chlorpromazine injection, or enucleation are rarely performed now because of improved CPC techniques.

3. References

[1] The Eye M,D, Association. Glaucoma In: Basic and Clinical Science Course; The American Academy of Ophthalmology: Copyright @2008. San Francisco LEO 2009; pp: 214-15.

[2] Kanski J. Glaucoma In Clinical Ophthalmology. 6th ed. Butherworth Heinmann Elsevier London, 2007. 429-431

[2] Youn J, Cox T, Herndon L, Allingham R, Shields M. (1998). A Clinical Comparison of Transscleral Cyclophotocoagulation with Neodymium: YAG and Semiconductor Diode Lasers. *Am J Ophthalmol, Vol.* 126, pp. 640-47.

[3] Kirwan J, Shah P, Khaw P. (2002) Diode Laser Cyclophotocoagulation: Role in the Management of Refractory Pediatric Glaucomas. *Ophthalmology, Vol.* 109, pp. 316-23.

[4] Semchyshyn T, Tsai J, Joos K. (2002) Supplemental Transscleral Diode Laser Cyclophotocoagulation after Aqueous Shunt Placement in Refractory Glaucoma *Ophthalmology*, Vol. 109, pp. 1078-84.

[5] Lai J, Tham C, Chan J, Lam D. (2005) Diode laser transscleral cyclophotocoagulation as primary surgical treatment for medically uncontrolled chronic angle closure glaucoma: long-term clinical outcomes. *Glaucoma*, Vol. 14, pp. 114-19.

[6] Waggle N, Freedman S, Buckley E, Davis J, Biglan A. (1998) Long-term outcome of Cyclocryotherapy for Refractory Pediatric Glaucoma. *Ophthalmology, Vol.* 105, pp. 1921- 27

[7] Vernon S, Koppens J, Menon J, Negi A. (2006) Diode laser cycloablation in adult a results of standard protocol and review of current literature. *Clinical and Experimental Ophthalmology, Vol.* 34, pp. 411-20.

[8] Agarwal H, Gupta V, Sihota R. (2004) Evaluation of contact versus non-contact Diode laser cyclophotocoagulation for refractory glaucomas using similar energy *Clin Exp Ophthalmol, Vol.* 32, pp. 33-38

[9] Bloom P, Tsai J, Sham K. Miller M. Rice N, Hitchings R. (1997) "Cycloid"Trans-scleral Diode laser cyclophotocoagulation in the treatment of advanced refractory glaucoma. *Ophthalmology, Vol.* 104, pp. 1519-29.

[10] Wong E, Chew P, Chee C, Wong J. (1997) Diode laser contact transscleral cyclophotocoagulation for refractory glaucoma in Asian patients. *Am J Ophthalmol, Vol.* 124, pp. 797-04.

[11] Goldenberg-Cohen N, Bahar I, Ostashinski M, Lusky M, Weinberger D, Gaton DD. (2005) Cyclocryotherapy versus transscleral Diode laser cyclophotocoagulation for uncontrolled intraocular pressure. *Ophthalmic Surg Lasers Imaging, Vol.* 36, pp. 272-9.

[12] Pastor S, Singh K, Lee D, Juzych M, Lin S, Netland P, et al. (2001) Cyclophotocoagulation A Report by the American Academy of Ophthalmology. *Ophthalmology*, Vol. 108, pp. 2130-36.

[13] Shalini Sood, MDa,b and Allen D. (2009) Cyclophotocoagulation versus sequential tube shunt as a secondary intervention following primary tube shunt failure in pediatric glaucoma, *J AAPOS*. Vol. 13, pp. 379–383.

[14] Cioffi G, Durcan J, Girkin C, Gross R, Netland P, Samples J, Samuelson T. (2009-2010) Surgical Therapy for Glaucoma, *American Academy of Ophthalmology*

[15] Murphy C, Spry P, Burnett C, Broadway C, Diamond D. (2003) Two centre study of the dose-response relation for transscleral Diode laser cyclophotocoagulation in refractory glaucoma. *Br J Ophthalmol, Vol.* 87, pp. 1252-1257

[16] Jimmy S. M. Lai, FRCS, FRCOphth,*† Clement C. Y. Tham, FRCS*§ Jonathan C. H. Chan, MRCSEd,*† and Dennis S. C. Lam, FRCS, FRCOphth*‡ (J Glaucoma 2005;14:114-119)

[17] Ness P, Khaimi M, Feldman R, Tabet R, Sarkisian S, Skuta G, Chuang A, and Mankiewicz K. Intermediate Term Safety and Efficacy of Transscleral Cyclophotocoagulation After Tube Shunt Failure. J Glaucoma 2011;00:000-000

[18] Hollander D, Lin S. Delayed therapeutic success with endoscopic cyclophotocoagulation in treating refractory post-penetrating keratoplasty glaucoma. Br J Ophthalmol 2003;87:791-803

[19] Mistlberger A, Liebmann J, Tschiderer H, Ritch R, Ruckhofer J, and Grabner G.Contact Diode laser transscleral cyclophotocoagulation is useful in eyes with refractory glaucoma in which the risks of outflow surgery are deemed, Journal of Glaucoma 10:288-293

[20] Lai J, Tham C, Chan J, and Lam D. Diode Laser Transscleral Cyclophotocoagulation in the Treatment of Chronic Angle-Closure Glaucoma: A Preliminary Study. *Journal of Glaucoma* 12:360-364

[21] Schlote T, Derse M, Rassmann K Nicaeus T, Dietz K, and Thiel H. Efficacy and Safety of Contact Transscleral Diode Laser Cyclophotocoagulation for Advanced Glaucoma.*Journal of Glaucoma* 10:294-301

[22] Lin S. Endoscopic and Transscleral Cyclophotocoagulation for the Treatment of Refractory Glaucoma. J Glaucoma 2008;17: 238-247

[23] S Lin.Endoscopic cyclophotocoagulation.Br J Ophthalmol 2002;86:1434-1438

[24] Hauber A, Scherer W. Influence of Total Energy Delivery on Success Rate after Contact Diode Laser Transscleral Cyclophotocoagulation: A Retrospective Case Review and Meta-analysis.*Journal of Glaucoma* 11:329-333

[25] S Ataullah, S Biswas, P H Artes, E O'Donoghue, A E A Ridgway, A F Spencer. Long term results of Diode laser cycloablation in complex glaucoma using the Zeiss Visulas II system Br J Ophthalmol 2002;86:39-42

[26] M E Iliev, S Gerber. Long-term outcome of trans-scleral Diode laser cyclophotocoagulation in refractory glaucoma. Br J Ophthalmol 2007;91:1631-1635.

[27] Hayreh S. Neovascular glaucoma.*Prog Retin Eye Res.* 2007 September; 26(5): 470-485 NVG is a severely blinding,

[28] McKelvie P, Walland M. Pathology of cycloDiode laser: a series of nine enucleated eyes. Br J Ophthalmol 2002;86:381-386

[29] Tham C, Lai J, Fung P, Chua J, Poon A, and Lam D. Physical Effects of Reuse and Repeated Ethylene Oxide Sterilization on Transscleral clophotocoagulation Laser G-Probes *Journal of Glaucoma* 11:21-25

[30] Bansal A, and Ramanathan.Potential Contamination of the G-probe Used for Transscleral CycloDiode(J Glaucoma 2008;17:157-158)

[31] Hla Myint Htoon, PhD,z Ching Lin Ho, MMed (Ophth), MMed(Paed), FRCS (Ed),*Tin Aung, MMed (Ophth), FRCS(Ed), PhD,*zy and Shamira Perera, MBBS, BSc, FRCOphth Ramli N,.Risk Factors for Hypotony After Transscleral Diode Cyclophotocoagulation., (J Glaucoma 2010;00:000-000)

[32] Alipanahi R. (2008) Long-Term Outcome of Transscleral Diode Laser Cyclophotocoagulation for Refractory Glaucoma. *Rawal Med J*, Vol. 33, pp. 173-175.

7

Controlled Cyclophotocoagulation

Paul-Rolf Preußner
University Eye Hospital, Langenbeckstr
Germany

1. Introduction

Glaucoma treatments which partially destroyed the ciliary body started already in the thirthies of the 20th century. Heat and cold were used for this purpose, delivered from different devices such as hot needles, cryo applicators, ultrasound generators or radiation devices. All these methods were successful in lowering introcular pressure, but many eyes were lost and ended in a phthisis. The reasons of such disastrous outcomes is not fully investigated in all details, but it is mostly assumed that the production of aqueous humor has been reduced too much. In summary, the methods were called "cyclodestructive", a wording primarily related to the destruction of tissue in the ciliary body, but also making graphical the high destructive potential to the eye.

With the invention of lasers, many CW-lasers were utilized for tissue coagulation of the ciliary body, and the new word "cyclophotocoagulation" was created, also to distinguish photo- from cryocoagulation (1–13).

For a long time, current opinion was to restrict cyclophotocoagulation to intractable cases due to severe complications which had been observed by several authors (e.g. (14–21)). Meanwhile, however, transscleral cyclophotocoagulation is proposed also as primary therapy (22; 23).

An improvement of the coagulation was achieved by the introduction of contact methods (24), however, efforts undertaken in the past to optimize therapy parameters (25–29) including aspects of radiation transport (30; 31) could not solve the principal problem that the laser burns cannot be observed directly.

Without information about coagulation success, dosage cannot be adjusted to the individual situation which shows a strong inter- and intraindividual variation of optical properties of the corresponding tissue (32). For the reasons mentioned, we had developed a real-time control system (33; 34) to solve this problem.

2. Controlling device

During coagulation of the tissue, chemical and physical effects are induced which change the optical properties, i.e. the transmission, absorption and reflection in this material (35). For the ciliary body, this effect cannot be observed directly. However, the transmitted laser radiation produces diffuse stray light which is partly reflected from the fundus and can be observed from outside the eye by a sensor. The principle of the corresponding device is illustrated in fig. 1. The light intensity monitored by the sensor during the laser exposure depends on many

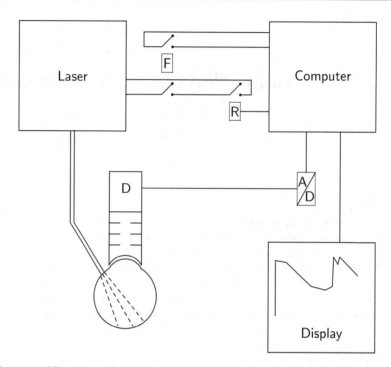

Fig. 1. Functional Diagram. *The laser radiation passing through sclera and ciliary body is partly reflected from the fundus and recorded by a detector* D. *The amplified electronical signal is digitized by an A/D-converter, recorded by a computer and displayed on a screen in real time. The whole process is initiated by pressing the foot-switch* F, *which starts the computer and closes* one *of the switches for the laser device. The* second one *is closed by a semiconductor-relay* R, *which is controlled by the computer. Exposure is stopped either if the operator (viewing the screen) releases his foot-switch* F *or if the computer opens the relay* R, *when the recorded signal has fulfilled certain programmable criteria.*

parameters such as fundus reflectivity, pupil width etc. and can therefore not be used directly as an *absolute* measure of the coagulation stage of the tissue. However, the coagulation process changes the light observed *as function of time* in any case. Therefore, this time dependence can be used to monitor the progress of coagulation. The electronic signal has to be normalized to its starting value, i.e., only *relative values* are used for further evaluation.

There are 2 ways the process can be controlled. First, the surgeon can interrupt the exposure if the displayed curve of changing transmission has a certain shape. This is possible, but difficult, because typical time scales are in the range of 0.1-0.5s, which is approximately the surgeon's own reaction time. As a second "operator", the computer can interrupt the exposure.

3. Physical parameters

3.1 Laser power
Laser power has to be adjusted in such a way that the target tissue is coagulated as selectively as possible, thereby saving all surrounding tissues. The physical parameters describing this

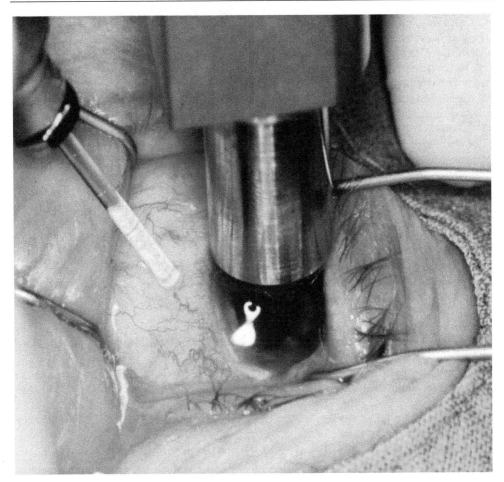

Fig. 2. Application to a Patient's Eye

in context are the *temperature gradient* and the *heat conduction*, which determine the *thermal relaxation time*. If laser power is too low, a long time is needed until coagulation starts. During this time, a high portion of heat is already dissipated into the surrounding tissue. This results in an unwanted large area of coagulated tissue, which can also be observed from the high value of the total energy, the product of power and time. A very high laser power, on the other hand, induces a steep temperature gradient with a higher risk of overheating parts of the target tissue before the rest is sufficiently coagulated. Such overheated tissue has a high probability of so-called "pop spots". A pop spot is a local overheating of the tissue in which the tissue membranes are disrupted by the steam pressure with an audible "pop" as in a pop corn.

As a compromise, we preferably use a laser power of 5W for the 810nm diode laser in Caucasian eyes and found the same value suitable for the 940nm laser in African eyes. Only in very rare cases of buphthalmos with very thin sclera this value has to be reduced to 3W.

3.2 Laser wavelength

The laser wavelength for transscleral cyclophotocoagulation must be selected in such a way that the laser light is *transmitted* through the conjunctiva, the sclera and the ciliary muscle, and that it is *absorbed* by the pigment epithelium of the ciliary body. These requirements, however, can only be fulfilled approximatively, depending on the spectral characteristics of the eye. Caucasian and African eyes strongly differ in the absorption and transmission of visible and infrared radiation. If the absorption is too high, the fraction of energy already absorbed in conjunctiva, sclera or ciliary muscle causes an unwanted overheating of these tissues. Absorption and transmission of ocular tissues show a strong wavelength dependence (36). The spectra shown is this paper are consistent with the fact that the flux density needed for the 1064nm Nd:YAG laser is approximately 2-fold higher than with the 810nm diode laser. They also show that the same behavior as with the 810nm laser in Caucasian eyes could be expected with a 940nm laser in African eyes. In a few African eyes treated with the 810nm laser in Mainz University Eye Hospital, the abovementioned real-time control did not work, i.e. many pop spots occured. Therefore, after tests with African cadaver eyes in Ghana (43), the 940nm laser was clinically established in Cameroun.

Applications of shorter wavelengths for transscleral cyclophotocoagulation in the visible red range have been reported only by Scandinavian authors for a population with very lightly pigmented eyes (8; 37; 38), again consistent with the spectra in (36).

3.3 Location

As location, we chose the transition region between pars plicata and pars plana of the ciliary body, i.e., 3-3.5mm posterior to the limbus. We intend to coagulate at least a part of the secreting tissue, but care should be taken of the ciliary muscle including fixation of zonula fibers (which could be disintegrated), because the procedure should also be applicable to phakic, accommodating eyes. The effectiveness of even higher limbus distances has been proven by other authors (39). Fortunately, our real-time control shows optimal performance just in the chosen limbus distance.

Normally, 360° are treated. The only exceptions are scleral lesions / thinned sclera, particularly the areas of previous trabeculectomies.

3.4 Optic of the laser applicator

The laser applicator (the tip directly pressed on the eye) should be designed in such a way that the optical power density at the conjunctiva is minimal and the power density in the target tissue (ciliary body) is maximal. Focussing therefore seems to be a reasonable procedure. Unfortunately, the outcome of focussing is rather poor. If a (spherical) lens is used, even for a material with a high refractive index a relatively long focal width results, because the refractive index of the sclera is similar to that of water, i.e., much larger than one. This problem could be solved in principle by a so-called "gradient index lens" (40), for which the focal width can be set to any position. But, our own measurements and calculations (31) also with such optical devices have shown that diffuse multiple scattering in scleral tissue largely neutralises the focussing effect. Fortunately, radiation transport can be optimised by an appropriate choice of the diameter of the optical tip. As shown in (31), this diameter should be larger than or at least equal to the thickness of the sclera. On the other hand, a smaller tip diameter theoretically causes a higher pressure on the sclera leading to an improved optical transmission (41; 42). Thus, both effects have to be balanced against each other by an optimal tip diameter. Tests in Caucasian and African cadaver eyes showed that a tip diameter of 1.5mm was optimal for Caucasian and of 1.95mm for African eyes.

3.5 Shape of transmission curves

Typical curves resulting from coagulation in porcine eyes, Caucasian cadaver eyes and in the eyes of Caucasian patients are in detail reported in (33), see fig.3 for an example. The curves of African eyes principally show the same shape, but with slightly different amplitudes from minimum to maximum which therefore needed different software settings.

The shape of these curves (see fig.3) corresponds to the temperature change in the target tissue: In the first, horizontal part (1), no irreversible chemical or physical effects occur, therefore the transmission in the tissue remains constant. The temperature may increase to about 45-50°C. In the second, decreasing part (2), the transmission is reduced mainly by shrinkage of the tissue. The temperature further increases to about 60-70°C. After that, only minor changes in the transmission occur (3), but the temperature increases to a value above 100°C. Trapped, overheated steam then disrupts tissue membranes in the "pop spot". Since for the "wanted" effect of irreversible coagulation, a temperature of about 55-60°C is sufficient, the process should be interrupted at the end of phase two. This is normally less than 1/3 of the time to pop spot, because at the beginning of the coagulation, the temperature raise is steeper than at the end due to heat dissipation to the neighbourhood. Fortunately, further heating above 60°C but well below 100°C is not critical, thus giving a relative safe "therapeutic window" before a pop spot occurs.

4. Clinical applications

4.1 Indication

Controlled cyclophotocoagulation is indicated in all open angle glaucomas in which eye drops do not effectively reduce the intraocular pressure. This includes cases of insufficient compliance in industrial countries as well as developing countries in which eye drops are not available or not effordable. In severe cases of hemorrhagical secondary glaucoma in blind eyes even repeated controlled cyclophotocoagulation may be insufficient and should be replaced by cryocoagulation.

4.2 Preoperative preparation and anesthesia

It is recommended to dilate the pupil preoperatively because it increases the signal-to-noise-ratio of the detector of the real time control, but when the pupil cannot be dilated, the procedure can be applied anyway.

Anesthesia can be a para- or retrobulbar injection, or a general anesthesia, or a combination of topical anesthesia by eye drops and general analgesia (e.g. Propofol combined with a short acting opioid). Topical anesthesia alone with eye drops is insufficient. In case of para- or retrobulbary injections, it should be kept in mind that the risk of these injections is higher than that of the controlled cyclophotocoagulation. Analgesia alone needs very high drug doses when the simulataneous topical anesthesia is omitted.

4.3 Treatment

Generally, 16 spots are applied over 360°. A larger number (24 spots) did not result in a significantly higher IOP reduction, but in a significantly higher and longer lasting

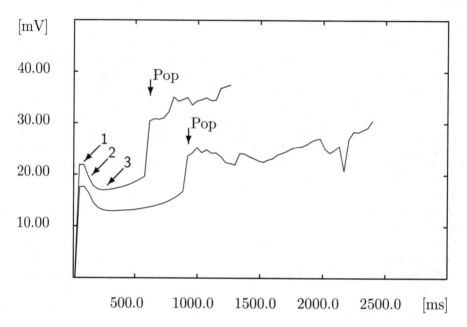

Fig. 3. Typical Transmission Curves. *The recordings are from porcine eyes. The numbers (1,2,3) and their meaning are explained in the text.*

inflammation reaction (cells).   An integrated instrument comprising laser source and computer and its application in Cameroun is shown in fig.4.

4.4 Postoperative medication

After surgery, local antibiotics are applied once in order to prevent infections based on minor (and prehaps overlooked) corneal or conjinctival lesions. Local steroids and Scopolamin or Homatropine are applied until there are no more signs of inflammation (cells) visible at the slitlamp.

4.5 Complications

Major complications such as intraocular bleedings, shallow anterior chamber, chorioideal detachment, ocular hypotension <7mmHg or phthisis have not been observed during more than 2000 treatments of Caucasian patients with the 810nm laser in the university eye hospital of Mainz, Germany, nor in more than 1000 treatments of African patients with the 940nm laser in the eye clinic at Acha Bafoussam, Cameroun. Such complications also did not come to our knowledge from other hospitals using this method.

Some minor complications can happen from time to time:

Conjunctival hemorrhages can occur at the locations where the tip is placed on the conjunctiva, particularly in patients with systemic anticoagulation.   Depending on the surgeons' experience and care also corneal erosions can be produced. Intraocular iritis (cells)

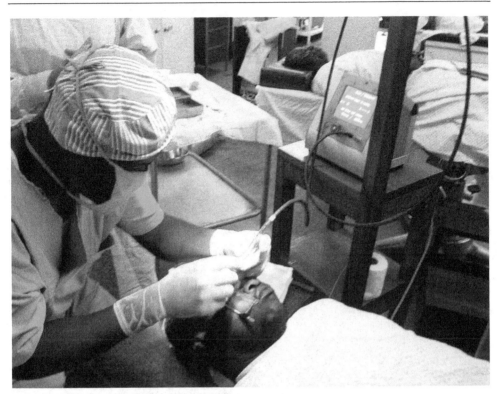

Fig. 4. Application in Camerounian Patients

mostly disappear after one or two days, and higher degrees of inflammation (fibrin exudation) is extremely rare (<1% of the treatments).

In our opinion, also pop spots should be looked at as complications. Even if the probability of pop spots is highly reduced by the real-time control of the coagulation, this probability is not zero. In Caucasian eyes one or more pop spots occur in ≈20% of the eyes, in African eyes in ≈30%.

Even if *visual acuity* as a measure of unwanted side effects has been recorded pre- and postoperatively, the data have not been evaluated systematically. They are often incomplete and biased by the often unknown refraction and by additional reasons (e.g. cataract) that worsens visual acuity. Nevertheless, a significant decrease following the treatment did not occur. It did, however, in Mainz University eye hospital in one case that was treated with 24 spots in the starting phase. The reason was a macula edema. With the generally recommended protocol of 16 spots no further macula edema was observed.

4.6 Influence on Intraocular Pressure (IOP)

4.6.1 Caucasian eyes

Despite the high treatment numbers in the University Eye Hospital Mainz, these patients could not be followed up systematically because of the deduction rules of the health insurance. Patients are referred from other doctors to the University Hospital, but seen again only in case of complications or isufficient treatment. Fig.5 shows the IOP of another German hospital which could do a systematic follow-up without selection bias.

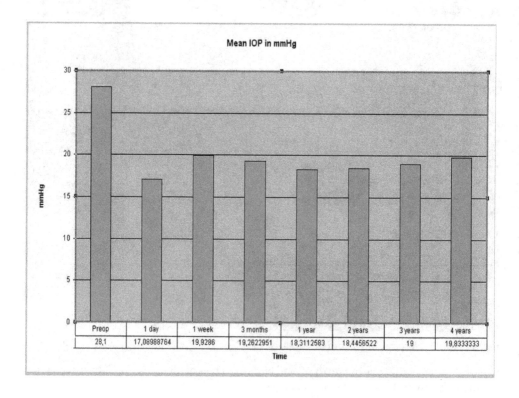

Mean IOP in mmHg

Time	Preop	1 day	1 week	3 months	1 year	2 years	3 years	4 years
	28,1	17,08988764	19,9286	19,2622951	18,3112583	18,4456522	19	19,8333333

Fig. 5. Intraocular Pressure in European Eyes. *The IOP of 40 eyes in which controlled cyclophotocoagulation was the 1st and only glaucoma surgery is shown as function of the follow-up time of 4 years. The numbers on the bottom of each column show the averages. (Picture by courtesy of Dr. Gerl, Dr. Schmickler, Augenklinik Ahaus, Germany)*

4.6.2 African eyes

272 eyes of 188 patients with primary open angle glaucoma were treated in the eye hospital of Bafoussam, Cameroun. Follow-ups were scheduled for 1 day, 1 week, 1 month, 3 months, 6 months and 1 year after surgery. But mostly, patients were unable to meet such fixed dates. Instead, if at all, they appeared more or less at random times after surgery. All individual IOP changes at all recording times are shown in figs. 6 and 7.

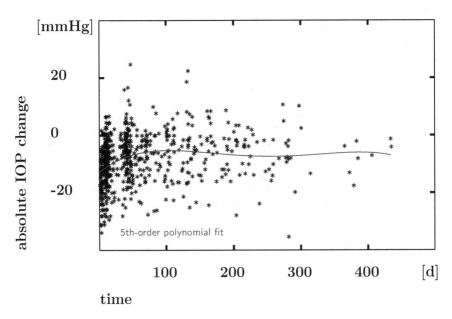

Fig. 6. Absolute Change in IOP *The average of the starting IOP was 28.5mmHg.*

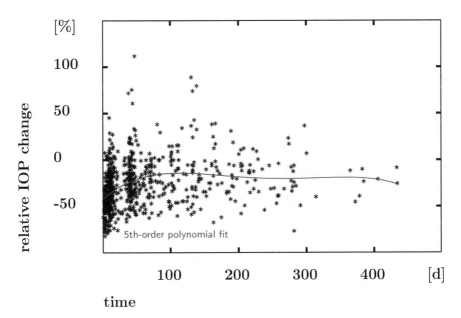

Fig. 7. Relative Change in IOP

5. Discussion

Controlled cyclophotocoagulation with the 810nm laser for Caucasian and with the 940nm laser for African glaucoma eyes is a method with nearly negligible complications. However, the individual IOP reduction is not predictable.

Re-treatments are possible, but an interval of at least 4 weeks is recommended, because a significant prostaglandine release for at least 2 weeks is an unavoidable concomittant of the coagulation (45). The maximum number of re-treatments performed so far was 13 in an eye in which no other glaucoma surgery was possible (only functioning eye of this patient, and this eye had already multiple surgeries). The function of the eye could be preserved at an IOP that finally reached 8mmHg. Even if not explicitly shown for humans, at least a partial recovery must be assumed for the coagulated tissue.

The low complication risk can be understood as a result of the low energy load compared with the uncontrolled coagulation. In Caucasian eyes, the energy per spot is $\approx$1.5J and in Africans $\approx$1.0J, which is to be compared with the much higher values reported from other authors: 3.6J (13) or 2.2J to 3.3J (30) in Caucasians and 2.25 to 3.125J in Africans (22). Nd:YAG-laser values are even higher (44).

In Africans, IOP reduction is obviously higher and complication rate lower compared to the uncontrolled coagulation with the 810nm laser (22).

As a consequence of the high power (5W) and low exposure time ($\approx$0.2s in Africans and $\approx$0.3s in Caucasians), the major fraction of energy is thermalized in the highest absorbing tissue, i.e. in the (black) pigmented ciliary epithelium, thus causing a selective coagulation of this target tissue.

As a major drawback, cyclophotocoagulation in general may result in conjunctival scarring which interferes with other procedures such as trabelectomy or shunt tube placement. However, the probability of such conjunctival scarring is reduced by a more selective approach.

To apply such a high power without the risk of very many pop spots, the real time control is an indispensable necessity of the device.

6. References

[1] Weekers R, Lavergne G, Watillon M, Gilson M, Legros AM (1961) Effects of photocoagulation of the ciliary body upon ocular tension. Am J Ophthalmol 52:156-163

[2] Beckman H, Kinoshita A, Rota AN, Sugar HS (1972) Transscleral ruby laser irradiation of the ciliary body in the treatment of intractable glaucoma. Trans Am Acad Ophthal Otol 76:423-436

[3] Beckman H, Sugar HS (1973) Neodymium laser cyclophotocoagulation. Arch Ophthalmol 90:27-28

[4] Hampton C, Shields MB, Miller KN, Blasini M (1990) Evaluation of a protocol for transscleral neodymium:YAG cyclophotocoagulation in one hundred patients. Ophthalmology 97:910-917

[5] Brooks AMV, Gillies WE (1991) The use of YAG cyclophotocoagulation to lower pressure in advanced glaucoma. Aust NZ J Ophthal 19:207-210

[6] Heidenkummer HP, Mangouritsas G, Kampik A (1991) Klinische Anwendungen und Ergebnisse der transskleralen Nd:YAG-Zyklophotokoagulation bei therapierefraktärem Glaucom. Klin Mbl Augenheilk 198:174-180

[7] Wright MM, Grajewski AL, Feuer WJ (1991) Nd:YAG cyclophotocoagulation: outcome of treatment for uncontrolled glaucoma. Ophthalmic Surg 22:279-283

[8] Immonen IJ, Puska P, Raitta C (1994) Transscleral contact krypton laser cyclophotocoagulation for treatment of glaucoma. Ophthalmology 101:876-882

[9] Brancato R, Carassa RG, Bettin P, Fiori M, Trabucchi G (1995) Contact transscleral cyclophotocoagulation with diode laser in refractory glaucoma. Eur J Ophthalmol 5:32-39

[10] Hamard P, Kopel J, Valtot F, Quesnot S, Hamard H, Haut J (1995) Traitement des glaucomes réfractaires par cyclophotocoagulation au laser à diode. J Fr Ophthalmol 18:447-454

[11] Hawkins TA, Stewart WC (1993) One-year results of semiconductor transscleral cyclophotocoagulation in patients with glaucoma. Arch Ophthalmol 111:488-491

[12] Hennis HL, Stewart WC (1992) Semiconductor diode laser transscleral cyclophotocoagulation in patients with glaucoma. Am J Ophthalmol 113:81-85

[13] Omofolasade K, Gaasterland DE, Pollack IP, Enger CL (1996) Long-term outcome of initial ciliary ablation with contact diode laser transscleral cyclophotocoagulation for severe glaucoma. Ophthalmology 103:1294-1302

[14] Maus M, Katz LJ (1990) Choroidal detachment, flat anterior chamber, and hypotony as complications of neodymium:YAG laser cyclophotocoagulation. Ophthalmology 97:69-72

[15] Smith RS, Stein MN (1969) Ocular hazards of transscleral laser radiation: II. Intraocular injury produced by ruby and neodymium lasers. Am J Ophthalmol 67:100-110

[16] Hamada M, Suzuki R, Kurimoto S (1991) Transient complete visual loss during transscleral cyclophotocoagulation. Jap J Clin Ophthalmol 45:949-951

[17] Edwards DP, Brown SV, Higginbotham E (1989) Sympathetic ophthalmia following Nd:YAG cycloptherapy. Ophthalmic Surg 20:544-546

[18] Bechrakis NE, Müller-Stolzenburg NW, Helbig H (1994) Sympathetic ophthalmia following laser cyclocoagulation. Arch Ophthalmol 112:80-84

[19] Geyer O, Neudorfer M, Lazar M (1993) Retinal detachment as a complication of neodymium:yttrium:aluminium garnet laser cyclocoagulation. Ann Ophthalmol 25:170-172

[20] Johnson SM (1998) Neurotrophic corneal defects after diode laser cycloablation. Am J Ophthalmol 126:725-727

[21] Sabry K, Vernon SA (1999) Scleral perforation following trans-scleral cyclodiode. Br J Ophthalmol 83:502-503

[22] Egbert PR, Fiadoyor S, Budenz DL, Dadzie P, Byrd S (2001) Diode laser transscleral cyclophotocoagulation as a primary surgical treatment for primary open-angle glaucoma. Arch Ophthalmol 119:345-350

[23] Kramp K, Vick HP, Guthoff R (2002) Transscleral diode laser contact cyclophotocoagulation in the treatment of different glaucomas, also as primary surgery. Graefes Arch Clin Exp Ophthalmol 240:698-703

[24] Federman JL, Ando F, Schubert HD, Eagle RC (1987) Contact laser for transscleral photocoagulation. Ophthalmic Surg 18:183-184

[25] Allingham RR, Kater AW de, Bellows AR, Hsu J (1990) Probe placement and power levels in contact transscleral neodymium:YAG cyclophotocoagulation. Arch Ophthalmol 108:738-742

[26] England C, Van der Zypen E, Fankhauser F, Kwasniewska S (1988) A comparison of optical methods used for transscleral cyclophotocoagulation in rabbit eyes produced with the Nd:YAG laser: a morphological physical and clinical analysis. Lasers Light Ophthalmol 2:87-102

[27] Kwasniewska S, Fankhauser F, Van der Zypen E, Rol P, Henchoz PD, England C (1988) Acute effects following transscleral contact irradiation of the ciliary body and the retina/choroid with the cw Nd:YAG laser. Lasers Light Ophthalmol 2:25-34

[28] Schuman JS, Noecker RJ, Puliafito CA, Jacobsson JJ, Shepps GJ, Wang N (1991) Energy levels and probe placement in contact transscleral semiconductor diode laser cyclophotocoagulation in human cadaver eyes. Arch Ophthalmol 109:1534-1538

[29] Takahashi H, Okisaka S (1991) Safety and effectiveness of contact transscleral cyclophotocoagulation with continuous-wave Nd:YAG laser. Jap J Clin Ophthalmol 45:1233-1237

[30] Roider J, Schmidt-Erfurth U, El-Hifnawi E, Herboth T, Hoerauf H, Birngruber R, Laqua H (1996) Zyklophotokoagulation mit dem Diodenlaser im Kontaktverfahren mit einer neuen fokussierenden Sonde. Ophthalmologe 93:576-580

[31] Preußner PR, Schwenn O (1995) Steps to optimize transscleral photocoagulation. Graefes Arch Clin Exp Ophthalmol 233:302-306

[32] Echelman DA, Stern RA, Shields SR, Simmons RB, Shields MB (1995) Variability of contact transscleral neodymium:YAG cyclophotocoagulation. Invest Ophthalmol Vis Sci 36:497-502

[33] Preußner PR, Boos N, Faßbender K, Schwenn O, Pfeiffer N (1997) Real-time control for transscleral cyclophotocoagulation. Graefes Arch Clin Exp Ophthalmol 235:794-801

[34] Preußner PR (1998) Kontrollierte Zyklophotokoagulation. Ophthalmologe 95:645-650

[35] Francis A. L'Esperance, Ophthalmic lasers, 3rd ed., Mosby, 1989.

[36] Geeraets WJ, Williams RC, Chan G, Ham WT, Guerry D, Schmidt FH (1960) The loss of light energy in retina and choroid. Arch Ophthalmol 64: 606-615

[37] Raivio VE, Immonen IJ, Puska PM (2001) Transscleral contact krypton laser cyclophotocoagulation for treatment of posttraumatic glaucoma. J Glaucoma 10:77-84

[38] Raivio VE, Vesaluoma MH, Tervo TM, Immonen IJ, Puska PM (2002) Corneal innervation, corneal mechanical sensitivity, and tear fluid secretion after transscleral contact 670nm diode laser cyclophotocoagulation. J Glaucoma 11:446-453

[39] Liu GJ,Mizukawa A, Okisaka S (1994) Mechanism of intraocular pressure decrease after contact transscleral continuous-wave Nd:YAG laser cyclophotocoagulation. Ophthalmic Res 26:65-79

[40] Schröder G (1990) Technische Optik. Kamprath-Reihe, Vogel, Würzburg, ISBN 3-8023-0067-X

[41] Rol P, Niederer P, Dürr U, Henchoz PD, Fankhauser F (1990) Experimental investigations on the light scattering properties of the human sclera. Laser and Light in Ophthalmol 3:201-212

[42] Vogel A, Dlugos C, Nuffer R, Birngruber R (1991) Die optischen Eigenschaften der menschlichen Sklera und deren Bedeutung für transsklerale Laseranwendungen. Fortschr Ophthalmol 88:754-761

[43] Holbach M, Fiadoyor S, Preußner PR. Controlled cyclophotocoagulation for the therapy of primary open angle glaucoma in African eyes. Presentation on the 101. congress of the Deutsche Ophthalmologische Gesellschaft (DOG), Berlin, 25.-28.09.2003

[44] Krott R, Diestelhorst M, Zollweg M, Krieglstein GK (1997) Zur Dosis-Wirkungs-Beziehung der transskleralen Kontaktzyklophotokoagulation. Ophthalmologe 94:273-276

[45] Nasisse MP, McGahan MC, Shields MB, Echelman D, Fleisher LN (1992) Inflammatory effects of continuous-wave neodymium:yttrium aluminum garnet laser cyclophotocoagulation. Invest Ophthalmol Vis Sci 33:2216-2223

8

Another Look on Cyclodestructive Procedures

Antonio Fea, Dario Damato,
Umberto Lorenzi and Federico M. Grignolo
Dipartimento di Fisiopatologia Clinica- Clinica Oculistica
University of Torino
Italy

1. Introduction

Cycloablation is a destructive procedure used to decrease the intra-ocular pressure (IOP) trough the ablation of the ciliary body that produces aqueous humour. Many destructive techniques, including diathermy, cryotherapy, ultrasounds, beta irradiation, and laser photocoagulation have been employed with a wide range of results and side effects. Although all above techniques can effectively destroy the ciliary body, only few of them have been used widely enough to convincingly demonstate their clinical usefulness and gain general acceptance. The ideal method of cyclodestruction should produce clinically useful and predictable reduction of intraocular pressure (IOP), with minimal complications and side effects. (Bartamian & Higginbotham, 2001). Ideally it should have a wide therapeutic window between insufficient and too aggressive treatment intensity, that can result in either insufficient IOP reduction or hypotony/phtisis. Cyclodestructive procedures are usually reserved for cases of glaucoma in eyes with little or no visual potential that proved refractory to medical treatment and outflow surgeries. (Lin, 2008) As an exception to this long established indication, cyclodestructive procedures performed with the 810 nm infrared diode laser transscleral cyclophotocoagulation have been successfully applied also in eyes with refractory glaucoma and good visual potential (Rotchford et al., 2010; Wilensky & Kammer, 2004) supporting an emerging notion that the indications for transscleral laser cyclophotocoagulation should not be limited to eyes with poor visual acuity or potential.

2. Background

Coagulation or destruction of the ciliary body to reduce aqueous production has been advocated in the treatment of glaucoma since the 1930s with the introduction of penetrating cyclodiathermy (Voght et al., 1936). In the 1950s, cyclocryotherapy was proven reasonably safe and effective to reduce IOP with less tissue destruction and better predictability compared to cyclodiathermy (Bietti, 1950). Problems still existed, however, including intense postoperative pain, intraocular pressure (IOP) rise, marked inflammation, hemorrhage, and a significant incidence of hypotony and visual loss. Ciliary ablation with ultrasounds was also briefly utilized, but it was eventually abandoned because of marked scleral thinning and ectasia at the treatment site (Coleman at al., 1985).

2.1 Laser cyclophotocoagulation

Laser cyclophotocoagulation has become the principal surgical method for reducing aqueous production. The first laser transscleral cyclophotocoagulation (TSCPC) was described by Beckam and Sugar in the early 1970s. Initially, they used the 694 nm ruby laser, but later reported that the 1064 nm infrared Neodymium : Yttrium-Aluminium-Garnet laser (Nd : YAG) was more effective due to its superior transmission through the sclera and absorption by the ciliary epithelium. The delivery of laser energy to the ciliary processes through the sclera may be performed either with an indenting contact probe or a noncontact projected beam. The development of the compact, portable 810 nm I.R. ophthalmic diode laser has made it more convenient to perform contact TSCPC. The same 810 nm I.R. diode laser beam can also be delivered inside the eye through an endoscope to directly photocoagulate the ciliary body under endoscopic guidance. This technique, named endoscopic cyclophotocoagulation (ECP), has become an increasingly important weapon in the glaucoma surgeon's armamentarium for the treatment of refractory glaucoma at the time of ocular surgery and may have some distinct advantages over the transscleral approach in eyes with visual potential. In 1976, Merritt described his method of transpupillary cyclophotocoagulation of the ciliary processes under indirect visualization via a gonioscopic laser lens. This interesting approach, potentially safer than the more invasive ECP, did not become popular because of the difficulty in visualizing and treating the ciliary processes through the gonio-lens, but it may still represent a good option for aniridic eyes.

Laser cyclo-destructive procedures can be divided as follows:

- Transpupillary CPC
- Transvitreal endophotocoagulation
- Transscleral CPC
    - Noncontact and contact 1064 nm Nd:YAG laser
    - Contact 810 nm diode laser
- Endoscopic 810 nm diode laser CPC

In the United States, CPC is used predominantly for refractory glaucoma difficult to control with conventional glaucoma filtration, such as neovascular glaucoma, traumatic glaucoma, glaucoma in aphakic eyes, advanced developmental glaucoma, inflammatory glaucoma, glaucoma associated with corneal transplantation, silicone oil-induced glaucoma, and glaucoma in eyes with conjunctival scarring from previous surgery. Cyclophotocoagulation is also used in eyes with limited visual potential, in urgent situations with dangerously elevated IOP, or for pain relief in eyes with no visual potential. It has uncommonly been used in patients who are not candidates for conventional glaucoma therapy due to poor compliance with care or poor postoperative follow-up. Cyclophotocoagulation has also been evaluated for use as primary surgical treatment in developing countries where conventional glaucoma therapy is not available (Egbert 2001).

3. Description of the various CPC procedures

3.1 Transpupillary cyclophotocoagulation

Direct transpupillary treatment of the ciliary processes with the argon laser (488/514 nm) is rarely used, because a clear visual axis and a well-dilated pupil are required to enable photocoagulation of the entire length of the ciliary processes. Clinical results have been poor when treatment was limited to the anterior most portions of the ciliary processes. Transpupillary CPC of the ciliary processes, exposed through peripheral iridectomy or a widely dilated pupil, can be effective. The mechanism may be related to a laser-induced retraction of the ciliary body.

3.2 Transvitreal endophotocoagulation

Transvitreal endophotocoagulation using a visible or infrared laser beam (514 nm argon, 532 nm solid-state or 810 nm diode) delivered through a vitreo-retinal endoprobe has been used with some success when performed in conjunction with a vitrectomy in the operating room. It requires clear media, aphakia or pseudophakia to directly treat the ciliary processes visible in the field of the operating microscope with scleral indentation. The laser power is titrated to produce a visible burn using continuous wave exposure durations that favour some thermal spread in the deeper layers of the ciliary processes.

3.3 Transscleral cyclophotocoagulation (TSCPC)

Due to the optical properties of the human sclera, TSCPC is performed with infrared emitting lasers, most commonly with the 810 nm Diode Laser delivered via a contact probe or with the 1064 nm Nd:YAG laser, delivered either with a non-contact projected beam or with a contact probe.

3.4 1064 nm Nd:Yag Laser Non-Contact TSCPC

Transscleral ciliary body ablation utilizing the Nd:YAG laser at 1064 nm wavelength has the theoretical advantage of better transmission through the scleral with less back scatter than shorter wavelengths, such as 514 nm argon and 810 nm diode lasers. Non-contact TSCPC was performed using the Nd:YAG laser in the free-running thermal mode (Microruptor III Lasag, Thun, Switzerland, no longer commercially available) for a duration of 20 msec, and the defocus setting number, which offsets the focal point of the 1064 nm infrared treating beam 3.6 mm posteriorly to the focal point of the red aiming beam. In this way, when the red aiming beam is focused on the conjunctiva, the infrared treatment beam is focused 3.6 mm below, supposedly within the ciliary processes. The laser energy is adjusted from 5 to 8 Joules (J) per application. Retrobulbar or peribulbar anaesthesia is given, and the patient is seated at the laser slit lamp. The treatment is directed parallel to the visual axis, focusing the aiming beam on the sclera, 1.5 mm posterior to the limbus, superiorly and inferiorly, and 1.0 mm posterior to the limbus nasally and temporally. A contact lens with 1.0 mm markings parallel to the limbus can be used to facilitate the placing of the applications, to hold the eyelids open and to bleach the conjunctiva. Alternatively, a lid speculum can be used to open the eyelids, and the red aiming beam can be focused on the centre of a 3 mm slit beam. Approximately eight to ten applications per quadrant are placed from 270 to 360 degrees. Treatment may be reduced to 180 degrees in patients judged to be clinically at risk for hypotony (Pastor et al., 2001).

3.5 1064 nm Nd:Yag Laser Contact TSCPC

Retrobulbar or peribulbar anaesthesia is given, the patient lies supine, and a eyelid speculum is placed. The anterior edge of the 2.2 mm sapphire tip of the delivery fibre optic handpiece (Surgical Laser Technologies, Inc., Malvern, PA) is placed 0.5 to 1.0 mm posterior to the limbus (the probe is centred 1.5 to 2.0 mm posterior to the limbus). Gentle pressure is applied with the probe, which is oriented perpendicular to the sclera. The laser energy setting is 5 to 9 Joules, for a duration of 0.7 seconds, with approximately eight spots per quadrant placed from 270 to 360 degrees. After the procedure, atropine and dexamethasone ointments are applied and the eye is patched. The patch may be removed in the evening and anti-glaucoma drops should be reinstituted. Prostaglandin analogues may be excluded in the short term if cystoid macular edema (CME) is a concern, and cholinergics should be temporarily discontinued to avoid increased anterior segment inflammation. Postoperative prednisolone acetate 1% is applied 4 times daily for 10 to 14 days and tapered according to inflammation (Lin, 2008).

3.6 810 nm Diode Laser Contact TSCPC

It is performed using a semiconductor diode laser system (IRIS Oculight SLx, IRIDEX Corp., Mountain View, CA), its 810 nm wavelength exhibits lower scleral transmission (35%) but considerably greater absorption by melanin than the 1064 nm wavelength. The laser energy is transmitted through a 600 μm diameter quartz fiber with a spherical protruding tip oriented by the footplate of the hand-piece called "G-Probe". Positioning the G-Probe parallel to the optical visual axis with the shorter edge of the footplate next to the anterior border of the limbus will centre the fibre optic tip 1.0-1.2 mm posterior to the corneoscleral limbus and direct the energy toward the ciliary processes. The tip protrudes 0.7 mm beyond the footplate contact surface, which indents the conjunctiva and sclera to enhance the transmission of the laser energy. The probe footplate is curved spherically to match the scleral curvature. Maximum settings from the system are 3.0 watts power and 9.9 seconds duration. Retrobulbar or peribulbar anesthesia is given and a lid speculum is placed. Duration is set at 2000 ms (2 seconds), and the initial power setting is 1750 mW. The power is increased in 250 mW increments to a maximum of 2500mW until an audible "pop" (caused by tissue explosion of the ciliary process, the iris root anteriorly or the retina posteriorly) is heard, then the power is reduced by 250 mW and treatment is completed at this power. Some surgeons recommend lower power and longer burn duration, for example 1250 mW at 4 seconds (5.0 Joules) in heavily pigmented eyes and 1500 mW at 3.5 seconds in lightly pigmented eyes (5.25 Joules). Six applications per quadrant are typically placed over 270 degrees involving the inferior, nasal and superior quadrants for a total of 18 applications per treatment. This is based on burns spaced half the width of the G-Probe footplate (2 mm), but various reports have used from 18 to 40 spots, with 180 to 360 degrees for the initial treatment (Pastor et al., 2001). Generally, the incidence of retreatment increases when a lower energy and/or a lower number of spots are applied. With all non-contact or contact TSCPC procedures, the outcome predictability is limited by the inability to visualize treated tissue. In lieu of direct visualization, trans-illumination may be used to identify the location of the ciliary body, especially in eyes with abnormal anatomy or in enlarged eyes (congenital glaucoma). An ocular trans-illuminator is placed against the posterior globe and directed towards the ciliary sulcus. In a darkened room, the diffuse illumination will demarcate the ciliary body, which can be marked externally (Sharkey & Murray, 1994).

3.7 810 nm diode laser endoscopic cyclophotocoagulation (ECP)

The laser unit for ECP (Endo Optiks, Little Silver, NJ) incorporates 1) a diode laser that emits 810 nm continuous-wave energy, 2) a 175W Xenon light source, 3) a Helium-Neon laser aiming beam, and 4) a video imaging and recording camera. All 4 optical elements are transmitted through a 18-gauge or 20-gauge fibre-optic probe, which is inserted into the eye. The optimal focus for the laser is 0.75 mm from the probe tip, and the endoscope provides a 70-degree field of view. The main unit is compact and portable with a maximum power output of 2.0 W. The laser power and the exposure duration (up to 9.99 seconds) are adjustable with the controls in the console. The foot pedal controls the laser firing, with the actual duration of each application determined by the exposure duration setting or by the pedal depression, whichever ends first. The 2 main approaches to reach the ciliary processes are via a limbal or a pars plana entry. The limbal approach is preferred to avoid the anterior vitrectomy and the associated risks for choroidal and retinal detachment. However, certain cases are more safely treated through the pars plana, for example, aphakic eyes with posterior synechiae limiting the access to the ciliary sulcus. In both situations, a retrobulbar block with lidocaine and bupivicaine is performed or general anaesthesia can be considered in selective cases. In the limbal approach, after dilation of the pupil with cyclopentolate 1% and phenylephrine 2.5%, a paracentesis is created and the anterior chamber is filled with viscoelastic agent, which is further used to expand the nasal posterior sulcus. This viscoelastic expansion of the posterior chamber allows for easier approach to the pars plicata with the ECP probe. A 2.2-mm keratome is then used to enter into the anterior chamber at the temporal limbus. After orientation of the probe image outside of the eye, the 18-gauge or 20-gauge endoprobe is inserted through the incision into the posterior sulcus. At this time, the ciliary processes are viewed on the monitor and treatment can begin. The laser is set at continuous-wave and power settings are 300 to 900 mW. Approximately a 180-degree span of ciliary processes is photocoagulated (more area can be treated if a curved probe is used). Laser energy is applied to each process until shrinkage and whitening occur. The ciliary processes are treated individually or in a "painting" fashion across multiple processes. If excessive energy is used, the process explodes with a "pop" sound due to bubble formation, leading to excessive inflammation and breakdown of the blood-aqueous barrier. After the nasal 180 degrees of ciliary processes are treated, a separate incision is created at the nasal limbus in a similar fashion as above. The temporal processes are then photocoagulated for a total of up to 360 degrees, if desired. Typically, 180 to 360 degrees are treated. Before closure of the wounds, the viscoelastic material is removed from the anterior chamber with irrigation and aspiration. In the pars plana approach, an infusion port is inserted through the inferior pars plana and 2 superior entries are created for vitrectomy and illumination. Only a limited anterior vitrectomy is performed to allow adequate and safe access to all of the ciliary processes. The ECP probe can be inserted through each superior entry for treatment of the opposite 180 degrees of processes. There may be a few superior processes that cannot be accessed because the entry ports are not exactly 180 degrees opposite to each other. Laser CPC is carried out with the same parameters and end points as described for the limbal approach. If the anterior segment surgeon has not had extensive experience in posterior segment surgery, assistance from a retinal surgeon should be sought for the establishment of the pars plana entry ports and the limited anterior vitrectomy. Risk of inadvertent choroidal and/or retinal detachment is a serious concern and should be minimized. In all patients, whether under local or general anaesthesia, retrobulbar bupivicaine is administered before or at end of the surgery to minimize postoperative pain. Sub-Tenon's injection of 1mL of triamcinolone (40 mg/mL) is also given for inflammation. On postoperative day 1, patients are placed on a regimen of topical antibiotics, steroids, nonsteroidal anti-inflammatory agents, cycloplegics, and their preoperative glaucoma medications except for miotics and prostaglandin analogues because these may exacerbate intraocular inflammation or its sequelae. Antibiotics are discontinued after 1 week, and the steroids, nonsteroidal anti-inflammatory agents, and cycloplegics are tapered as inflammation subsides. Glaucoma medications are removed according to the intraocular pressure (IOP) requirements. Administration of acetazolamide during the evening of surgery may be used to prevent a spike in IOP from underlying glaucoma, inflammation, or possible retained viscoelastic (Lin, 2008).

4. Published results

It is difficult if not impossible to compare studies that have different entry criteria and definitions of success. In fact, "success" in cyclophotocoagulation procedures has been defined as achieving IOP < 21 or 22 mmHg, and/or an IOP reduction of 20% or 30%; some study considered IOP < 5 mmHg as hypotony and, thus, a failure. Most studies allow the postoperative use of medications to achieve this definition of success.

4.1 Transscleral cyclophotocoagulation
4.1.1 1064 nm Nd:Yag Laser Non-Contact TSCPC

In a retrospective study, Youn et al. (Youn et al., 1996) reviewed 479 patients in a follow-up period of 3-75 months (mean 22 months). The range of laser energy settings was 4 to 8 J. Postoperative IOP was between 5 and 20 mmHg in 52% of the patients. Forty percent of the patients lost two or more Snellen visual acuity lines. Visual deterioration was significantly associated with neovascular glaucoma, African descent, post-treatment hypotony, and more than 6 months of follow-up. Phthisis was encountred in 14% of treated patients. Noncontact Nd:YAG cyclophotocoagulation enhances the risk of graft failure in patients with previous penetrating keratoplasty. In a prospective, unmasked randomized trial, Shields et al. (Shields et al., 1993) assigned two groups of 89 patients to two energy settings, 4 J (range 3.7 to 4.5 J) for the Group A and 8 J (range 7 to 8.5 J) for the Group B, with 30 applications utilizing a contact lens. Among the patients who did not require further surgery, better success (75% versus 60%) and fewer retreatments (25% versus 40%) were observed in the higher energy. Among those patients who received no further surgery, vision loss was 56% of patients in Group A (4 J) versus 42% of patients in group B (8 J). There was no significant difference between the two groups. Mean follow-up was 12.6 months, ranging from 5 to 20 months. Delgado et al. (2003) studied the results of Nd:YAG laser non-contact TSCPC on neovascular glaucoma. Mean follow-up was 27 months (range 1 – 148), 115 eyes were evaluated using 7.8 J energy setting (20 to 40 application over 270 degrees) and the success rate was 65%, 49.8% and 34.8% after 1, 3 and 6 years respectively. There were 11.5% phtisis and 39.1% eyes had a loss of two or more Snellen visual acuity lines. An interesting retrospective study (Ayyala et al., 1998) attempted to compare mitomycin C trabeculectomy, glaucoma drainage device (GDD) and Nd:YAG non-contact TSCPC in the glaucoma management after penetrating keratoplasty. This was a non-comparative case series with fewer than 20 patients in each group. Mean follow-up was 12.9 months. There was no statistically significant difference in successful IOP control between mitomycin C trabeculectomy (77% success), GDD (80% success), or non-contact TSCPC (63%). There was no significant difference in the rate of failure of the corneal graft following trabeculectomy (15%), GDD (0%), or TSCPC (17%) that compared fairly with the 11% to 65% failure rate of the corneal graft following glaucoma surgery reported in the literature. (Pastor et al., 2001). As the criteria for success varied in the different studies, it is not surprising that the rate of success spanned from 35% to 83%. The most common complications included the loss of two or more Snellen visual acuity lines in up to 40% of patients, phthisis in 0 to 14%, hyphema in 0 to 4%, and corneal oedema in 0 to 6% of patients. Sympathetic ophthalmia has also been reported as an extremely rare complication. (Bechrakis et al., 1994).

STUDY	LASER TYPE	GLAUCOMA	F-UP (mo)	N (eyes)	VA LOSS (%)	N. TREAT	POWER	DEGREES	N. SPOTS	SUCCESS (%)	SUCCESS CRITERIA
Delgado et al., 2003	nc YAG	neovascular	27	115	39	1,4	7,8 (J)	270	20-40	50	IOP<22; no pthysis; no further surgery
Youn et al., 1998	nc YAG	all	10,4	46	0	1,13	5,21 to 7,5 (J)	360	32	83	5<IOP<21
Shields et al., 1993	nc YAG	all	12	45	26	1	4 (J)	360	30	60	no additional glaucoma surgery
Shields et al., 1993	nc YAG	all	12	44	36	1	8 (J)	360	30	75	no additional glaucoma surgery
Youn et al., 1996	nc YAG	all	22	479	40	1	6 (J)	N/A	25	52	5<IOP<20
Lin et al., 2004	c YAG	all	67	68	16	1,4	7 to 9 (W)	360	32 - 40	60,3(1 yr.); 48,5 (10 yrs.)	3<IOP<25; no other TCP
Schuman et al., 1992	c YAG	all	19	116	31	1,27	7 to 9 (W)	N/A	32 - 40	65	3<IOP<22

Table 1. Nd: YAG Laser

4.1.2 1064 nm Nd:Yag laser contact TSCPC

There are fewer studies (see Table 1) reporting the use of Nd:YAG laser contact TSCPC than there are reporting non-contact TSCPC. Schuman et al. (Schuman et al., 1992) reported retrospectively on a series of 116 eyes of 114 patients with a mean follow-up of 1 year (range 6-19 months). Treatment consisted of 32 to 40 applications, for a total of 7 to 9 W of power delivered for 0.7 seconds. IOP control of 3 to 22 mmHg was achieved in 65% of eyes. Twenty-seven percent were retreated. Hypotony with less than 3 mmHg occurred in nine eyes, six of which were phthisical. Nineteen eyes (16%) lost light perception, and 47% of eyes with V.A. of 20/200 or better lost two or more Snellen visual acuity lines (17 of 36 eyes). Lin et al (Lin et al., 2004) in 2004 reported similar results about a series of 68 eyes with a mean follow-up of 5.58 years (range 0.1 – 10 years). Treatment consisted of 32 to 40 applications, for a total of 7 to 9 watts of power delivered for 0.7 seconds. Intraocular pressure control of 3 to 25 mmHg was achieved in 60 % of eyes after one year and in 48% after ten years with only one treatment. 40% of patient where retreated, and this has been considered a failure. Hypotony less than 3 mmHg was seen in 3 eyes, none of which were phthisical. Eleven eyes worsened their visual acuity.

4.1.3 810 Nm diode laser contact TSCPC

For a variety of reasons, mainly clinical effectiveness and practicality, 810 nm diode laser contact TSCPC has been universally adopted to the point to become the standard of care for specific conditions. As a result, there are more publications in the literature on 810nm diode TSCPC (see Table 2) than on any other CPC modality, although many of them are only retrospective. As indicated in Table 2, the mean number of eyes reported in the studies was 55.82 (SD =+/- 58.26) (Standard Deviation) eyes with a variety of diagnoses and of laser treatment parameters. Laser power ranged from 1.25 to 3 watts (mean 1.94 W) for a mean exposure time of 2.16 seconds, for a mean number of applications of 22.10 (SD=+/- 7.02) over 180 to 360 degrees, sometimes adjusting the power for pops and sometimes not. Mean follow-up was 19.86 months (SD=+/- 12.71). Mean success rate was 67.26% (SD=+/- 15.70), but this cannot be a good indicator, because the definition of success was heterogeneous (see Table 2). Mean number of medication was 2.52 (SD=+/- 0.63) pre-operatively and 1.62 (SD=+/- 0.71) post-operatively. Mean loss of visual acuity was 24.74% (SD=+/- 16.78). Retreatment rate was 1.48 (SD=+/- 0.45). Complications were, hypotony (0 to 25%), phthisis (0 to 11%), AS inflammation (0 to 27%), choroidal detachment (0 to 10%), cataract progression (0 to 40%), atonic pupil (0 to 70%) and hyphema (0 to 13%). Rarely reported complications were endophthalmitis, failure of corneal graft, CMO, bullous keratopathy, band keratopathy, persistent ocular pain. Rarely reported complications included necrotizing scleritis (Ganesh et al., 2006), scleral perforation (Kwong at al., 2005), iris retraction and retroflexion (Sony et al., 2003) and malignant glaucoma (Azuara-Blanco et al., 1999). Table 2 stratifies the outcomes among various types of glaucoma. In Neovascular Glaucoma success rate ranges from 40% to 64% with a mean follow up from 9 to 60 months; in Silicon Oil Glaucoma success rate ranges from 44% to 82% with a mean follow up from 4 to 22 months; in Pediatric Glaucoma success rate ranges from 67% to 72% with a mean follow up from 20 to 21 months; in Chronic Angle Closure Glaucoma (CACG) success rate ranges from 86% to 92% with a mean follow up from 12 to 26 months; and in Keratoprosthesis Glaucoma success rate is 66% with a mean follow up of 26.6 months. 810 nm Diode Laser Contact TSCPC has also been used in 49 eyes with a good visual acuity (20/60 or better).

STUDY	GLAUCOMA	F-UP (mo)	N (eyes)	N. TREAT	POWER (W)	TIME (s)	DEGREES	N. SPOTS	SUCCESS CRITERIA	SUCCESS (%)	VA LOSS (%)
Spencer et al., 1999	all	21,5	58	1,6	2,00	2	270	14	IOP <= 22	81	20,7
Yildirim et al., 2009	nv	24	33	1	1,50	2	270	17	5<IOP<21	61	18,2
Ghosh et al., 2010	nv	9	14	1	2,00	2	180-270	25	30% IOP reduction	64	21,4
Preussner et al., 2010	africans	6	75	N/A	5,00	0,2	360	20	N/A	N/A	N/A
Malik et al., 2006	all	35	28	2	2,12	2	360	24	6<IOP<21	64	46,4
Semchyshyn et al., 2002	all	26,9	21	1,38	2,00	2	270	21,9	5<IOP<=21	66	52,4
Schlote et al., 2000	inflammatory	12	22	2	2,00	2	270	12,5	5<IOP<21 in va>0,02 or IOP<30% in va<0,02	77,3	36,4
Rotchford et al., 2010	good vision	60	49	1,73	2,00	2	N/A	14,4	IOP<=21	89,8	61,2
Sood et al., 2009	pediatric	19,8	9	1	1,25	3,5	180-270	17,4	IOP<22;no complications; no further surgery	66,7	20,0
Kirwan et al., 2009	pediatric	21	77	2,3	1,50	1,5	300	40	IOP<22 or 30% IOP reduction	72	7,5
Lai et al., 2002	CACG	12	14	1,14	2,00	2	270	16,3	IOP < 21	85,7	0,0
Lai et al., 2005	CACG	26,5	13	1,15	2,00	2	270	17,5	IOP < 21	92,3	38,5
Han et al., 1999	silicon oil	12	11	1,18	2,00	2	360	23,5	IOP <=21	81,8	18,2
Agarwal et al., 2004	all types	15,8	30	1,2	1,50	2	360	40	IOP < 22	94	6,7
Rivier et al., 2009	keratoprotesis	26,6	18	1,3	1,87	2	270	17,5	lowering digital pressure	66	38,9
Noureddin et al., 2006	all	13,69	36	1,25	2,25	2	360	28	IOP<=21	72,2	22,2
Sivagnanavel et al., 2005	silicone oil glaucoma	21,8	18	1,5	2,00	1,5	180	25	IOP < 22	44	55,6
Egbert et al., 2001	all	13,2	40	1,22	1,50	1,5	360	20	IOP <=22	48	25,0
Egbert et al., 2001	all	13,2	39	1,22	1,25	2,5	360	20	20% IOP reduction	46	20,5

Table 2. (continues on next page) 810 nm diode laser contact TSCPC

STUDY	GLAUCOMA	F-UP (mo)	N (eyes)	N. TREAT	POWER (W)	TIME (s)	DEGREES	N. SPOTS	SUCCESS CRITERIA	SUCCESS (%)	VA LOSS (%)
Ansari et al., 2007	all	12,5	74	1,01	2,00	2	360	30	30% IOP reduction	82	13,0
Kaushik et al., 2008	all	14,3	66	1,16	2,00	2	270	18	5<IOP<22	78,8	4,5
Nabili et al., 2004	diabetic neovascular glaucoma	N/A	20	1,45	2,00	2	270	15	5<IOP<22	40	40,0
Kramp et al., 2002	all	13,9	193	1,3	1,60	2	360	27	10<IOP<22	76,4	N/A
Grueb et al., 2006	all	24	90	1,3	2,00	2	180	17,5	4<IOP<18; 20% IOP reduction	36,7	11,1
Iliev et al., 2007	all	30,1	131	1,54	2,00	2	270	22	6<IOP<21 or IOP reduction >30%	69,5	26,0
Schlote et al., 2007	aphakic and posttraumatic	42	46	2,58	2,00	2	180	20	5<IOP<21	43,8	63,0
Heinz et al., 2006	juvenile idiopathic arthritis	10,1	21	2,15	2,00	2	180	25	IOP<=21	32	14,3
Ocakoglu et al., 2005	all	11,4	32	1,68	2,50	2	270-300	22	IOP<=22	72	0,0
Murphy et al., 2003	all	17	263	1,5	N/A	N/A	N/A	N/A	5<IOP<22 or 30% IOP reduction	79,5	19,4
Walland, 1998	all	10,1	22	1	1,50	1,5	360	40	IOP<22	54,5	31,8
Walland, 1998	all	11,4	8	1	1,50	1,5	180	20	IOP<22	62,5	31,8
Frezzotti et al., 2010	all	17	124	1,26	2,00	2	180-270	15	5<IOP<21 or pain relief	67,3	12,9
Leszcynski et al., 2009	neovascular	60	30	2,4	1,75	10	270	17,5	N/A	N/A	10,0
Raivio et al., 2008	all	26	60	1,4	0,43	2	180	20	8<IOP<21	80	30,0
Gangwani et al., 2010	silicon oil	4	9	2,34	1,87	2	270	30	IOP<21	66,7	11,1
Youn et al., 1998	all	10,4	49	1,2	2,37	2	360	24,63	5<IOP<22	71	8,2
Brancato et al., 1995	all	20,7	68	N/A	2,60	2	360	18	2<IOP<=21	70,8	N/A

Table 2. (continued) 810 nm diode laser contact TSCPC

The success rate on pressure reduction (IOP <21) was 90%, but 60% of eyes lost 1 Snellen visual acuity line and 30% of the eyes lost more than 2 Snellen visual acuity lines. 810 nm Diode Laser Contact TSCPC has been compared to Ahmed Valve implantation by Yildirim et al. (Yildirim et al., 2009) who found a success rate of 61% for TSCPC vs. 59% for Ahmed Valve with a mean follow up of 24 months. In a similar study Sood et al (Sood et al., 2009) compared 810 nm Diode TSCPC to Ahmed Valve implantation in Pediatric Glaucoma and found a success rate of 66.7% for TSCPC vs 62.5% for Ahmed Valve with a mean follow up of 19.8 and 26.3 months respectively. Malik et al (Malik et al., 2006) compared 810 nm Diode TSCPC to Molteno tube shunt and found a success rate of 64% for TSCPC vs 81% for Molteno tube shunt with a mean follow up of 35 months. Youn et al (Youn et al., 1998) compared non-contact TSCPC with 1064 nm Nd:YAG and 810 nm diode lasers in a prospective, randomized, unmasked trial. Mean follow-up was 10.4 months. Success was 83% and 71% of the YAG and diode patients, respectively, (no statistically significant difference). Retreatment in the YAG group was lower (8.7%; 4/46) than the diode group (18%; 6/49). Although not statistically significant, the Nd:YAG group had a slightly higher success. In clinical practice the 1064 nm Nd:YAG laser in the free-running thermal mode is not commercially available anymore and most clinicians have elected to use the more compact and user-friendly 810 nm diode laser with the contact G-Probe. Agarwal et al (Agarwal et al., 2004) compared the 830 nm Diode Laser contact TSCPC to the 830 nm Diode Laser non-contact TSCPC 830 and found a success rate of 94% for Contact vs. 90% for Non-Contact after a mean follow up of 15.8 months. Although there is not a general agreement, most studies have found that the amount of energy used for 810 nm diode laser contact TSCPC seems to correlate with treatment success rate, without implying a higher complication or vision loss rate.

4.2 Endoscopic cyclophotocoagulation
4.2.1 810 Nm diode laser endoscopic cyclophotocoagulation (ECP)
810 nm diode laser ECP is a relatively new method for CPC, and this is reflected in the relatively smaller number of publications (see Table 3). It's very difficult to compare such studies because laser parameters are different or not well specified. In Table 3 we summarized six studies that evaluated a 33.3 mean number of patients (SD=+/- 18.3) range 12 - 68, with various types of glaucoma, including pediatric glaucoma, for a mean follow-up of 11.9 months (SD=+/- 5.5) range 4.5-21.3 and with different definition of success. Mean success rate was 59.1% (SD=+/- 23.7) range 17-82.9%. Mean pre- and post-operative number of medication was 2.2 (SD=+/- 0.5) and 1.5 (SD=+/- 0.5) respectively. Mean visual acuity loss of two or more Snellen lines was 9% (SD=+/- 8) range 0-22% and retreatment rate was 1.16 (SD=+/- 0.2). Complications were hypotony (0 to 8%), phthisis (0 to 3%), anterior segment inflammation (0 to 6%), hyphema (0 to 9%), and RD (0 to 8%). In pediatric glaucoma (refractory glaucoma with corneal opacities) the success rate (IOP <21mmHg without complication and further surgery) was 17% at 13 months of follow up. (Al-Haddad et al., 2007). The authors attributed the poor results to the surgical difficulties of refractory pediatric glaucoma. Lima et al (Lima et al., 2004) compared ECP to Ahmed Valve implantation in 6\8 patients and found a success rate of 73.5% vs 70.6% (p = 0.7) respectively (mean follow up of 21.3 and 19.8 months respectively). Complications were different: ECP reported more cases of hypotony, phthisis, anterior segment inflammation, while Ahmed valve reported more cases of endophthalmitis, choroidal detachment and

STUDY	GLAUCOMA	F-UP (mo)	N (eyes)	VA LOSS (%)	N. TREAT	DEGREES	SUCCESS (%)	SUCCESS CRITERIA
Lima et al., 2004	all	21,3	68	9	1	210	73,5	6<IOP<21
Yip et al., 2009	all	15,9	29	17	1	270	48,3	IOP<20%, no medications added
Kahook et al., 2007 (1 site)	all	4,5	15	0	1	240-300	47	IOP reduction of 3 mmHg at least; 1 medication reduction
Kahook et al., 2007 (2 sites)	all	4,5	25	0	1	240-300	92	IOP reduction of 3 mmHg at least; 1 medication reduction
Al-Haddad et al., 2007	pediatric	13,0	12	8	1,17	270	17	IOP<=21; no complications; no further surgery
Carter et al., 2007	aphakic and pseudophakic children	12	34	N/A	1,8	180-270	53	IOP<24; no complications; no further surgery
Murty et al., 2009	all	12,3	50	22	N/A	270-360	82,9	IOP<22

Table 3. 810 nm diode laser ECP

retinal detachment. Kahook et al (Kahook et al., 2007) compared 2-incision ECP to 1-incision ECP, finding a success rate of 92% for 2-incision vs. 47% for 1-incision. No major complications have been reported.

5. Personal considerations and role of anti-VEGF and panfotocoagulation

We personally have experience with cyclocryotherapy, contact diode TSCP and ciliary ablation with ultrasound. We long ago abandoned the US ciliary ablation due to the difficulties of the treatment and some serious adverse events related to the difficulty of centering the ultrasound beam exactly on the ciliary body. We are not using anymore cyclocryotherapy mainly because of the inflammatory processes related to this method. Inflammatory processes might be present with diode laser TSCP as well if the treatment is not titrated. We are very concerned of possible adverse events related to cycloddestruction and with the diode laser we prefer to stay on the safe side at the eventual price of retreatment rather than risk serious complications. Our current protocol with the diode laser is to treat 180 degrees using the G-probe. The time is pre-set at 2 seconds and we generally start with a 1800 mW power. We increase the power until a bob can be appreciated and then we decrease the power by 100 mW and we continue the treatment. We pay a lot of attention to keep the probe strongly pressed on the globe in order to achieve a better conduction through the sclera. The number of applications is titrated on the basis of the IOP level and on the type of glaucoma. We generally give more applications if the IOP is elevated with the exception of uveitic and neovascular glaucoma where we never apply as first treatment more than 14 applications, because we fear that in this forms of secondary glaucoma there might coexist a lower acqueous production. Concerning the use of anti-VEGF, Although there are several reports that claim a resolution of IOP elevation, we cannot confirm these findings. Probably the patients that come to our Department present long standing forms of iris neovascularisation. Although some of our patients did not present a complete angle occlusion at gonioscopy, we never had a complete normalization of IOP by using intravitreal injections. In a few cases intravitreal ant-VEGF injection, nevertheless, allowed for a partial recovery of the glaucoma with some clearing of the cornea, which allowed us for starting a pan-retinal photocoagulation. Retinal cryotherapy is always added whenever the panretinal photocoagulation is impossible due to corneal decompensation, cataract or vitreous hemorrage.

6. Summary

Both 810 nm diode laser TSCPC and ECP are effective procedures for the treatment of refractory glaucoma. TSCPC is an extra-ocular procedure that has mainly been used in eyes that had received prior filtration surgeries or that had very limited visual potential. However, more recently, there has been a trend toward using 810 nm diode laser TSCPC as the primary surgery in eyes with relatively good vision. ECP is an intra-ocular surgery that has also been used as a primary procedure, often combined with phacoemulsification cataract extraction, but should probably be considered almost exclusively in eyes that have good potential vision. These relative indications for each type of CPC are guided by the possible complications of each procedure. TSCPC is a "blind" procedure that has significant rates of success, but also hypotony and/or phthisis, which may relate to its external approach. Greater energy is generally required to penetrate the sclera as compared with the

STUDY	PROCEDURE	GLAUCOMA	F-UP (mo)	N (eyes)	VA LOSS (%)	N. TREAT	POWER (J)	DEGREES	N. SPOTS	SUCCESS (%)	SUCCESS CRITERIA
Yildirim et al., 2009	TCP diode vs	neovascular	24	33	18	1	>1,5	270	17	61,2	5<IOP<21, no further surgery
Yildirim et al., 2009	ahmed valve	neovascular	24	33	27	N/A	N/A	N/A	N/A	59,2	5<IOP<21, no further surgery
Malik et al., 2006	TCP diode vs	all	35	28	46	2	1,75 - 2,5	360	24	64	6<IOP<21
Malik et al., 2006	molteno tube	all	35	26	54	N/A	N/A	N/A	N/A	81	6<IOP<21
Sood et al., 2009	TCP diode vs	pediatric	19,8	9	20	1	1 - 1,5	180-270	17	66,7	IOP<22, no complications; no further surgery
Sood et al., 2009	ahmed valve	pediatric	26,3	8	75	N/A	N/A	N/A	N/A	75 (12mo); 62,5 (24mo)	IOP<22, no complications; no further surgery
Agarwal et al., 2004	C TCP diode 830 nm vs.	all	15,8	30	6	1,2	1,5	360	40	94	IOP < 22
Agarwal et al., 2004	NC TCPdiode 830 nm	all	15,8	30	6	1,6	1,5	360	40	90	IOP < 23
Youn et al., 1998	TCP YAG vs.	all	10,4	46	0	1,13	5,21 - 7,5	360	32	83	5<IOP<21
Youn et al., 1998	TCP diode	all	10,4	49	8	1,2	1,75 - 3	360	25	71	5<IOP<22

Table 4. Comparing procedures

endoscopic approach. EPC allows the photocoagulation of the ciliary processes under direct visualization, but can also lead to the overtreatment of the ciliary tissues and surrounded structures, including the vascular structure of ciliary process, the pars plana, and the iris root, all of which may potentially predispose to phthisis or hypotony. The major disadvantage of ECP is that it is an intra-ocular procedure. Endophthalmitis, choroidal haemorrhage, and retinal detachment are rare, but remain potential serious complications. New transscleral 810 nm laser applications over the pars plana with a new micropulse laser emission mode, have been reported to result in effective IOP lowering, while avoiding most collateral problems of 810 nm continuous wave diode laser TSCPC and EPC (Tan et al., 2010).

7. References

Agarwal, H.C.; Gupta, V. & Sihota, R. (2004). Evaluation of contact versus non-contact diode laser cyclophotocoagulation for refractory glaucomas using similar energy settings. *Clin Experiment Ophthalmol.* Feb; 32(1):33-8.

Ansari, E. & Gandhewar, J. (2007). Long-term efficacy and visual acuity following transscleral diode laser photocoagulation in cases of refractory and non-refractory glaucoma. *Eye (Lond).* Jul; 21(7):936-40.

Ayyala, RS.; Pieroth, L.; Vinals, AF.; et al. (1998). Comparison of mitomycin C trabeculectomy, glaucoma drainage device implantation, and laser neodymium: YAG cyclophotocoagulation in the management of intractable glaucoma after penetrating keratoplasty. *Ophthalmology.* 105:1550–6.

Azuara-Blanco, A. & Dua, H.S. (1999). Malignant glaucoma after diode laser cyclophotocoagulation. *Am J Ophthalmol.* Apr; 127(4):467-9.

Bartamian, M. & Higginbotham, E.J. (2001). What is on the horizon for cycloablation? *Curr Opin Ophthalmol.* Apr; 12(2):119-23. Review.

Bechrakis, N.E.; Müller-Stolzenburg, N.W. ; Helbig, H. & Foerster, M.H. (1994). Sympathetic ophthalmia following laser cyclocoagulation. *Arch Ophthalmol.* Jan; 112(1):80-4. PubMed PMID: 8285899.

Bietti, G. (1950). Surgical intervention on the ciliary body: new trends for the relief of glaucoma. *JAMA.* 142:889–897.

Brancato, R.; Carassa, R.G.; Bettin, P.; Fiori, M. & Trabucchi, G. (1995). Contact transscleral cyclophotocoagulation with diode laser in refractory glaucoma. *Eur J Ophthalmol.* Jan-Mar; 5(1):32-9.

Carter, B.C.; Plager, D.A. Neely, D.E.; Sprunger, D.T.; Sondhi, N. & Roberts, G.J. (2007). Endoscopic diode laser cyclophotocoagulation in the management of aphakic and pseudophakic glaucoma in children. *J AAPOS.* Feb; 11(1):34-40.

Coleman, D.J.; Lizzi, F.L.; Driller, J. et al. (1985). Therapeutic ultrasound in the treatment of glaucoma. I. Experimental model. *Ophthalmology* 92:339–46.

Delgado, M.F.; Dickens, C.J.; Iwach, A.G.; Novack, G.D.; Nychka, D.S.; Wong, P.C. & Nguyen, N. (2003). Long-term results of noncontact neodymium:yttrium-aluminum-garnet cyclophotocoagulation in neovascular glaucoma. *Ophthalmology.* May; 110(5):895-9.

Egbert, P.R.; Fiadoyor, S.; Budenz, D.L. et al. (2001). Diode laser transscleral cyclophotocoagulation as a primary surgical treatment for primary open-angle glaucoma. *Arch Ophthalmol.* 119:345–50.

Frezzotti, P.; Mittica, V.; Martone, G.; Motolese, I.; Lomurno, L.; Peruzzi, S. & Motolese, E. (2010). Longterm follow-up of diode laser transscleral cyclophotocoagulation in the treatment of refractory glaucoma. *Acta Ophthalmol.* Feb; 88(1):150-5.

Ganesh, S.K. & Rishi, K. (2006). Necrotizing scleritis following diode laser trans-scleral cyclophotocoagulation. *Indian J Ophthalmol.* Sep; 54(3):199-200.

Gangwani, R.; Liu, D.T.; Congdon, N.; Lam, P.T.; Lee, V.Y.; Yuen, N.S. & Lam, D.S. (2011). Effectiveness of diode laser trans-scleral cyclophotocoagulation in patients following silicone oil-induced ocular hypertension in Chinese eyes. *Indian J Ophthalmol.* Jan-Feb; 59(1):64-6.

Ghosh, S.; Singh, D.; Ruddle, J.B.; Shiu, M.; Coote, M.A. & Crowston, J.G. (2010). Combined diode laser cyclophotocoagulation and intravitreal bevacizumab (Avastin) in neovascular glaucoma. *Clin Experiment Ophthalmol.* May; 38(4):353-7.

Grueb, M.; Rohrbach, J.M.; Bartz-Schmidt, K.U. & Schlote, T. (2006). Transscleral diode laser cyclophotocoagulation as primary and secondary surgical treatment in primary open-angle and pseudoexfoliatve glaucoma. Long-term clinical outcomes. *Graefes Arch Clin Exp Ophthalmol.* Oct; 244(10):1293-9.

Han, S.K.; Park, K.H.; Kim, D.M. & Chang, B.L. (1999). Effect of diode laser trans-scleral cyclophotocoagulation in the management of glaucoma after intravitreal silicone oil injection for complicated retinal detachments. *Br J Ophthalmol.* Jun; 83(6):713-7.

Heinz, C.; Koch, J.M. & Heiligenhaus, A. (2006). Transscleral diode laser cyclophotocoagulation as primary surgical treatment for secondary glaucoma in juvenile idiopathic arthritis: high failure rate after short term follow up. *Br J Ophthalmol.* Jun; 90(6):737-40.

Iliev, M.E. & Gerber, S. (2007). Long-term outcome of trans-scleral diode laser cyclophotocoagulation in refractory glaucoma. *Br J Ophthalmol.* Dec; 91(12):1631-5.

Kahook, M.Y.; Lathrop, K.L. & Noecker, R.J. (2007). One-site versus two-site endoscopic cyclophotocoagulation. *J Glaucoma.* Sep; 16(6):527-30.

Kaushik, S.; Pandav, S.S.; Jain, R.; Bansal, S. & Gupta, A. (2008). Lower energy levels adequate for effective transcleral diode laser cyclophotocoagulation in Asian eyes with refractory glaucoma. *Eye (Lond).* Mar; 22(3):398-405.

Kirwan, J.F.; Shah, P. & Khaw, P.T. (2002). Diode laser cyclophotocoagulation: role in the management of refractory pediatric glaucomas. *Ophthalmology.* Feb; 109(2):316-23.

Kramp, K.; Vick, H.P. & Guthoff, R. (2002). Transscleral diode laser contact cyclophotocoagulation in the treatment of different glaucomas, also as primary surgery. *Graefes Arch Clin Exp Ophthalmol.* Sep; 240(9):698-703.

Kwong, Y.Y.; Tham, C.C.; Leung, D.Y. & Lam, D.S. (2006). Scleral perforation following diode laser trans-scleral cyclophotocoagulation. *Eye (Lond).* Nov; 20(11):1316-7.

Lai, J.S.; Tham, C.C.; Chan, J.C. & Lam, D.S. (2003). Diode laser transscleral cyclophotocoagulation in the treatment of chronic angle-closure glaucoma: a preliminary study. *J Glaucoma.* Aug; 12(4):360-4.

Lai, J.S.; Tham, C.C.; Chan, J.C. & Lam, D.S. (2005). Diode laser transscleral cyclophoto-coagulation as primary surgical treatment for medically uncontrolled chronic angle closure glaucoma: long-term clinical outcomes. *J Glaucoma.* Apr; 14(2):114-9.

Lee, R.M.; Al Raqqad, N.; Gomaa, A.; Steel, D.H.; Bloom, P.A. & Liu, C.S. (2011). Endoscopic cyclophotocoagulation in osteo-odonto-keratoprosthesis (OOKP) eyes. *J Glaucoma.* Jan; 20(1):68-9; author reply 69.

Leszczyński, R.; Domański, R.; Formińska-Kapuścik, M.; Mrukwa-Kominek, E. & Rokita-Wala, I. (2009). Contact transscleral cyclophotocoagulation in the treatment of neovascular glaucoma: a five-year follow-up. *Med Sci Monit.* Mar; 15(3):BR84-7.

Lima, F.E.; Magacho, L.; Carvalho, D.M.; Susanna, R. Jr., & Avila, M.P. (2004). A prospective, comparative study between endoscopic cyclophotocoagulation and the Ahmed drainage implant in refractory glaucoma. *J Glaucoma*. Jun; 13(3):233-7.

Lin, P.; Wollstein, G.; Glavas, I.P. et al. (2004). Contact transscleral neodymium:yttrium-aluminum-garnet laser cyclophotocoagulation long-term outcome. *Ophthalmology*. 111:2137-2143. [Erratum in: *Ophthalmology*. 2005; 112:446.]

Lin, P.; Wollstein, G.; Glavas, I.P. & Schuman, J.S. (2005). Contact transscleral neodymium:yttrium-aluminum-garnet laser cyclophotocoagulation Long-term outcome. *Ophthalmology*. Nov; 111(11):2137-43. [Erratum in: Ophthalmology. 2005 Mar; 112(3):446.]

Lin, S.C. (2008). Endoscopic and transscleral cyclophotocoagulation for the treatment of refractory glaucoma. *J Glaucoma*. Apr-May; 17(3):238-47. Review.

Malik, R.; Ellingham, R.B.; Suleman, H. & Morgan, W.H. (2006). Refractory glaucoma--tube or diode? *Clin Experiment Ophthalmol*. Nov; 34(8):771-7.

Murphy, C.C.; Burnett, C.A.; Spry, P.G.; Broadway, D.C. & Diamond, J.P. (2003). A two centre study of the dose-response relation for transscleral diode laser cyclophotocoagulation in refractory glaucoma. *Br J Ophthalmol*. Oct; 87(10):1252-7.

Murthy, G.J.; Murthy, P.R.; Murthy, K.R.; Kulkarni, V.V. & Murthy, K.R. (2009). A study of the efficacy of endoscopic cyclophotocoagulation for the treatment of refractory glaucomas. *Indian J Ophthalmol*. Mar-Apr; 57(2):127-32.

Nabili, S. & Kirkness, C.M. (2004). Trans-scleral diode laser cyclophoto-coagulation in the treatment of diabetic neovascular glaucoma. *Eye (Lond)*. Apr; 18(4):352-6.

Noureddin, B.N.; Zein, W.; Haddad, C.; Ma'luf, R. & Bashshur, Z. (2006). Diode laser transscleral cyclophotocoagulation for refractory glaucoma: a 1 year follow-up of patients treated using an aggressive protocol. *Eye (Lond)*. Mar; 20(3):329-35.

Ocakoglu, O.; Arslan, O.S. & Kayiran, A. (2005). Diode laser transscleral cyclophotocoagulation for the treatment of refractory glaucoma after penetrating keratoplasty. *Curr Eye Res*. Jul; 30(7):569-74.

Pastor, S.A.; Singh, K.; Lee, D.A.; Juzych, M.S.; Lin, S.C.; Netland, P.A. & Nguyen, N.T. (2001). Cyclophotocoagulation: a report by the American Academy of Ophthalmology. Ophthalmology. 2001 Nov; 108(11):2130-8.

Preussner, P.R.; Ngounou, F. & Kouogan, G. (2010). Controlled cyclophotocoagulation with the 940 nm laser for primary open angle glaucoma in African eyes. *Graefes Arch Clin Exp Ophthalmol*. Oct; 248(10):1473-9. Epub 2010 May 2.

Raivio, V.E.; Immonen, I.J. & Puska, P.M. (2001). Transscleral contact krypton laser cyclophotocoagulation for treatment of glaucoma in children and young adults. *Ophthalmology*. Oct; 108(10):1801-7.

Raivio, V.E.; Puska, P.M. & Immonen, I.J. (2008). Cyclophotocoagulation with the transscleral contact red 670-nm diode laser in the treatment of glaucoma. *Acta Ophthalmol*. Aug; 86(5):558-64.

Rivier, D.; Paula, J.S.; Kim, E.; Dohlman, C.H. & Grosskreutz, C.L. (2009). Glaucoma and keratoprosthesis surgery: role of adjunctive cyclophotocoagulation. *J Glaucoma*. Apr-May; 18(4):321-4.

Rotchford, A.P.; Jayasawal, R.; Madhusudhan, S.; Ho, S.; King, A.J. & Vernon, S.A. (2010). Transscleral diode laser cycloablation in patients with good vision. *Br J Ophthalmol*. Sep; 94(9):1180-3.

Schlote, T.; Derse, M. & Zierhut, M. (2000). Transscleral diode laser cyclophotocoagulation for the treatment of refractory glaucoma secondary to inflammatory eye diseases. *Br J Ophthalmol*. Sep; 84(9):999-1003.

Schlote, T.; Grüb, M. & Kynigopoulos, M. (2008). Long-term results after transscleral diode laser cyclophotocoagulation in refractory posttraumatic glaucoma and glaucoma in aphakia. *Graefes Arch Clin Exp Ophthalmol.* Mar; 246(3):405-10.

Schuman, J.S.; Bellows, A.R.; Shingleton, B.J. & al. (1992). Contact transscleral Nd:YAG laser cyclophotocoagulation. Midterm results. *Ophthalmology.* 99:1089–94; discussion 1095.

Semchyshyn, T.M.; Tsai, J.C. & Joos, K.M. (2002). Supplemental transscleral diode laser cyclophotocoagulation after aqueous shunt placement in refractory glaucoma. *Ophthalmology.* Jun; 109(6):1078-84.

Sharkey, J.A. & Murray, T.G. (1994). Identification of the ora serrata and ciliary body by transillumination in eyes undergoing transscleral fixation of posterior chamber intraocular lenses [letter]. *Ophthalmic Surg.* 25:479–80.

Shields, M.B.; Wilkerson, M.H. & Echelman, D.A. (1993). A comparison of two energy levels for noncontact transscleral neodymium-YAG cyclophotocoagulation. *Arch Ophthalmol.* Apr; 111(4):484-7.

Sivagnanavel, V.; Ortiz-Hurtado, A. & Williamson, T.H. (2005). Diode laser trans-scleral cyclophotocoagulation in the management of glaucoma in patients with long-term intravitreal silicone oil. *Eye (Lond).* Mar; 19(3):253-7.

Sony, P.; Sudan, R.; Pangtey, M.S.; Khokhar, S. & Kumar, H. (2003). Iris retraction and retroflexion after transscleral contact diode laser photocoagulation. *Ophthalmic Surg Lasers Imaging.* Nov-Dec; 34(6):470-1.

Sood, S. & Beck, A.D. (2009). Cyclophotocoagulation versus sequential tube shunt as a secondary intervention following primary tube shunt failure in pediatric glaucoma. *J AAPOS.* Aug; 13(4):379-83.

Spencer, A.F. & Vernon SA. (1999). "Cyclodiode": results of a standard protocol. *Br J Ophthalmol.* Mar; 83(3):311-6.

Tan, A.M.; Chockalingam, M.; Aquino, M.C.; Lim, Z.I.; See, J.L. & Chew, P.T. (2010). Micropulse transscleral diode laser cyclophotocoagulation in the treatment of refractory glaucoma. *Clin Experiment Ophthalmol.* Apr; 38(3):266-72.

Vogt, A. (1936). Versuche zur intraokularen druckherabsetzung mittelst diathermieschädigung des corpus ciliare (Zyklodiathermiestichelung). *Klin Monatsbl Augenheilkd.* 97:672–3.

Walland, M.J. (1998). Diode laser cyclophotocoagulation: dose-standardized therapy in end-stage glaucoma. *Aust N Z J Ophthalmol.* May; 26(2):135-9.

Wilensky, J.T. & Kammer, J. (2004). Long-term visual outcome of transscleral laser cyclotherapy in eyes with ambulatory vision. *Ophthalmology.* Jul; 111(7):1389-92.

Yildirim, N.; Yalvac, I.S.; Sahin, A.; Ozer, A. & Bozca, T. (2009). A comparative study between diode laser cyclophotocoagulation and the Ahmed glaucoma valve implant in neovascular glaucoma: a long-term follow-up. *J Glaucoma.* Mar; 18(3):192-6.

Yip, L.W.; Yong, S.O.; Earnest, A.; Ji, J. & Lim, B.A. (2009). Endoscopic cyclophotocoagulation for the treatment of glaucoma: an Asian experience. *Clin Experiment Ophthalmol.* Sep; 37(7):692-7.

Youn, J.; Cox, T.A.; Allingham, R.R. & Shields, M.B. (1996). Factors associated with visual acuity loss after noncontact transscleral Nd:YAG cyclophotocoagulation. *J Glaucoma.* 5:390–4.

Youn, J.; Cox, T.A.; Herndon, L.W.; et al. (1998). A clinical comparison of transscleral cyclophotocoagulation with neodymium: YAG and semiconductor diode lasers. *Am J Ophthalmol.* 126: 640–7.

Part 2

Clinical Concepts – Specific Glaucoma Entities

9

Congenital Glaucoma

Jair Giampani Junior and Adriana Silva Borges Giampani
Federal University of Mato Grosso,
Brazil

1. Introduction

1.1 Terminology, epidemiology and heredity

Congenital glaucoma is a major cause of blindness in children, despite its low incidence (1:10,000 births)[1]. This category includes isolated congenital glaucoma (also called primary congenital glaucoma) and glaucomas associated with other developmental anomalies, either systemic or ocular.

Juvenile glaucoma is the term used to designate cases in which the pressure rise develops after the third birthday but before the age of 16 years.[2] The enlargement of the eye (buphthalmos) is least common, despite the elevated intraocular pressure. Gonioscopy is normal or reveals trabeculodysgenesis. This condition may simulate the primary open-angle glaucoma.

The eyes with primary congenital glaucoma have an isolated maldevelopment of the trabecular meshwork not associated with others developmental ocular anomalies or ocular diseases that can raise intraocular pressure. It's most common glaucoma of infancy, occurring in about 1: 30,000 live births[1].

Primary congenital glaucoma is a bilateral disease in about 75% of cases, with males accounting for approximately 65% of cases. [2] Most cases are sporadic in occurrence, with no evident hereditary pattern. In approximately 10% in which a hereditary pattern is evident, it generally is believed to be autosomal recessive. Many authors believe the inheritance pattern is polygenic.[1]

1.2 Pathogenesis

Clinical evidence supports the theory that the obstruction to aqueous flow, with a resultant increase in intraocular pressure, is located at the trabecular sheets. This obstruction is caused by maldevelopment of the anterior chamber angle, unassociated with any other major ocular anomalies (isolated trabeculodysgenesis).[2]

Clinically, trabeculodysgenesis is characterized by absence of the angle recess, with the iris inserted into the surface of the trabeculum in one of two configurations:[2]

a. Flat iris insertion: the iris inserts flatly into the thickened trabeculum at or anterior to the scleral spur.
b. Concave iris insertion: is less common. The plane of the iris is well posterior to the normal position of the scleral spur. However, the anterior iris stroma continues upward and over the trabecular meshwork, obscuring the scleral spur and the others angular structures.

1.3 Clinical presentation

Frequently, the first symptoms of primary congenital glaucoma are epiphora, photophobia and blepharospasm. These symptoms occur secondary to the corneal epithelial edema caused by elevated intraocular pressure.

The elevated intraocular pressure also causes an enlargement of the eye (buphthalmos) (Figure 1), mainly at the corneoscleral junction. Stretching of the zonules can cause lens subluxation.[3]

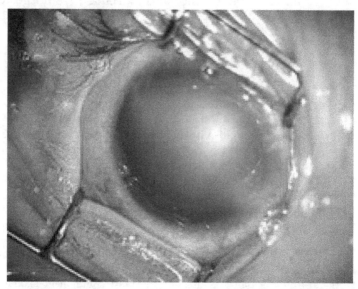

Fig. 1. Buphthalmos and corneal edema (Courtesy Prof. Augusto Paranhos Jr.)

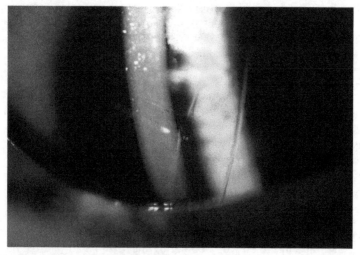

Fig. 2. Haab's striae (Courtesy Prof. Ernst Oltrogge)

As the cornea stretches, ruptures of the Descemet´s membrane allow influx of aqueous into the corneal stroma and epithelium, causing an increase in edema and haze. The breaks in Descemet´s membrane (Haab´s striae - Figure 2) are single or multiples, and appear as elliptical parallel ridges on the posterior cornea.[3] The Haab's striae are usually horizontal or oblique in contrast to traumatic Descemet's tears that are vertically oriented. Progressive myopia may occur if the elevated intraocular pressure persists.

Pain is unusual in the older child with glaucoma, unless corneal erosion or ulceration appear.

In contrast to the adult eye, the scleral canal in the infant eye enlarges as part of the generalized enlargement of the globe, and the lamina cribrosa may bow posteriorly, in response to elevated intraocular pressure. Therefore, cup size may be increased from neuronal loss, enlargement of the scleral canal, or both.[2]

1.4 Initial evaluation and follow-up (Flowchart 1)

Depending on the patient's age and ability to cooperate, either an office examination or an examination using general anesthesia with intravenous ketamine is required to evaluate the child with glaucoma.[3]

Examination of the corneal diameter should be undertaken first, followed by applanation tonometry, slit lamp examination, gonioscopy and evaluation of the optic discs.

a. corneal diameter should be measured in both vertical and horizontal meridians with calipers. The horizontal diameter is usually easier to measure and more accurate than the vertical, due an excessive corneal limbus stretching in this meridian. A diameter > 12 mm prior to the age of one year should be viewed with suspicion.[4]

b. Intraocular pressure could be measure with a Goldmann tonometer, Perkins tonometer or Tono-Pen. Elevated intraocular pressure by itself, unless extreme, is not sufficient to confirm a diagnosis of glaucoma. It is necessary to depend on signs such as increased corneal diameter and corneal thickness, increased cup-disc ratio or evidence of trabeculodysgenesis to confirms the diagnosis.

    The normal intraocular pressure in children under general anesthesia is unknown. Some authors consider glaucoma suspects children with IOP above 14 mm Hg.[4] Nevertheless, its important to remember the major of anesthetics reduces the intraocular pressure, while ketamine may increase intraocular pressure.[4]

c. The slit lamp examination may reveal corneal edema, haze and ruptures of the Descemet´s membrane (Haab´s striae). The anterior chamber is deep, with iris hypoplasia sometimes showing the iris pigment epithelium.[4] Stretching of the zonules can cause lens subluxation.

d. Gonioscopy should be performed with a Koeppe lens or one of the others goniolenses. Gonioscopy of the eye with congenital glaucoma reveals an anterior insertion of the iris directly into the trabecular meshwork. This insertion most commonly is flat (Figure 3), although a concave insertion may also be seen. The level of the iris insertion may vary at different areas of the angle. No pigment band is present, but a thin section of ciliary body can be seen through the thickened trabeculum. The peripheral iris may show a thinning of the anterior stroma.

e. Opthalmoscopy of the eye with congenital glaucoma may be impossible in some cases, due corneal edema and/or haze. The infant glaucomatous cup usually has a configuration different from that of an adult glaucomatous cup. It's more commonly round, steep walled and central.[1] The cup tends to enlarge circumferentially with progression of the glaucoma. In the very young, cupping can decrease after intraocular pressure is brought under control. To provide records for future comparison, it is best to take photographs of the optic nerve head, whenever possible.

f.   Auxiliary exams: the measurement of axial length by A-scan ultrasonography has been recommended by some authors for routine use in the diagnosis and follow-up of congenital glaucoma.[4] The eyes with congenital glaucoma commonly present an elevated axial length due the elevated intraocular pressure.

Fig. 3. Gonioscopy showing the flat iris configuration (Courtesy Prof. Augusto Paranhos Jr.)

The standard automated perimetry may be useful in the diagnosis and follow-up of congenital glaucoma patients above 7 years old.[4] Unfortunately, there is not adequate software to analyze children in any automated perimeters.

Patients with congenital glaucoma require follow-up examinations for life. The IOP measure, ophthalmoscopy and visual field analysis, when it is possible, must be realized at least every 3 to 6 months, depending the glaucoma severity. The long-term prognosis for intraocular pressure control in successfully treated cases of congenital glaucoma appears excellent. However, the visual outcome and IOP control in unsuccessfully treated cases after one or two surgical procedures, may be poor.

1.5 Differential diagnosis

Many conditions may confuse the primary congenital glaucoma diagnosis and present corneal edema, epiphora, corneal enlargement or elevated intraocular pressure. [2]

a.   Cloudy cornea at birth: trauma with breaks in the Descemet´s membrane, intrauterine rubella, metabolic disorders (mucopolysaccharidoses) and congenital hereditary endothelial dystrophy.

b.   Corneal enlargement: megalocornea and high myopia.

c.   Epiphora: congenital obstruction of the nasolacrimal duct.

d.   Secondary infantile glaucoma: trauma, ectopia lentis, uveitis, tumors, retinopathy of prematurity and persistent hyperplastic primary vitreous, corticosteroid-related glaucoma.

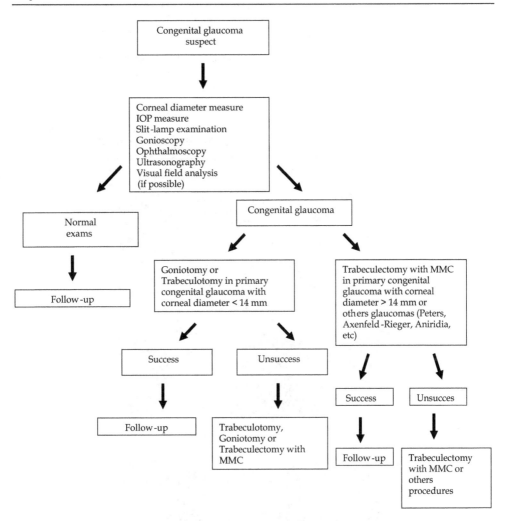

Flowchart 1. congenital glaucoma management and follow-up

1.6 Management

Congenital glaucoma is essentially a surgical disease, in which surgery must be performed as early as possible. Goniotomy and trabeculotomy are usually the first procedures of choice (Flowchart 1).[1] Both are safe and have a low incidence of complications. Factors that can decrease the success rate of initial trabeculotomy are the association of CG with others ocular anomalies (Peters, Sturge-Weber, Aniridia, etc.) and a corneal diameter of > 14 mm.[2] Usually, trabeculectomy is the option when previous goniotomies or trabeculotomies failed. Glaucoma drainage implants, non-penetrating surgery and cyclodestructive procedures are options also.

Surgery is preferred for several reasons, including problems with compliance to medications, lack of knowledge about the systemic effects of medications in the infant and poor response to clinical treatment in infants. Moreover, surgery has a high success rate and low incidence of complications.

Neither goniotomy nor trabeculotomy should be performed by surgeons inexperienced with the procedure. The first operation, whether goniotomy or trabeculotomy, has the greatest chance of success.

a) Goniotomy

Goniotomy is a very safe procedure when performed skillfully. Goniotomy is commonly the procedure of choice when corneal transparency permits adequate visualization of the angle (Figures 4 and 5). Corneal clouding only rarely prevents performance of goniotomy, particularly if cloudy epithelium is removed.[4]

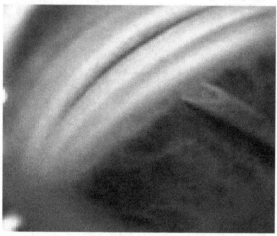

Fig. 4. Goniotomy (Courtesy Prof. Augusto Paranhos Jr.)

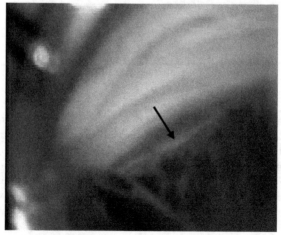

Fig. 5. Goniotomy: see the iris configuration after incision (arrow) (Courtesy Prof. Augusto Paranhos Jr.)

It is necessary a goniolenses, like the Worst lens, to performed the goniotomy through direct visualization of the angle.

Shaffer[5] reported in a study on a series of 287 eyes, one or two goniotomies cured 94% of patients diagnosed between 1 month and 24 months of age. Goniotomy is unlikely to be effective if corneal diameter exceeds 14 mm, since in such eyes the Schlemm´s canal is obliterated.[2]

b) Trabeculotomy

Trabeculotomy may be necessary if corneal clouding prevents visualization of the angle (Figures 6 and 7). It was described initially by Burian in 1964, and posteriorly improved by Harms and Machensen.[4]

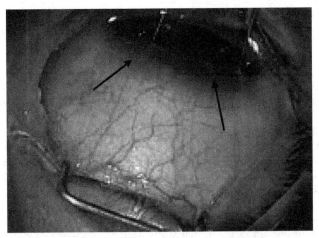

Fig. 6. Trabeculotomy: see the enlargement of the corneoscleral junction (arrows) (Courtesy Prof. Augusto Paranhos Jr.)

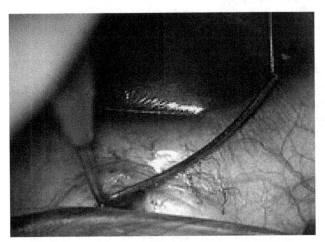

Fig. 7. Trabeculotomy: see the trabeculotome position (Courtesy Prof. Augusto Paranhos Jr.)

Trabeculotomy also has a high success rate, with most studies citing an 80% to 90% success rate.[6] The incidence of complications is low, and includes hyphema, tears in Descemet´s membrane, ciclodialysis, iridodialysis and synechiae.[3]

c) Update in trabeculectomy in congenital glaucoma

Usually, trabeculectomy is the option when previous goniotomies or trabeculotomies failed. It has been reported that trabeculectomy without adjunctive antimetabolites in pediatric patients (less than 18 years of age) has a successful outcome in 30 % to 50% of cases.[7-9] The 50% rate is from a study with relatively short follow-up (mean 15.5 months).[7] Studies with longer follow-up report a success rate of 30% to 35%. [8-9]

Mitomycin C (MMC) is a more potent inhibitor of fibroblast proliferation comparing to 5-fluorouracil, and can be used intraoperatively, making it an attractive alternative for children in which previous surgery have failed. Clinical studies comparing the two antifibrotic agents have demonstrated a greater success rate and a greater degree of IOP with MMC.[10-13]

Susanna et al. [14] had an overall success rate of 67% with a mean follow-up of 17 months in a series of 56 patients (79 eyes) with primary congenital glaucoma or developmental glaucomas underwent to trabeculectomy and adjunctive MMC. This success rate is better than it described for Giampani Jr et al.[15] (55.26 %), probably because their longer follow-up (61.16 months).

Beck et al.[16] described a success rate of 58% after 24 months follow-up, although they had a large number of aphakic patients and a mean age of 91.2 months (7.6 years old). Sidoti et al. [17] showed a success rate of 59% in a case series with 29 eyes, with a mean follow-up time of 25.1 +/- 16 months. Giampani Jr et al.[15] described a success rate of 90.2 % at 24-month, 78.7% at 36-month, 60.7 % at 48-month and 50.8 % at 60-month.

A very high success rate (95%) was described by Mandal et al. in a series of 19 mitomycin C trabeculectomies (Table 1).[18] However, this study had only one patient under 1 year of age, which may be an important factor in that study's superb success rate. Miller and Rice also showed a better prognosis for surgeries performed in older children.[19]

Susanna et al. noted no changes in success rate when comparing eyes that had previous glaucoma surgery with those eyes that had no prior surgery.[14] They suggested that the results of the group that had no prior glaucoma surgery were skewed by the presence of more eyes with poor prognoses, namely Axenfeld-Rieger syndrome, Sturge-Weber syndrome, and Aniridia. Beck et al.[16] demonstrated a lower success rate for the group that had prior glaucoma surgery (55% compared with 70%), but without statistically significant difference. Giampani Jr et al. observed that the success rate was also higher in the group with no previous glaucoma surgery (64.28% compared with 51.21 %), but without statistically significant difference also (p= 0.32).[15]

Endophthalmitis is a major complication associated with trabeculectomy, and it has been reported in children who have had trabeculectomy with mitomycin C.[20] Giampani Jr et al. observed eight eyes with endophthalmitis in a total of 164 operated eyes (4.88 %).[15] Beck and associates[16] reported a higher endophthalmitis rate (8%), while Susanna et al[14] reported one case in 79 eyes, and Wallace and associates[21] noted one case in a series of 16 eyes. Mandal et al. had no cases of endophthalmitis in 19 eyes.[18] Sidoti et al. described the highest infection complication rate of any reported series (10% of blebitis and 7% of endophthalmitis).[17] Probably, the higher MMC concentration utilized for them (0.5 mg/mL) explained, in part, that rate. In adults, the endophthalmitis rate after use of antimetabolites range from 2% to 9%.[22-24]

Others complications, like overfiltration and hypotony maculopathy, are rarely observed after trabeculectomy with adjunctive mitomycin C in primary congenital glaucomas.[15]

Authors	Success rate (%)	Follow-up (months)
Giampani Jr. et al.[15]	55.26%	61.16
Beck et al [16]	58%	24
Sidoti et al.[17]	59%	25.1
Susanna et al.[14]	67%	17
Mandal et al.[18]	95%	19.52

Table 1. Trabeculectomy success rate in congenital glaucoma

a) Aqueous drainage device surgery in congenital glaucoma

Aqueous drainage devices were recommended in congenital glaucoma treatment when others procedures, like goniotomy, trabeculotomy and trabeculectomy failed (Figures 8 and 9). Unfortunately, the long-term successful rate is generally poor.[4]

O´Malley et al. described, in a chart review including 38 eyes with congenital glaucoma, a success rate about only 42% after 10 years follow-up.[25] Khan et al. observed, in a small sample of 11 eyes with congenital glaucoma, a success rate of 90.9% after 2 years follow-up, using the silicone Ahmed valve.[26] A long –term study using this device is needed to determine whether or not silicone as a good option in congenital glaucoma patients.

The most common complications in congenital glaucoma patients are tube malpositioning with corneal touch, tube exposure, endophthalmitis, retinal detachment and ocular motility abnormalities.[27]

b) Cyclodestructive procedures

Cyclocryotherapy may be used when repeated surgery to improve outflow has failed. Transscleral cyclophotocoagulation has been used to produce thermal damage to the ciliary body and processes to decrease aqueous production. This method can have the advantage of less pain and inflammation than with cyclocryotherapy, but it still usually is reserved for cases in which surgery to improve aqueous outflow has failed.[3]

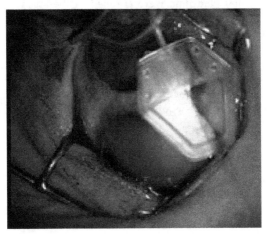

Fig. 8. Ahmed valve in primary congenital glaucoma (Courtesy Augusto Paranhos Jr.)

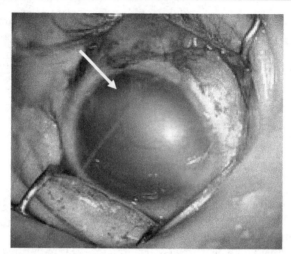

Fig. 9. Ahmed valve: see the tube in the anterior chamber (arrow) (Courtesy Augusto Paranhos Jr.)

c) Novel surgical procedures

Viscocanalostomy was recently described as a novel surgical procedure to improve the aqueous outflow in congenital glaucoma patients. Kay et al. reviewed 39 eyes that underwent dilation and probing of Schlemm´s canal and viscocanalostomy. Surgical success was achieved in 27 of 39 eyes (69%) with an average follow-up of 22 months. In patients without history of previous surgery and the diagnosis of primary congenital or juvenile glaucoma, surgical success was achieved in 17 of 19 eyes (89%) with an average follow-up of 20 months. There were no serious surgical complications associated with this procedure in this study.[28]

Nouredin et al. studied the effectiveness of viscocanalostomy in patients with primary congenital glaucoma and compared it with trabeculotomy ab externo. Eight patients with bilateral primary congenital glaucoma were enrolled in the study. After establishing the diagnosis, the more severely affected eye was randomly selected to undergo either trabeculotomy ab externo or viscocanalostomy, whereas the second eye underwent the other surgery 2 weeks after the first. The mean standard deviation (SD) follow-up period was 12.5 (1.86) months. A drop in IOP was noted in both groups at week 1, month 6 and at the last follow-up visit (p<0.001).[29] Viscocanalostomy proved to be as effective as trabeculotomy ab externo in lowering IOP in this small sample study. Nevertheless, long-term follow-up studies using viscocanalostomy are required to determine it as a good option in congenital glaucoma patients.

2. Glaucomas associated with congenital anomalies

2.1 Iridocorneal dysgenesis

Iridocorneal dysgenesis consists of overlapping rare congenital disorders involving the cornea and the iris, some of which may be associated with glaucoma. These conditions occur as a result of abnormal neural crest cell development and are: Axenfeld-Rieger syndrome, Peters anomaly and aniridia.[30]

a) Axenfeld-Rieger syndrome

This syndrome is characterized by a mesodermal dysgenesis with different degrees of presentation. The Axenfeld anomaly shows a prominent and anteriorly displaced Schwalbe´s line (called posterior embryotoxon) onto which are attached strands of peripheral iris tissue (Figure 10). The secondary glaucoma is rare in this condition. On the other hand, the Rieger anomaly is an autosomal dominant condition with a high degree of penetrance, where mutations in PITX2 and FOXC1 genes were described.[31] Involvement is usually bilateral but not always symmetrical. The slit-lamp biomicroscopy may show posterior embryotoxon, iris stromal hypoplasia, corectopia, pseudopolycoria and ectropion uveae (Figure 11). The gonioscopy in mild cases shows Axenfeld anomaly. In severe cases, broad leaves of the iris stroma adhere to the cornea anterior to Schwalbe´s line. Glaucoma develops in about 50% of cases, usually during the early childhood.[4]

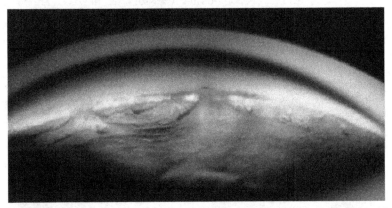

Fig. 10. posterior embryotoxon onto which are attached strands of peripheral iris (Courtesy Prof. Ernst Oltrogge)

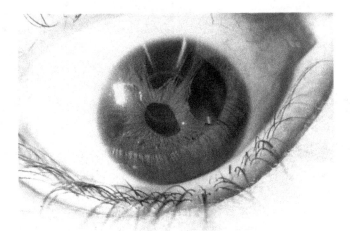

Fig. 11. Rieger´s anomaly showing corectopia and pseudopolycoria (Courtesy Prof. Celso Antonio de Carvalho)

The Rieger´s syndrome consists of Rieger´s anomaly in association with systemic malformations, like hypodontia (a decrease in the number of teeth), microdontia (a decrease in the teeth size) and facial malformations, including hypoplasia of the maxilla, a broad flat nasal bridge, telecanthus (a lateral displacement of the medial canthus) and hypertelorism (an increased distance between the bony orbits).[30] Others anomalies include redundant paraumbilical skin.

Some authors proposed the term Axenfeld-Rieger syndrome for all clinical variations within this spectrum of developmental disorders.[4]

The glaucoma treatment is surgical in the most cases of these disorders. Options of incisional surgery include goniotomy, trabeculotomy and trabeculectomy. The first two procedures have been used in infants with limited success. Trabeculectomy with adjunctive mitomycin C is the surgical procedure of choice for most patients with glaucoma associated with Axenfeld-Rieger syndrome. The long-term successful rates, however, are poor.[14,15]

b) Peters anomaly

This anomaly is characterized by a congenital central cornea leukoma associated with a defect in the corresponding posterior stroma and Descemet´s membrane, with synechiae extending from the central iris to the periphery of the corneal opacity (Figure 12).[32] Some patients may have a central keratolenticular adherence with shallowing of the anterior chamber, whereas others may have an anterior polar cataract. A variety of less commonly associated ocular findings include microcornea, microphthalmia, cornea plana, aniridia, sclerocornea and corectopia. An association between Peters anomaly and the systemic alterations seen in Axenfeld-Rieger syndrome is not uncommon.[4]

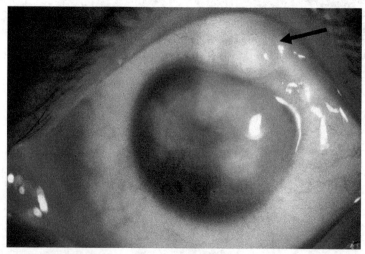

Fig. 12. Peters anomaly after trabeculectomy with MMC (see the bleb – arrow) (Courtesy Prof. Ernst Oltrogge)

Most cases are sporadic, although autosomal recessive inheritance and chromosomal defects have been described. About 80% percent of cases are bilateral. The pathogenesis involve a defect neural crest cell migration in the sixth to eight weeks of fetal development, during which time the anterior segment of the eye is formed.[30]

Glaucoma occurs in 50% to 70% of cases. Elevated intraocular pressure unresponsive to topical medications should be treated surgically, before penetrating keratoplasty is performed. Trabeculectomy with use of antimetabolites is the procedure of choice in these cases.[32] Unfortunately, the long-term visual outcome and glaucoma control are usually poor.[4]

c) Aniridia

It is a bilateral condition with life-threatening associations. It occurs as a result of abnormal neuroectodermal development secondary to a mutation in the PAX6 gene linked to 11p13.[30] This gene controls the development of a number of structures, hence the broad nature of ocular and systemic manifestations. The inheritance is autosomal dominant in most cases.

The aniridia is variable in severity, ranging from minimal to total (Figure 13). However, even eyes with total involvement usually show a residual iris tissue in the angle on gonioscopy. Others ocular findings include corneal lesions (leukomas, microcornea and sclerocornea), cataract, aphakia and lens subluxation, foveal hypoplasia, choroidal coloboma and optic nerve hypoplasia. The systemic manifestations include Wilm's tumor, genitourinary anomalies, mental retardation and cerebellar ataxia.

Glaucoma occurs in approximately 2/3 of cases and usually presents in late childhood and adolescence.[4] The intraocular pressure control is usually difficult, and the medical therapy is inadequate in most cases. The surgical procedures, like goniotomy and trabeculotomy, show poor long-term results. The trabeculectomy with adjunctive antimetabolites is the procedure of choice is most cases. However, the long-term results are also disappointing.[14-16]

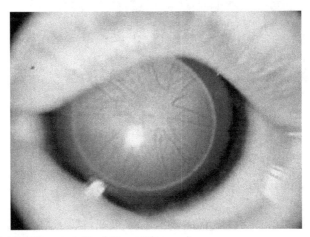

Fig. 13. Total aniridia (Courtesy Prof. Ernst Oltrogge)

2.2 Phacomatoses

The Phacomatoses are characterized by the formation of hamartias and hamartomas in the eye, central nervous system, skin and viscera. They are hereditary disorders with variable penetrance and expressivity.

a) Sturge-Weber syndrome

Also called encephalotrigeminal angiomatosis is characterized by facial haemangioma (naevus flammeus –Figure 14), choroidal haemangioma and intracranial meningeal angiomata. The haemangioma usually involves the first and second divisions of the trigeminal nerve. The disease has little familial tendency, and no sexual or racial predisposition. Chromosomal abnormalities have been reported in some patients, and the disorder may be a dominant trait with incomplete penetrance.[33]

Glaucoma develops in about 30% of patients, ipsilateral to the facial haemangioma, especially if the lesion affects the upper eyelid.

The glaucoma pathogenesis involves a trabeculodysgenesis and an elevated episcleral venous pressure. The medical treatment with prostaglandin analogues (enhancing uveo-scleral outflow) may be useful in some cases. Nevertheless, surgical approach is necessary in most cases. The goniotomy may be successful in eyes with angle anomalies (trabeculodysgenesis). The combined trabeculotomy-trabeculectomy gives good results in early-onset cases, before the buphthalmos appearing. Surgery always carries a high risk of choroidal effusion and suprachoroidal haemorrhage. Adverse consequences of this may be minimized by performing a posterior sclerotomy before opening the eye.[34]

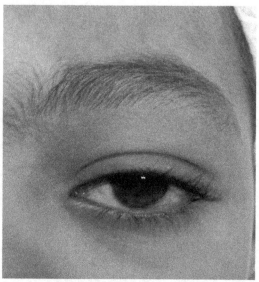

Fig. 14. Naevus flammeus in Sturge-Weber syndrome

b) Neurofibromatosis

It is a neuroectodermal dysplasia characterized by tumor-like formations (neurofibromas) derived from the proliferation of peripheral nerve elements. The neurofibromas can occur in the central nervous system, central and peripheral nerves, as well in skin and mucus membranes. Inheritance is autosomal dominant with irregular penetrance and variable expressivity. Glaucoma is uncommon, usually unilateral and congenital. Classically, neurofibromatous involvement of the upper lid is present. Glaucoma is present in 50% of all eyes with plexiform neuroma.[4]

Many mechanisms have been postulated as causes of glaucoma in neurofibromatosis. The elevated intraocular pressure may occur secondary to obstruction of aqueous outflow by neurofibromatous tissue, developmental angle anomaly or angle closure caused by neurofibromatous thickening of the ciliary body or synechiae.

Many surgical procedures, like goniotomy, trabeculotomy, trabeculectomy and cyclodestructive procedures have been reported for the glaucoma treatment. [35] However, the overall rate of success of surgery in literature is much lower than that for primary congenital glaucoma.[33]

3. Secondary infantile glaucoma

The secondary infantile glaucomas may be associated with non-hereditary congenital diseases, trauma or intraocular tumors. The secondary glaucoma after congenital cataract surgery is usually a disease with poor visual outcome. Fortunately, the modern cataract surgery and the novels topical anti-inflammatory drugs reduced the complications after congenital cataract surgery, like vitreous loss, retinal detachment and glaucoma. Nevertheless, the treatment of elevated intraocular pressure after congenital cataract surgery is usually difficult and a trabeculectomy with adjunctive antimetabolite may be necessary. [4] Others secondary infantile glaucoma causes include persistent hyperplastic primary vitreous, retrolental fibroplasia, corticosteroid-related glaucoma and retinoblastoma.

4. References

[1] Dickens CJ., Hoskins JR HD. Epidemiology and Pathophysiology of Congenital Glaucoma. In The Glaucomas. Ritch R, Shields MB, Krupin T. Mosby, second edition, 729-738; 1996.

[2] Kanski J. J. Primary Congenital Glaucoma. In Clinical Ophthalmology. Butterworth-Heinemann, fifth edition, 245-248; 2003.

[3] Dickens CJ, Hoskins JR HD. Diagnosis and Treatment of Congenital Glaucoma. In The Glaucomas. Ritch R, Shields MB, Krupin T. Mosby, second edition, 739-749; 1996.

[4] Betinjane, AJ. Glaucoma Infantil. In Glaucoma. Susanna Jr R. Cultura Médica. 145-179; 1999.

[5] Shaffer RN. Prognosis of goniotomy in primary infantile glaucoma. Trans Am Ophthalmol Soc 80:321; 1982.

[6] Anderson DR. Trabeculotomy compared to goniotomy for glaucoma in children. Ophthalmology 90: 805; 1983.

[7] Beauchamp GR, Parks MM. Filtering surgery in children: barriers to success. Ophthalmology 1979, 86: 170-80.

[8] Inaba Z. Long-term results of trabeculectomy in the japanese: an analysis by life-table method. Jpn J Ophthalmol 1982, 26: 361-73.

[9] Gressel MG, Heuer DK, Parrish II RK. Trabeculectomy in young patients. Ophthalmology 1984, 91: 1242-6.

[10] Katz GJ, Higginbotham EJ, Lichter PR et al. Mitomycin C versus 5-fluorouracil in high-risk glaucoma filtering surgery. Ophthalmology 1995; 102: 1263-9.

[11] Kitazawa Y, Kawase K, Matsushita H, Minobe M. Trabeculectomy with mitomycin. A comparative study with Fluorouracil. Arch Ophthalmol 1991; 109: 1693-8.

[12] Lamping KA, Belkin JK. 5-Fluorouracil and Mitomycin C in pseudophakic patients. Ophthalmology 1995; 102: 70-5.

[13] Prata JA Jr, Minckler DS, Baerveldt G et al. Trabeculectomy in pseudophakic patients: postoperative 5-fluorouracil versus intraoperative mitomycin C antiproliferative therapy. Ophthalmic Surg 1995; 26: 73-7.

[14] Susanna R, Oltrogge EW, Carani JCE, Nicolela MT. Mitomycin as adjunct chemotherapy in congenital and developmental glaucoma. J Glaucoma 1995; 4: 151-7.

[15] Giampani J; Borges-Giampani AS; Carani JC; Oltrogge EW; Susanna R. Efficacy and safety of trabeculectomy with mitomycin C for childhood glaucoma: a study of results with long-term follow-up. Clinics 63(4): 421-6; 2008.

[16] Beck AD, Wilson WR, Lynch MG, Lynn MJ, Noe R. Trabeculectomy with adjunctive mitomycin C in pediatric glaucoma. Am J Ophthalmol 1998; 126: 648-57.

[17] Sidoti PA, Belmonte SJ, Liebmann JM, Ritch R. Trabeculectomy with Mitomycin-C in The Treatment of Pediatric Glaucomas. Ophthalmology 2000; 107: 422-9.

[18] Mandal AK, Walton DS, John T, Jayagandan A. Mitomycin C-augmented trabeculectomy in refractory congenital glaucoma. Ophthalmology 1997; 104: 996-1001.

[19] Miller MH, Rice NS. Trabeculectomy combined with β-irradiation for congenital glaucoma. Br J Ophthalmol 1991; 75: 584-90.

[20] Wahee US, Ritterband DC, Greenfield DS, Liebmamm JM, Sidoti AO, Ritch R. Bleb-related ocular infection in children after trabeculectomy with mitomycin C. Ophthalmology 1997; 104: 2117-20.

[21] Wallace DK, Plager DA, Synder SK, Raiesdana A, Helveston EM, Ellis FD. Surgical results of secondary glaucomas in childhood. Ophthalmology 1998; 105: 101-111.

[22] Wolner B, Liebmann JM, Sassani JW, Ritch R, Speaker M, Marmor M. Late bleb-related endophthalmitis after trabeculectomy with adjunctive 5-fluorouracil. Ophthalmology 1991; 98: 1053-60.

[23] Higginbotham EJ, Stevens RK, Musch DC, et al. Bleb-related endophthalmitis after trabeculectomy with mitomycin C. Ophthalmology 1996; 103: 650-6.

[24] Greenfield DS, Suver IJ, Miller MP, Kangas TA, Palmberg PF, Flynn HW. Endophthalmitis after filtering surgery with mitomycin. Arch Ophthalmol 1996; 114: 943-9.

[25] O'Malley Schotthoefer E; Yanovitch TL; Freedman SF. Aqueous drainage device surgery in refractory pediatric glaucomas: I. Long-term outcomes. AAPOS; 12(1): 33-9; 2008.

[26] Khan AO; Al-Mobarak F. Comparison of polypropylene and silicone Ahmed valve survival 2 years following implantation in the first 2 years of life. Br J Ophthalmol; 93(6):791-4; 2009.

[27] Khan AO; Al-Mobarak F. Comparison of polypropylene and silicone Ahmed valve survival 2 years following implantation in the first 2 years of life. Br J Ophthalmol 93(6): 791-4; 2009.

[28] Kay JS; Mitchell R; Miller J. Dilation and Probing of Schlemm´s Canal and Viscocanalostomy in Pediatric Glaucoma. J Pediatr Ophthalmol Strabismus 48(1): 30-7; 2011.

[29] Noureddin BN; El-Haibi CP; Cheikha A; Bashshur ZF. Viscocanalostomy versus trabeculotomy ab externo in primary congenital glaucoma: 1-year follow-up of a prospective controlled pilot study. Br J Ophthalmol; 90(10): 1281-5; 2006.

[30] Kanski JJ. Iridocorneal dysgenesis. In Clinical Ophthalmology. Butterworth-Heinemann, fifth edition, 248-252; 2003.

[31] Borges AS, Susanna Jr. R, Carani JCE, Betinjane AJ, Alward WL, Stone EM, Sheffield VC, Nishimura DY. Genetic analysis of PITX2 and FOXC1 in Rieger Syndrome patients from Brazil. J Glaucoma 11(1): 51-56; 2002.

[32] Shottenstein EM. Peters anomaly. In The Glaucomas. Ritch R, Shields MB, Krupin T. Mosby, second edition, 887-897; 1996.

[33] Weiss JS, Ritch R. Glaucoma in the Phacomatoses. In The Glaucomas. Ritch R, Shields MB, Krupin T. Mosby, second edition, 899-924; 1996.

[34] Bellows AR. Choroidal effusion during glaucoma surgery in patients with prominent episcleral vessels. Arch Ophthalmol 97: 793; 1979.

[35] Bost M. Congenital glaucoma and von Recklinghausen disease. Pediatrie 40:207; 1985.

10

Primary Angle Closure Glaucoma

Michael B. Rumelt

Washington University Deparment of Ophthalmology and Visual Sciences
St. Louis, Missouri
USA

1. Introduction

Glaucoma, a leading cause of blindness world wide, may be classified into two main types based on the anatomy of the anterior chamber angle: open angle, which is generally a chronic disease and narrow angle glaucoma, which can be an acute medical emergency. An acute primary angle closure glaucoma attack presents with a painful, inflamed eye, cloudy cornea, fixed mid dilated pupil, reduced vision, high intraocular pressure, and possibly nausea and vomiting. If not diagnosed or untreated promptly and appropriately, the attack can result in severe damage and possibly blindness.

2. Epidemiology

It is estimated that by 2020 in the United States 3 million persons will have glaucoma, approximately 10% to 16% will have narrow angle glaucoma. World wide by 2020 it is estimated almost 80 million persons will have glaucoma. Angle closure glaucoma accounts for as much as half of blindness from glaucoma cases in other nations (particularly Asian countries). Four million are bilaterally blind. (1)

Risk is higher older individuals, individuals with high hyperopic refractive error (2), and diabetes.

The ethnic risks for acute angle closure glaucoma is approximately 1 in 1000 for Caucasians (3-11), 1 in 100 for Hispanics and Asians (12-20); 2-4 in 100 for Inuits (21-23). Primary narrow angle closure glaucoma is three times more frequent in Caucasian females over age fifty, less frequent in African Americans or native Americans, and is very common in India with intumescent lenses a frequent component.

3. Genetics

Genetics may play a role in the genesis of primary angle closure glaucoma in some situations. Autosomal dominant nanophthalmos (NNO1) with high hyperopia and angle closure glaucoma (51) maps to chromosome 11. An autosomal recessive form of nanophthalmos has been found in an Amish-Mennonite family (NNO2) and analysis found the mutation to be a frameshift insertion, 1143C in the membrane frizzled-related protein (MFRP) gene is located at cytogene location (11q23.3) and encodes a member of the frizzeled related proteins family, some of which may play a role in eye development.

Axenfeld–Rieger ocular dysgenesis is associated with mutations of the Human Pituitary Homeobox 2 (PITX2) and forkhead box C1 (FOXC1) genes (52).

3.1 Classification of angle closure glaucoma

A new definition and classification of angle closure glaucoma based on population and epidemiologic studies has been developed to allow comparison between the studies. It has the following types: Primary Angle closure suspect; Primary angle closure; Primary Angle closure glaucoma; Primary Acute Angle Closure Glaucoma Crisis attack. The term glaucoma is not applied unless there is glaucomatous optic nerve damage, characteristic visual field changes, and specific gonioscopic criteria. The terms chronic, intermittent, and subacute are eliminated.

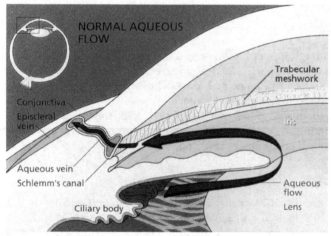

Fig. 1. Normal angle anatomy

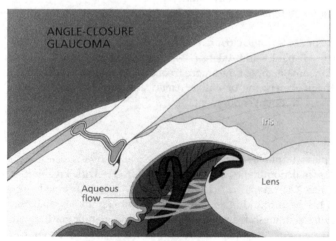

Fig. 2. Anatomy of primary angle closure glaucoma

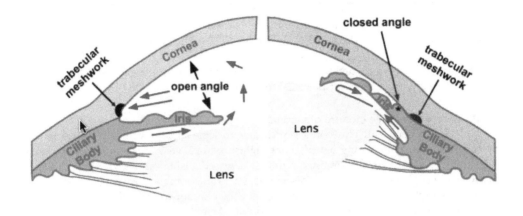

Fig. 3. The perheral iris in apposition to the trabecular meshwork blocking flow with an resultant increase intraocular pressure

3.2 Primary angle closure suspect

Anatomically narrow angles, normal IOP, absence of peripheral anterior synechiae, absence of glaucomatous optic neuropathy, and normal visual fields. (25) Patients should be warned of the symptoms of angle closure, drugs that may precipitate an attack, and the importance of a prompt evaluation by an ophthalmologist. They should be followed at appropriate intervals determined by the clinical expertise of the ophthalmologist, with gonioscopy and intraocular pressure monitoring performed at each visit, at least once a year. (56) If the patient is to be traveling to or living in a remote area where medical and/or ophthalmological may be unavailable for lengthy periods of time or transportaion may be delayed if an emergency arises, consideration of prophylactic laser peripheral iridotomies may be discussed with the patient (along with risks of the procedure).

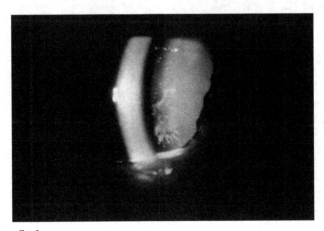

Fig. 4. Glauckomaflecken

Primary angle closure glaucoma: narrow angles, peripheral anterior synechiae, iris changes, glaucomaflecken, elevated intraocular pressure, excessive pigmentation in the trabeculum, no optic nerve damage, and normal visual fields. (26-28) They should be followed at least annually.

Primary angle closure glaucoma narrow angles, peripheral anterior synechiae, glaucomatous optic neuropathy, and characteristic visual findings. (29)

3.3 Primary acute angle closure glaucoma crisis attack presentation

About 10% of patients with closed angles present with acute angle closure crises characterized by sudden ocular pain, seeing halos around lights, red eye, very high intraocular pressure (>30 mmHg), nausea and vomiting, sudden decreased vision, and a fixed, mid-dilated pupil. Acute angle closure is an ocular emergency. Primary angle closure glaucoma occurs when the peripheral iris blocks the access of aqueous humor to the trabecular meshwork. Continued production of aqueous humor results in elevated intraocular pressure and damage to the nerve. In plateau iris, mild dilation of the pupil results in similar blockage of the angle. If not diagnosed promptly and treated appropriately, severe damage or blindness may result with either anatomical condition. (30)

An attack may present with headache and vomiting, and can be misdiagnosed as neurological or gastrointestinal in origin. If the attack occurs in a setting where either the patient can't communicate or an ophthalmologic consultation is unavailable or delayed, damage to the eye may be severe. Examples are demented patients in a nursing home, in post operative recovery, or the intensive care unit where the patient is sedated or receiving pain medication. Patients may choose self-diagnosis or treatment with over the counter medications to reduce healthcare costs and thus delay diagnosis and treatment.

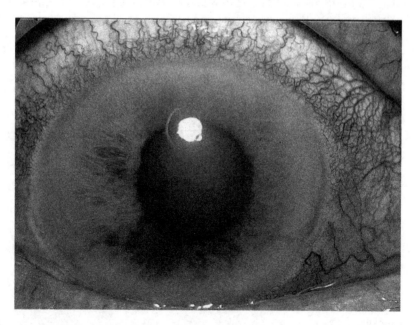

Fig. 5.

3.4 Example of a medical treatment regimen for acute primary angle closure glaucoma crisis attack

1. Topical brimonidine tartrate (Aphagan P®) x1 and timolol maleate-dorzolaminde HCL (Cosopt®) x1 (and an instruction for bid, unless there are contraindications).
2. IV acetazolamide (Diamox®) 500 mg (and an instruction for acetazolamide 250 mg tid).
3. PO glycerol 50% 100cc (1.5gr/kg) or isosorbide 25% for patients without diabetes mellitus.
4. In IOP below 60 mm Hg adding topical pilocarpine 2% x1.
5. IOP measurement after 30 min. If the IOP decreased, adding an instruction for pilocarpine 2% qid.
6. Massage with glass rod over the center of the cornea to force aqueous into the angle.
7. Analgesics and an antiemetic if necessary for pain and vomiting respectively up to every 4-6 hours.
8. Nd:YAG laser iridotomy in both eyes a day after. Adding topical apraclonidine (Iopidine®) 0.25% x1 and prednisolone acetate (Pred Forte®) qid for a week.
9. Indentation: it may be possible to break an attack by pressing with a four-mirror gonioscope lens, which may deepen the chamber angle and break peripheral anterior synechiae by hydraulic forces. Alternatively one may press firmly with a muscle hook or glass rod to accomplish the same goal: to flatten the cornea and compress aqueous humor into the anterior chamber angle to release fresh peripheral anterior synechiae. This may decrease the likelihood of developing chronic angle closure glaucoma.
10. Corneal edema may preclude gonioscopy and thus oral glycerin or topical glycerin may be useful in clearing the cornea.
11. The use of miotics like pilocarpine should be delayed until there is a drop in iop, generally less than 40 mm Hg so ischemia of the pupillary sphincter can resolve and the pupillary sphincter can function. Miotics may cause thickening of ciliary body and forward displacement of the ciliary body, thus worsening pupillary block but its use is still recommended.

If intervention is rapid enough, the attack may be broken and vision saved.

An attack that doesn't resolve may require filtering surgery, but operating on an inflamed eye with high intraocular pressure can be fraught with severe complications, including malignant glaucoma.

3.5 Etiology of angle closure
3.5.1 Primary angle closure

Pupillary block

Anatomically narrow angle: iris bombe, chronic progressive angle closure in which peripheral anterior synechiae gradually occlude the angle generally in an asymptomatic fashion and thus may be mis-diagnosed as open angle glaucoma if gonioscopy is omitted.

Ciliary block

Pan retinal photocoagulation can cause swelling of the ciliary body, scleral buckles, some drugs.

Plateau iris has a relatively deep mid anterior chamber with narrowing at the angle the severity of potential apposition or closure depending upon where the iris root inserts on the angle structures.

3.5.2 Secondary angle closure

Due to forces that pull the iris-lens diagphragm foreward such as uveitis with iris bombe, diabetic neovascular glaucoma, forces pushing iris lens forward such as swollen lens, tumor, and malignant glaucoma following intraocular surgery. Malignant glaucoma first described by von Graefe (31) in 1869 in the classical form has elevated intraocular pressure, shallow or flat anterior chamber in the presence of a patent iridectomy. It occurs rarely after filtering surgery for angle closure glaucoma, with an incidence of 0.6 to 4%. The mechanism proposed is blockage of aqueous flow at the iris lens anterior vitreous face. Aqueous is misdirected into the vitreous cavity and displaces the iris-lens diaphragm forward resulting in shallow or flat anterior chamber. A newer theory (32) postulates that choroid expansion is involved. Many entities have been associated with malignant glaucoma: intraocular surgery, glaucoma drainage devices, various laser surgeries, (Neodynium-doped Yttrium Garnet) Nd:YAG cyclophotocoagulation, and other causes. Diagnosis is facilitated by Ultrasound BioMicroscopy). Treatment consists of phenylephrine to tighten zonules, topical beta-blockers, alpha agonists, and carbonic anhydrase inhibitors (topical and systemic) to reduce aqueous production. Prostaglandin analogues may be helpful by increasing uveoscleral outflow with reduction of intraocular pressure. If medical therapy fails, Nd:YAG laser might disrupt the vitreious face and allow normal flow of aqueous. If that fails, pars plana vitrectomy with or without lensectomy may disrupt the anterior vitreous face restoring normal flow. In pseudophakic patients, lens remnants should be removed and the vitreous face disrupted.

3.5.3 Secondary angle closure due to lens factors such as intumescent cataracts.

Drug induced angle closure glaucoma.

Anticholinergic are the most common for inducing "pupillary block" angle-closure glaucoma adrenergic agents, certain beta(2)-adrenergic agonists and anticholinergic agents may induce pupillary dilation and precipitate angle-closure glaucoma in susceptible patients: locally administered phenylephrine drops, nasal ephedrine, nebulized salbutamol or systemically administered (epinephrine for anaphylactic shock). Other drugs that can induce pupillary dilation and precipitate angle-closure glaucoma due to anticholinergic effects include tropicamide and atropine drops, tri and tetracyclic antidepressants, antihistamines, mydriatics, and phenothiazines. A novel anticholinergic form follows the use of periocular botulinum toxin diffusing back to the ciliary ganglion inhibiting the pupillary sphincter.

Sulfa based drugs (33) (acetazolamide, hydrochlorothiazide, cotrimoxazole, and topiramate (34)) induce "non-pupillary block" angle-closure glaucoma as an idiosyncratic reaction to the drug, cause swelling of the ciliary body with anterior rotation of the iris-lens diaphragm, and lead to the development of angle-closure glaucoma.

4. History of gonioscopy and concepts of angle closure glaucoma

In the modern eye clinic, the ease of use of the slit lamp microscope and various diagnostic contact lenses can lead one to take for granted the technological advance that each represents. Examination of the anterior chamber by gonioscopy, described in 1907, only became commonly used in the 1950's. It is instructive to learn about the history of gonioscopy and evolving understanding of the pathophysiology of angle closure. The work of Dellaporta(36) provides an excellent review and source of much of the following information.

Until the middle of the twentieth century, glaucoma was classified into congestive and non-congestive. Treatment included bleeding, purging, leeches, counter-irritation and injecting mercury into an eye with chronic glaucoma to cause systemic inflammation, which would hopefully counteract the inflammation caused by glaucoma.

Herman von Helmholtz revolutionized the field of ophthalmology in 1851 with the invention of the ophthalmoscope.

Albrect von Graefe noted in 1856 that scleral ectasias in glaucoma often became smaller after iridectomy. He deduced that IOP could be lowered by this procedure.

Examination of the anterior chamber angle dates back to 1875 when Alexios Trantas, a Greek ophthalmologist living in Istanbul until 1922 when he was forced to resettle in Athens due to political repression, was the first to examine the angle in a living person. In a 1907 presentation to the French Ophthalmological Society, he described his observations of the angle and his method, direct gonioscopy, that used digital pressure on the limbal area to indent the eye and allow visualization of the angle with a direct ophthalmoscope and a plus lens, power ranging from plus four to plus fourteen diopters. The term gonioscopy (which derives from the Greek and means observe the angle (36)) was first used by him, in the body of a paper (not the title) published in 1915 (35), but lost until after the end of the First World War.

Maximilian Salzmann's papers on gonioscopy and the angle, were published independently of Trantas in 1915. He tried direct ophthalmoscopy first but then found indirect ophthalmoscopy with a contact lens to be more satisfactory. He initially used Adolf Eugen Fick's scleral contact lens, first described in a paper published in 1888 (37). Salzmann later used a customized Zeiss scleral contact lens with a smaller diameter, that made gonioscopy easier.

In 1893 Theodor Leber (38-39) showed that the aqueous flows from the posterior chamber to the anterior chamber through the pupil. He and his collaborators injected various substances, including fine India ink, into the vitreous or anterior chamber of freshly enucleated eyes or those scheduled to undergo medically necessary enucleation and demonstrated the materials in the anterior chamber, iris, and Schlemm's canal.

The development of the slit lamp microscope by Zeiss in 1920 further advanced gonioscopy. Leonhard Koeppe examined patients sitting at the slit lamp with the contact lens he developed, held in position by a bandage, allowing viewing of the nasal and temporal aspects of the angle.

Later Karl Wolfgang Ascher examined patients in the supine position, and used the Keoppe lens, thus adding views of the superior and inferior angle. Ascher also identified episcleral veins near the limbus which carried clear fluid and when compressed with a small glass rod demonstrated the flow of aqueous from the anterior chamber into the blood vessels. He subsequently named them "aqueous veins".

In 1920, Edward James Curran described relative pupillary block and its treatment by peripheral iridectomy for the first time. Edward James Curran's observations were not accepted for many years.

Manuel Uribe Tronosco in 1925 invented a self illuminating monocular gonioscope (40), developed a version of the Koeppe lens made of polymethylmethacrylate rather than glass, and then a binocular microscope. In 1947 Edward James Curran published a book on gonioscopy.

Little progress was made until the 1936 publication of Otto Barkan's landmark paper, "On the Genesis of Glaucoma" (41), based on his observations made possible by modifications to the technique of gonioscopy, that allowed him to differentiate glaucoma into open angle and narrow angle glaucoma. His appreciation of the importance of pupillary block to angle closure glaucoma was a vital advance in gonioscopy and the understanding of the mechanism of glaucoma. Otto Barkan's ingenious innovation was to combine a handheld Zeiss binocular microscope suspended from the ceiling, an intensely bright source of illumination, the Koeppe lens, and finally the patient in a supine position. This process allowed great mobility, direct visualization of the entire angle, and manipulation of the eye. As important as Barkan's method of gonioscopy was, the widespread adoption by non glaucoma eye care specialists, was limited by the cumbersome details of the setup. Barkan also invented goniotomy for congenital glaucoma, facilitated by direct ophthalmoscopy using a special lens flattened on one edge to allow passage of a goniotomy knife

Because it was not efficient to apply direct gonioscopy to every patient, it became necessary to triage which patient would be examined. Wiliam van Herick (42) devised a method to identify patients with possibly narrow angles. He described positioning the slit beam at the temporal limbus angled sixty degrees to the side of the observer. If the space between the anterior iris stroma and the corneal endothelium was less than one fourth of the thickness of the cornea, those individuals would receive direct gonioscopy.

The development of the Goldmann indirect gonioscope lens (43), a contact lens incorporating one or more mirrors allowed examination of the entire angle with a patient seated before the slit lamp microscope. Two artifacts impact the utility of the lens: the requirement to use methylcellulose gel to eliminate air bubbles and if the lens was tiled, it could possibly indent the globe and falsely indicate a narrowing of the angle. The Koeppe lens won't indent the globe unless tilted and pressure applied, but with the patient in the supine position the chamber could deepen under the influence of gravity.

The development of the Zeiss 4-mirror and other similar lenses (44) which incorporated mirrors facilitated examination of the entire anterior chamber angle because these lenses were smaller in diameter than the cornea, used the tear film rather than methylcellulose to allow placement of the lens on the cornea, and had a handle which allowed indentation of the cornea to determine if apposition of the peripheral iris to the trabecular meshwork was permanent with synechiae or temporary and whether pressing with the contact lens could open the angle.

The technique of indenting the cornea was taught by Bernard Becker and Robert Moses at Washington University School of Medicine (45). Bernard Becker demonstrated the reduction of intraocular pressure by acetazolamide in 1954, a major advance in the treatment of glaucoma.

Glaucoma was officially divided into wide and narrow-angle types at the American Academy of Ophthalmology in 1948.

In the 1950s many advances in understanding angle closure glaucoma were made: Paul Chandler rediscovered Edward James Curran's work, and advanced the concept of pupillary block; Joseph Haas and Harold Scheie described angle opening after peripheral iridectomy and postulated resistance to the forward flow of aqueous lead to bowing of the peripheral iris; Otto Barkan supported Edward James Curran and Paul Chandler's concept; Chandler, Shaffer and Barkan described malignant glaucoma; and Tornquist described plateau iris.

Gerd Myer-Schwikerath in 1956 introduced Xenon photocoagulation of the iris but corneal and lens damage limited its use. It was replaced by laser iridotomies, first with the ruby, then with development of Argon and Neodynium-doped Yttrium aluminium garnet (ND:YAG) lasers. Iridectomy became noninvasive and moved from the operating room to the office.

The 1980's and 1990's saw the development of the concept of pupillary block, the concept of complete and incomplete plateau iris syndrome and the advent of laser iridoplasty, to shrink the peripheral iris to open the angle.

In the 2000's produced advances in instrumentation capable of non-contact anterior segment biometry: ultrasonic Biomicroscopy (UBM) (which does not require a clear cornea), ocular coherence tomography (OCT), and Pentascan using the Scheimpflug principle.

5. Examination of the angle to assess risk of closure

Gonioscopy

Because of total internal reflection of light, it is impossible to see angle structure and anatomy without other means. To overcome this problem, special contact lenses called goniocopy lenses are utilized. The examiner must be careful not to incorrectly estimate angle depth when illumination passes through the pupil because miosis might deepen the angle.

Direct gonioscopy

One looks through a contact lens to the meridian of interest in the eye with a Koeppe lens, requires methylcellulose, supine position, an assistant to hold lens in place with a q-tip, after the examination, vision may be blurred due to methylcellulose.

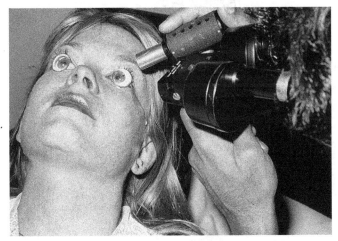

Fig. 6. Koeppe lens, hand held illuminator, microscope, supine patient

Indirect gonioscopy

To see a particular meridian of the angle, a contact lens with a mirror or series of mirrors is used. Examination of the angle anatomy is done at the slit lamp with either a Zeiss four mirror gonioscopy lens or a Goldmann lens, which requires methylcellulose gel to eliminate air bubbles and can blur vision after the exam for a period of time. Goldmann lenses are larger than the diameter of cornea and may be uncomfortable for the patient. Zeiss or Posner four mirror lenses do not require methylcellulose and rely on the tear film to allow placement of the lens without air bubbles. They have a smaller diameter compared to other type of contact lens and can be used to do indentation gonioscopy to determine if a narrowed angle can be opened or synechiae can be broken.

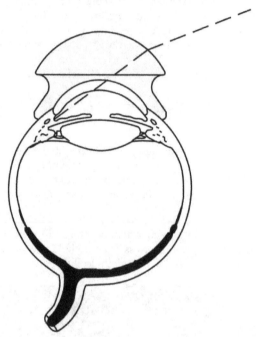

Fig. 7. Illustration of koeppe lens

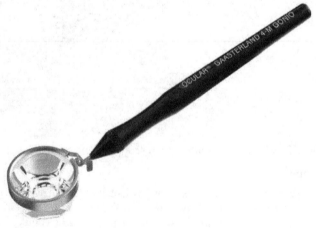

Fig. 8. Mirror gonioscope lens

5.1 Grading the anterior chamber depth with gonioscopy

At the bedside with the flashlight test, a flashlight beam is directed parallel to the iris from the temporal side. If the crescentic iris shadow thus formed is less than half to one-third or no shadow the eye is considered to have a narrow angle and merit further examination.

At the slit lamp William van Herick's (42) method of grading peripheral anterior chamber depth at the slit lamp consists of placing the slit beam at an angle of 60 degrees, just inside limbus, magnification 15, low to medium illumination, observe the space between corneal endothelium and front surface of iris. If the space (PAC) was less than one fourth of the thickness of the cornea (CT) the angle was considered possibly narrow and should be evaluated with gonioscopy.

Van Herick grading (42)

Grade 4 angle is wide open	PAC >CT
Grade 3 angle is narrow	PAC= 1/4 to 1/2 CT
Grade 2 angle dangerously narrow	PAC=1/4 CT
Grade 1 angle narrow or closed	PAC<CT

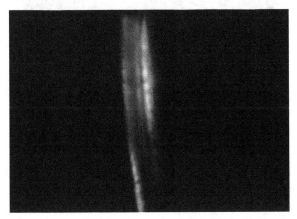

Fig. 9. Van Herick grade 1

Scheie grading (46)

Scheie proposed a grading system in which Roman numerals describe the degree of angle closure based upon the examiner's visualization of the anterior chamber angle's structures;

Grade I	all structures visible
Grade II	iris root visible
Grade III	posterior trabeculum obscured
Grade IV	only Schwalbe's line visible

Shaffer grading (47)

Shaffer graded the angle of iris insertion with plane of trabecular meshwork:

Grade 4	45 to 35 degree angle	wide open
Grade 3	35 to 20 degree angle	wide open
Grade 2	20 degree angle	narrow
Grade 1	<10 degree angle	extremely narrow
Slit	0 degree angle	narrowed to slit

Shaffer grading system of depth of anterior chamber showing angle between iris and trabeculum

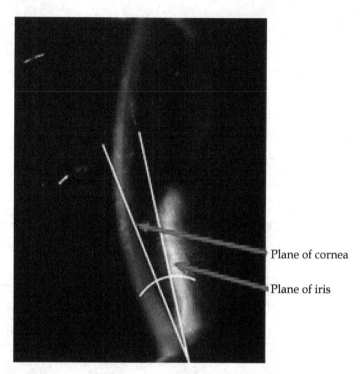

Plane of cornea

Plane of iris

Fig. 10.

Spaeth's grading (48)

Spaeth's grading scheme is as follows
Iris insertion
A   anterior to Schwalbe's line
B   between Schwalbe's line and slceral spur
C   scleral spur visibile
D   deep with ciliary body visible
E   very deep with >1 mm of ciliary body visible
Peripheral iris
F   flat
B   bowed anteriorly
P   pleateau iris
C   concave
Pigmentation of trabecular meshwork
0   no pigment
1+   minimal
2+   mild
3+   moderate
4+   intense

Provocative testing such as dark room prone provocative testing is rarely utilized. A positive test is helpful, but a negative test does not guarantee that a particular individual with narrow angles will not suffer a future attack.

Optical coherence tomography of the anterior segment (OCT) is a non contact imaging system that can show detailed images of the anatomy including the anterior chamber angle. It can't acquire images behind the heavily pigmented posterior iris epithelium because the coherent light is absorbed by the iris pigment epithelium and thus may not be adequate for study of the ciliary body, zonules, posterior chamber, or anterior vitreous. The size of the pupil may be affected by ambient light and constrict falsely indicating a deeper chamber. The following illustration demonstrates crowding of the angle by peripheral iris with a dilated pupil.

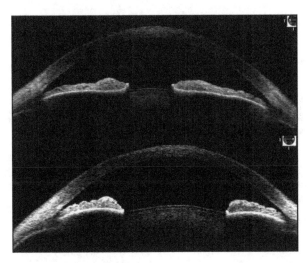

Fig. 11.

High resolution ultrasonography of the anterior segment, known as Ultrasound BioMicroscopy (UBM), is a contact imaging technique that can assess and display anterior chamber depth, configuration of the angle, lens position, iris thickness, and the ciliary body which may be thickened, rotated forward, have masses or cysts, or other anomalies presenting with angle closure in the presence of a cloudy cornea. UBM uses a higher frequency transducer (20-80 Mhz) than A-scan or B-scan (10 Mhz). Modifications in the system to apply the probe to the cornea eliminate the acoustic dead zone in front of the probe and allow the study to be performed sitting or supine.

Recent studies have suggested that increased iris thickness and cross-sectional area are associated with increased risk of angle closure glaucoma, there may be increased accumulation of proteins in iris in other cases. Another study comparing gonioscopy and UBM assessment of anterior chamber depth in Asian and Indian eyes found a very close correlation.

Central corneal thickness will affect Goldmann tonometry, since a thicker than "normal" cornea may be associated with a falsely higher pressure measurement and conversely measuring the intraocular pressure in a patient with a thinner cornea may underestimate the true intraocular pressure (49). A study comparing Pentacam Scheimpflug camera with ultrasonic pachymetry and noncontact specular microsopy in measuring central corneal thickness showed the values obtained are similar but the methods are not interchangeable (50).

A-scan biometry of the axial length of the eye will reveal those eyes that are very short such as in nanophthalmos and at risk of angle closure glaucoma.

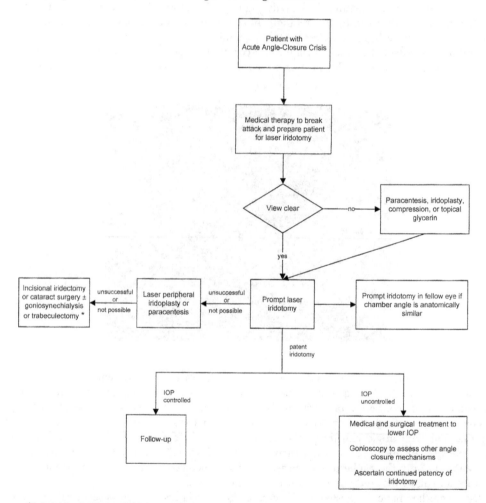

* Indicated for extensive synechial closure or optic nerve damage.

Fig. 12. Algorithm for the management of patients with acute angle-closure crisis American Academy of Ophthalmogy preferred practice pattern 2010

6. Management of chronic angle-closure glaucoma (CACG)

The first step in the chronic angle-closure glaucoma (CACG) is often a surgical procedure to open up, as far as possible, those segments of the drainage angle that are appositionally closed or narrow. Options may include laser peripheral iridotomy, argon laser peripheral iridoplasty, and lens extraction. Intraocular pressure (IOP) may, however, remain increased after these procedures, which may be the result of extensive residual synechial angle closure. IOP-lowering medications are indicated if a safe IOP level cannot be reached after angle-opening procedures. In the past, timolol and pilocarpine were extensively used in CACG. Once-daily prostaglandin analogue regimes are generally well tolerated by patients with CACG, and have become an important member in the medical arsenal against CACG. If the intraocular pressure remains elevated, or there is evidence of optic nerve damage, and/or significant visual field defects, then follow up intervals are similar to those when following an open angle glaucoma patient.

7. Medications available to treat elevated intraocular pressure

It is important to have a thorough knowledge of the patient's allergies, medical and surgical history, and a list of current medications to anticipate drug interactions or harmful side effects.

Alpha2-adrenergic receptor agonists: brimonidine tartrate 0.2%, 0.5%, 0.1% (Alphagan®, (Alphagan®P®), apraclonidine 0.5%, 1% (Iopidine®).

These medications may decrease IOP by reducing aqueous humor production and increase uveoscleral outflow.

The recommended dose is one drop of Alphagan®P® in the affected eye(s) twice daily, approximately 12 hours apart.

Use with precautions in coronary insufficiency, chronic renal failure, recent myocardial infarction, cerebrovascular disease, Raynaud disease, thromboangiitis obliterans, and patients with depression. A moderate risk of allergic response to this drug exists. Caution should be used in individuals who have developed an allergy to Iopidine. The brand Alphagan-P contains the preservative Purite and has been shown to be much better tolerated than its counterpart Alphagan. Coadministration with topical beta blockers may further decrease intraocular pressure; tricyclic antidepressants may decrease effects of brimonidine; CNS depressants such as barbiturates, opiates, and sedatives may potentiate effects of brimonidine. Contraindications if documented hypersensitivity and patients receiving Monoamine Oxidase Inhibitors inhibitors therapy.

Beta-adrenergic blocking agents: timolol maleate 0.25%,0.5% (Timoptic® Timoptic-XE®, Betimol®, Istalol®), levobunolol 0.25%, 0.5% (Betagan®), carteolol 1% (Ocupress®).

Beta-adrenergic receptor antagonists decrease aqueous humor production by the ciliary body and possibly increased outflow.

Treatment can be initiated at one drop of 0,25% Timoptic® solution in each affected eye twice a day.

These medications may cause bradycardia, bronchospasm, obstructive pulmonary disease, cardiac failure, may contain sulfites and cause allergic reactions. Use with caution in patients with cerebrovascular insufficiency; in myasthenic syndromes, may potentiate muscle weakness; patients with an anaphylactic reaction may be unresponsive to usual dose of epinephrine. The product may cause depression, confusion, hallucinations, and psychosis, especially in the elderly. These effects may occur suddenly and are typically reversible upon discontinuation; some have sulfites, which may cause allergic-type reactions in susceptible patients. Punctal occlusion after dosing may reduce systemic absorption.

Topical carbonic anhydase inhibitors: brinzolamide 1%(Azopt®) dorzolamide 2%(Trusopt®). Dosage is 1 drop in affected eye tid.

The mechanism of action is to reduce secretion of aqueous humor by inhibiting carbonic anhydrase in ciliary body, causing a decrease in intraocular pressure. May use concomitantly with other topical ophthalmic drug products to lower intraocular pressure.

Local ocular adverse effects, primarily conjunctivitis and lid reactions may occur with chronic administration.

Systemic carbonic anhydase inhibitors: acetzolamide 125mg, 250 mg tablet (Diamox®), 500mg extended release capsule (Diamox Sequels®); 25 mg, 50mg methazolamide) Neptazane®).

Dosage Acetazolamide tablet (Diamox®) dosage 250 mg tablet qDay/bid/tid/qid; (Diamox Sequels®) 500 mg po bid; 25, 50 mg Methazolamide (Neptazane®) dosage 50-100 mg po bit/tid.

Systemic absorption can affect carbonic anhydrase in the kidney, reducing hydrogen ion secretion at renal tubule, and increasing renal excretion of sodium, potassium bicarbonate, and water.

Systemic administration of carbonic anhydrase inhibitors may have potential serious side effects. They may decrease levels of lithium, alter excretion of amphetamines, quinidine, phenobarbital, and salicylates by alkalinizing urine. Derived chemically from sulfa drugs. Boxed warning: rare fatalities have occurred because of severe reactions to sulfonamides resulting in Stevens-Johnson syndrome, toxic epidermal necrolysis, fulminant hepatic necrosis, agranulocytosis, aplastic anemia, and other blood dyscrasias; reports of anorexia, tachypnea, lethargy, coma, and death with concomitant high-dose aspirin may cause substantial increase in blood glucose in some diabetic patients; may result in loss of potassium.

Miotic agents (parasympathomimetics): pilocarpine ophthalmic 0.5%, 1%,2%,4%, Gel; 4% (Isopto Carpine®, Pilopine HS Gel®).

Dosage is 1 gtt tid/qid, gel apply 0.5 inch ribbon in lower cul de sac q hs.

A naturally occurring alkaloid, pilocarpine mimics muscarinic effects of acetylcholine at postganglionic parasympathetic nerves, directly stimulate cholinergic receptors in the eye, decreasing resistance to aqueous humor outflow. Miotics cause the pupilary sphincter to contract, mechanically pulling the aris away from the trabecular meskwork and open the angle, and cause the ciliary muscle to contract increasing trabecular outflow. They may be ineffective when used concomitantly with nonsteroidal anti-inflammatory agents, are contraindicated with documented hypersensitivity and acute inflammatory disease of anterior chamber. In pregnancy, the risk to fetus not established or studied in humans but may be used if benefits outweigh risk to fetus. Use with caution in acute cardiac failure, peptic ulcer, hyperthyroidism, GI spasm, bronchial asthma, Parkinson disease, recent MI, urinary tract obstruction, and hypertension or hypotension.

Prostaglandin analogs: travoprost 0.004% (Travatan®, Travatan Z®), latanoprost 0.005% (Xalatan®), bimatoprost 0.01%,0.03% (Lumigan®).

Dosage 1 gtt in affected eye a Day.

Exact mechanism of action unknown but believed to reduce IOP by increasing uveoscleral outflow. Another mechanism of action may be through induction of metalloproteinases in ciliary body, which breaks down extracellular matrix, thereby reducing resistance to outflow through ciliary body.

Commonly causes ocular hyperemia; may cause permanent increases in brown pigment in iris and eyelid; eyelash growth may increase; bacterial keratitis may occur; use with caution in uveitis or macular edema (Prostaglandins may aggravate or induce cystoid macular edema); do not instill if wearing contact lenses. Co-administration with eye drops, containing the preservative thimerosal, may reduce effects (administer at intervals of 5 min between applications. Contraindicated if there is documented hypersensitivity; signs of inflammation. Use with caution in pregnant patients.

Topical hyperosmotic agents: glycerin (Ophthalgan®) One or two drops of applied to the cornea prior to gonioscopy may facilitate gonioscopy by clearing corneal edema.

Systemic hyperosmotic agents: mannitol (Osmitrol®), Ismotic® (isosorbide) Solution 45% w/v, glycerin (Osmoglyn®)

Prior to intravenous administration, assess for adequate renal function in adults by administering a test dose of 200 mg/kg IV over 3-5 min. Should produce a urine flow of at least 30-50 mL/h of urine over 2-3 h. If safe to administer, then administer 1.5-2 g/kg body weight IV over 30-60 minutes;

Isosorbide 45% soution, (Ismotic®) oral dosage 1-2 gm/kg body weight (55);

Glycerin (Osmoglyn®) oral dosage 1 ml/kg body weight (55).

Osmotic agents lower IOP by creating an osmotic gradient between ocular fluids and plasma.

Assess for adequate renal function in adults or children. Carefully evaluate cardiovascular status before rapid administration of mannitol since a sudden increase in extracellular fluid may lead to fulminating congestive heart failure; If blood is given simultaneously with mannitol, add at least 20 mEq of sodium chloride to each liter of mannitol solution to avoid pseudoagglutination. Consultation with specialists in internal medicine is strongly advised.

8. Neuroprotective agents

The use of neuroprotective agents may facilitate recovery of function or at least attenuation of damage. The results of studies of brimonidine and memantidine as potential neuroprotective agents are encouraging (54).

9. Surgical treatment

Surgical treatment may consist of laser iridotomies, laser iridoplasties to shrink the peripheral plateau iris, surgical iridectomies, and filtering procedures.

Argon laser peripheral iridotomy in eyes with light blue or green irides includes the following steps. After informed consent is obtained, Topical anesthetic (proparacaine 0.5%), topical alpha-agonist (apraclonidine or brimonidine), and pilocarpine 1% are placed on the eye. To perform laser peripheral iridotomy (LPI). Either the Abraham lens or equivalent lens, is placed on the cornea with the magnifying bubble rotated to an upper nasal position and the patient instructed to fixate with the opposite on an appropriate target. The lenses stabilize the eye, act as a speculum, reduce power due to the magnifying portion of the lens, and absorb heat to reduce the chances of burning of the cornea. The location of the treatment should be upper and nasal near the arcus sinelis in a spot where the iris appears thinner, such as an iris crypt. By placing the spot thusly, one may avoid annoying optical effects due to light entering the iridotomy, a rare occurrence requiring a large iridotomy opening or extremely observant patient. Suggested starting settings for the Argon laser are as follows:

Spot size - 50 mm Duration - 0.03-0.04 seconds Power - 900 mW. These may be adjusted depending on iris color and thickness of the iris stroma. Each surgeon should determine appropriate parameters for each clinical situation and adjust them accordingly. Prednisolone acetate 1% is started (4 times a day for 5-7 d). Follow up examination is in one hour to avoid missing any spike in intraocular pressure, which must be treated appropriately. The patient is seen in one week, one month, then at three to six months, then at least annually.

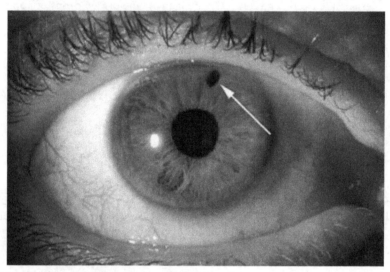

Fig. 13. Argon laser peripheral iridotomy is illustrated

ND: Yag laser peripheral iridotomy is indicated in eyes that have thick dark brown irides. After similar preparatory steps as above, the proposed treatment site is thinned with the Argon laser, and then the iris perforated with the ND:Yag with starting settings: power 1.7-3 mJ, pulses per burst 2. Follow up examination in one hour to avoid missing any spike in intraocular pressure, which must be treated appropriately. The patient is seen in one week, one month, then at three to six months.

The number of surgical iridectomies has declined dramatically with the introduction of laser procedures which are noninvasive and thus avoid the potential and real complications of intraocular surgery. Lensectomy with posterior chamber intraocular lenses for intumescent or dislocated cataracts has been reported to have good clinical results with deepening of the anterior chamber. However, results of clinical trials to determine the true value of this procedure are pending.

One type of patient with narrow angles deserves special attention: the rare individual with nanophthalmos. These highly hyperopic eyes with very short axial lengths and proportionally large lenses, are prone to very serious complications during and after intraocular surgery such as vitreous loss during surgery and post operative hypotony with effusions in the suprachoroidal space culminating in huge choroidal detachments that in extreme cases seem to fill the eye. Corrective surgery is difficult and may involve vitrectomy, removing sclera surrounding vortex veins, and drainage of the choroidals. Posterior sclerotomy prior to trabeculectomy has some but does have not widespread support. (58)

10. Financial cost of glaucoma

In the United States of America in 2006, approximately eighty five thousand laser iridotomies and three thousand laser iridoplasties were reimbursed by Medicare for payment (53).

The total financial burden of adult major visual disorders is estimated to be 25.4 billion, with more than $2.9 billion due to glaucoma. Outpatient medical and pharmaceutical costs accounted for the bulk of glaucoma expenditure. In 1996 the cost of Social Security benefits, lost income tax revenues, and healthcare expenditures was considered to be 1.5 billion dollars (USD). In 2003 it was estimated that blindness and vision loss were responsible $2.14 billion in non eye related costs.

There is also a cost to society in terms of quality of life and supportive care for the blind. Individuals with impared vision are at risk of falls, auto accidents, require more care, and may have reduced life expectancy.

Should the fellow eye be treated if it has not suffered an attack? It is usually warranted since both angles usually have similar structures. In the United States of America, medical liability may be a risk for not treating the fellow eye for blinding condition. The management of patients who are anatomically at risk who have not suffered an attack presents a dilemma: should they be treated or should treatment be delayed until the attack occurs. The cost of treatment must be factored into the decision with the knowledge that failure to diagnose primary angle closure glaucoma carries a risk of harm to the patient and malpractice litigation.

11. Prognosis

11.1 Acute angle closure

After the the acute attack is over, eyes should be examined for degree of angle closure, presence of peripheral anterior synechiae (PAS), and optic disc and visual field damage. Intraocular pressure (IOP) should be checked often to detect asymptomatic rise in IOP. The second eye should be assessed and treated to prevent attack. (59)

The prognosis is favorable if the IOP can be controlled. IOP is reported to be controlled with laser peripheral iridotomy alone in 42% to 72%, in whites more often then in Asians. (60) (61)

11.2 Angle closure glaucoma

Progressive visual deterioration may be prevented if control of the IOP can be achieved. Whether or not peripheral iridotomy alone can control the IOP depends the underlying mechanism and the stage of the disease when diagnosed. (62)

If more PAS, a higher IOP, and a larger cup-to-disc ratio are found, there is a likelyhood of poor pressure control following iridotomy. (63) Once glaucomatous optic neuropathy has developed most patients will require further treatment to control IOP. (64)

Clinical clues for non-ophthalmologists that an individual may be having an attack of angle closure glaucoma. If a patient, who may or may not be able to communicate, has an inflamed eye with oval pupil and hazy cornea with loss of clarity, the diagnosis of angle closure glaucoma should be entertained. If the patient wears thick glasses that magnify objects, the patient may be far sighted or hyperopic with a small eye at risk of angle closure glaucoma. The flashlight test may point to narrow angles if a bright light is positioned to shine on the eye from the ear side and only a temporal crescent is lit up and the rest of the iris is in shadow, instead of the entire iris being illuminated. A detailed medical is important to learn of prior eye problems, a family history of glaucoma, prior eye surgery, and a complete list of all medications both prescription and over the counter.

12. Summary

A significant number of individuals world wide are at risk of blindness from angle closure glaucoma. Acute angle closure glaucoma crises attacks are relatively easy to diagnose. The challenge is identification and examination of patients at risk of angle closure glaucoma, those with anatomically narrow angles who have not suffered an acute attack, those with evidence of subclinical attacks, symptoms of headache, blurry vision, halos around lights, narrowed angles, peripheral anterior synechiae, and the fellow eye of one that has suffered an attack of acute angle closure. Signs of a prior attack to look for include glaukomaflecken, Iris atrophy, ovoid pupil, and peripheral anterior synechiae.

The methods of grading the depth of the anterior chamber at the slit lamp (van Herick), indirect gonioscopy (Shaffer, Spaeth), and new non contact methods (UBM, anterior segment OCT, Scheimpflug, Pentascan) can be helpful in identifying patients who may be at risk of angle closure glaucoma and treated before they progress to optic nerve damage, visual field defects, and blindness.

13. Future directions in diagnosis and management of patients at risk of or suffering from angle closure glaucoma

The large numbers of individuals at risk of developing or those with eyes already damaged demonstrate the need for early detection and treatment, particularly in underdeveloped countries. A hand held self contained UBM or OCT would greatly facilitate the identification of those at risk. Such a portable device could scan the eye and wirelessly transmit data to a smart phone to store and display the results. The information could then be uploaded to a central health agency's website for further action.

To facilitate iridotomies in the field a hand held self contained portable ND:Yag laser would useful.

Current imaging methods analyze the optic nerve, nerve fiber layer, and other structures. Perhaps a future method could image nerve impulses traveling along the ganglion cell axons to provide information about their functional status, identify unhealthy ones, allow mapping, and help suggest when appropriate treatment should be started.

Study of the genetic machinery involved in the embryologic development of the eye might identify the genes and other process involved and enable restarting the genetic machinery in damaged or blind eyes to regenerate or rebuild damaged retina and optic nerves. This assumes that the genes involved are turned on for a period of time, then silenced, are not removed from the genome, but persist in all cells and could be restarted.

14. References

[1] Quigley H. A. Number of people with glaucoma worldwide. Br J Ophthalmolol. 1996, 80: 389-393.

[2] Noecker, Robert J., and Lauri Graham. "Acute Angle-Closure Glaucoma." *eMedicine Consumer Health.* Eds. Richard W. Alliinson, et al. 18 Nov. 2005. Medscape. 30 Oct. 2009.

[3] Bonomi L., Marchini G., Marraffa M., et al. Prevalence of glaucoma and intraocular pressure distribution in a defined population. The Egna-Neumarkt Study. Ophthalmology 1998; 105:209-15.

[4] Mitchell P., Smith W., Attebo K., Healey P. R. Prevalence of open-angle glaucoma in Australia. The Blue Mountains Eye Study. Ophthalmology 1996; 103:1661-9.

[5] Bankes JL, Perkins ES, Tsolakis S, Wright JE. Bedford glaucoma survey. Br Med J 1968; 1:791-6.

[6] Coffey M., Reidy A., Wormald R., et al. Prevalence of glaucoma in the west of Ireland. Br J Ophthalmol 1993; 77:17-21.

[7] Hollows F. C., Graham P. A. Intra-ocular pressure, glaucoma, and glaucoma suspects in a defined population. Br J Ophthalmol 1966; 50:570-86.

[8] Wensor M. D., McCarty C. A., Stanislavsky Y. L., et al. The prevalence of glaucoma in the Melbourne Visual Impairment Project. Ophthalmology 1998; 105:733-9.

[9] Klein B. E., Klein R., Sponsel W. E., et al. Prevalence of glaucoma. The Beaver Dam Eye Study. Ophthalmology 1992; 99:1499-504.

[10] Dielemans I., Vingerling J. R., Wolfs R. C., et al. The prevalence of primary open-angle glaucoma in a population-based study in The Netherlands. The Rotterdam Study. Ophthalmology 1994; 101:1851

[11] Bengtsson B. The prevalence of glaucoma. Br J Ophthalmol 1981; 65:46-9.

[12] Casson R. J., Newland H. S., Muecke J., et al. Prevalence of glaucoma in rural Myanmar: the Meiktila Eye Study. Br J Ophthalmol 2007; 91:710-4.

[13] Salmon J. F., Mermoud A., Ivey A., et al. The prevalence of primary angle closure glaucoma and open angle glaucoma in Mamre, western Cape, South Africa. Arch Ophthalmol 1993; 111:1263-9.

[14] Dandona L., Dandona R., Mandal P., et al. Angle-closure glaucoma in an urban population in southern India. The Andhra Pradesh eye disease study. Ophthalmology 2000; 107:1710-6.

[15] Bourne R. R., Sukudom P., Foster P. J., et al. Prevalence of glaucoma in Thailand: a population based survey in Rom Klao District, Bangkok. Br J Ophthalmol 2003; 87:1069-74.

[16] Vijaya L., George R., Arvind H., et al. Prevalence of angle-closure disease in a rural southern Indian population. Arch Ophthalmol 2006; 124:403-9.

[17] Ramakrishnan R., Nirmalan P. K., Krishnadas R., et al. Glaucoma in a rural population of southern India: the Aravind comprehensive eye survey. Ophthalmology 2003; 110:1484-90.

[18] Rahman M. M., Rahman N., Foster P. J., et al. The prevalence of glaucoma in Bangladesh: a population based survey in Dhaka division. Br J Ophthalmol 2004; 88:1493-7.

[19] Shiose Y., Kitazawa Y., Tsukahara S., et al. Epidemiology of glaucoma in Japan--a nationwide glaucoma survey. Jpn J Ophthalmol 1991; 35:133-55.

[20] Yamamoto T., Iwase A., Araie M., et al. The Tajimi Study report 2: prevalence of primary angle closure and secondary glaucoma in a Japanese population. Ophthalmology 2005; 112:1661-9.

[21] Van Rens G. H., Arkell S. M., Charlton W., Doesburg W. Primary angle-closure glaucoma among Alaskan Eskimos. Doc Ophthalmol 1988; 70:265-76.

[22] Arkell S. M., Lightman D. A., Sommer A., et al. The prevalence of glaucoma among Eskimos of northwest Alaska. Arch Ophthalmol 1987; 105:482-5.

[23] Bourne R. R., Sorensen K. E., Klauber A., et al. Glaucoma in East Greenlandic Inuit--a population survey in Ittoqqortoormiit (Scoresbysund). Acta Ophthalmol Scand 2001; 79:462-7.

[24] Seah S. K., Foster P. J., Chew P. T., et al. Incidence of acute primary angle-closure glaucoma in Singapore. An island-wide survey. Arch Ophthalmol 1997; 115:1436-40.

[25] Weinreb R. N., Friedman D. S., eds. Angle Closure and Angle Closure Glaucoma. World Glaucoma Association Consensus Series-3. The Netherlands: Kugler Publications, 2006.

[26] Anderson D. R., Jin J. C., Wright M. M. The physiologic characteristics of relative pupillary block. Am J Ophthalmol 1991;111:344-50.Tiedeman JS. A physical analysis of the factors that determine the contour of the iris. Am J Ophthalmol 1991; 111:338-43.

[27] Jin J. C., Anderson D. R. The effect of iridotomy on iris contour. Am J Ophthalmol 1990; 110:260-3.

[28] Seah S. K., Foster P. J., Chew P. T., et al. Incidence of acute primary angle-closure glaucoma in Singapore. An island-wide survey. Arch Ophthalmol 1997; 115:1436-40.

[29] American Academy of Ophthalmology Glaucoma Panel. Preferred Practice Pattern® Guidelines. Primary Open-Angle Glaucoma. San Francisco, CA: American Academy of Ophthalmology; 2010. Available at: www.aao.org/ppp.

[30] Aung T., Husain R., Gazzard G., et al. Changes in retinal nerve fiber layer thickness after acute primary angle closure. Ophthalmology 2004; 111:1475-9.

[31] von Graefe, A.,Beitragezur Pathol und Therapiedes Glaucoma, Arch. f. Ophth., 15:i 8,i869.

[32] Quigley H. A., Angle-Closure Glaucoma-Simpler Answers to Complex Mechanisms: LXVI Edward Jackson Memorial Lecture. Am J Ophthalmol 2009; 118:657-669. Panday V. A, Rhee D. J.

[33] Review of sulfonamide-induced acute myopia and acute bilateral angle-closure glaucoma. Compr Ophthalmol Update 2007; 8:271-6.

[34] Fraunfelder F. W., Fraunfelder F. T., Keates E. U. Topiramate-associated acute, bilateral, secondary angle-closure glaucoma. Ophthalmology 2004; 111:109-11.

[35] A. Trantas: Sur la gonioscopie (Ophtal- moscopie de l'angle iridocorneen). Arch Ophtalmol (Paris) 45:616, 1928.

[36] Dellaporta A. Historical notes on gonioscopy. Surv Ophthalmol 1975; 20:137-49.

[37] Salzmann M. Nachtrag zu ophthalmoskopie der kammerbucht. Z Augenheilk 1915; 34: 160-2.

[38] Blum, M., et al, Theodor Leber: a founder of ophthalmic research, Surv Ophthalmol, 1992: p. 83-8.

[39] Jaeger, W. The foundation of experimental ophthalmology by Theodor Leber. Doc Ophthal. 1988 Jan-Feb; 68:71-7.

[40] Troncoso M. U. Gonioscopy with the Electric Ophthalmoscope. New York, NY: New York Academy of Medicine; 1921.

[41] Barkan O., Boyle S. F., Maisler S. On the genesis of glaucoma. An improved method based on slit lamp microscopy of the angle of the anterior chamber. Am J Ophthalmol 1936; 19:209–15.

[42] Van Herick W., Shaffer R. N., Schwartz A. Estimation of width of angle of anterior chamber. Incidence and significance of the narrow angle. Am J Ophthalmol 1969; 68:626–9.

[43] Goldmann H. Zur Technik der Spaltlampenmikroskopie. Ophthalmologica 1938; 96:90–7.

[44] Allen L, Braley A. E, Thorpe H. E. An improved gonioscopic contact prism. AMA Arch Ophthalmol 1954; 51:451–5.

[45] Forbes M. Gonioscopy with corneal indentation. A method for distinguishing between appositional closure and synechial closure. Arch Ophthalmol 1966; 76:488–92.

[46] Scheie H. G. Width and pigmentation of the angle of the anterior chamber; a system of grading by gonioscopy. AMA Arch Ophthalmol 1957; 58:510–2.

[47] Shaffer R. N. Stereoscopic Manual of Gonioscopy. St. Louis, MO: Mosby; 1962.

[48] Spaeth G. L. The normal development of the human anterior chamber angle: a new system of grading. Trans Ophthalmol Soc UK 1971; 91:709–39.

[49] James D. Brandt, M. D., 1 Julia A. Beiser, M. S., 2 Michael A. Kass, M. D., 2 Mae O. Gordon, PhD,2and the Ocular Hypertension Treatment Study (OHTS). Group Central Corneal Thickness in the Ocular Hypertension Treatment Study (OHTS). *Ophthalmology 2001*; 108: 1779–1788

[50] Fujioka M., Nakamura M., Tatsumi Y., Kusuhara A., Maeda H., Negi A. Comparison of Pentacam. Scheimpflug camera with ultrasound pachymetry and noncontact specular m.icroscopy in measuring central corneal thickness. Curr Eye Res. 2007 Feb; 32:89-94.

[51] M. I. Othman, S. A. Sullivan, G. L. Skuta, D. A. Cockrell, H. M. Stringham, C. A. Downs, A. Forne, A. Mick M. Boehnke, 2 D. Vollrath, and J. E. Richards, Autosomal Dominant Nanophthalmos (*NNO1*) with High Hyperopia and Angle-Closure Glaucoma Maps to Chromosome 11. Am. J. Hum. Genet. 63:1411–1418, 1998.

[52] Fred B. Berry, Matthew A. L., J. Martin, Tim Footz D. Alan Underhill, Philip J. Gage and Michael A. Walter, Functional interactions between FOXC1 and PITX2 underlie the sensitivity to FOXC1 gene dose in Axenfeld-Rieger syndrome and anterior segment dysgenesis. Human Molecular Genetics, 2006, Vol. 15, No. 6 doi: 10.1 093/hmg/ddl008

[53] Jordana K. Schmier, M. A; David W. Covert, M. B. A; Edmund C. Lau, M. S; Alan L. Robin, M. D. Trends in Annual Medicare Expenditures for Glaucoma Surgical Procedures From 1997 to 2006. *Arch Ophthalmol.* 2009; 127:900-905.

[54] R H W Funk E-M Kniep and C Röhlecke. Detecting the effects of neuroprotection in living cells. *Eye* (2007) 21, S38–S41; doi:10.1038/sj.eye.6702887

[55] Kolker, A. E. Symposium on glaucoma The Association for Research in Ophthalmology and the National Society for the Prevention of Blindness.

[56] Hyperosmotic agents in glaucoma. Investigative Ophthalmology Volume 9 Number 6 June 1970 418-423.

[57] Primary Angle Closure Preferred Practice Pattern October 2010.

[58] Eibschitz-Tsimhoni M, Lichter P, Del Monte M, et al. Assessing the need for posterior sclerotomy at the time of filtering surgery in patients with Sturge-Weber syndrome. *Ophthalmology* 2003; 110:1361-1363.

[59] Hollows F. C, Graham P. A. Intra-ocular pressure, glaucoma, and glaucoma suspects in a defined population. Br J Ophthalmol. 1966; 50:570-586.

[60] Wishart P. K., Atkinson P. L. Extracapsular cataract extraction and posterior chamber lens implantation in patients with primary chronic angle-closure glaucoma: effect on intraocular pressure control. Eye. 1989; 3:706-712.

[61] Gunning F. P., Greve E. L. Lens extraction for uncontrolled glaucoma. J Cataract Refract Surg. 1998; 24:1347-1356.

[62] Ang L. P., Aung T., Chua W. H., et al. Visual field loss from primary angle-closure glaucoma: a comparative study of symptomatic and asymptomatic disease. Ophthalmology. 2004; 111:1636-1640.

[63] Salmon J. F. Long-term intraocular pressure control after Nd:YAG laser iridotomy in chronic angle-closure glaucoma. J Glaucoma. 1993; 2:291-296.

[64] Rosman M., Aung T., Ang L. P., et al. Chronic angle-closure with glaucomatous damage: longterm clinical course in a North American population and comparison with an Asian population. Ophthalmology. 2002; 109:2227-2231.

11

Normal-Tension (Low-Tension) Glaucoma

Tsvi Sheleg

Department of Ophthalmology, Western Galilee – Nahariya Medical Center, Nahariya, Israel

1. Introduction

Normal-tension glaucoma, also known as low-tension glaucoma, is defined as glaucomatous damage to the optic nerve and visual fields with normal diurnal values of intraocular pressure (IOP). The term 'low-tension glaucoma' is not often used because in most patients with normal-tension glaucoma, the IOP is within the higher range of normal values and rarely low. The diagnosis is insidious in many cases and requires a complete and thorough work-up to exclude other causes for optic disc and visual field abnormalities. The definition is problematic because the normal limits of IOP have a wide Gaussian curve range and their effect on the development of glaucoma varies. Some patients may retain a high IOP for many years without any glaucomatous damage, while others with low values of IOP may suffer from ongoing progressive glaucomatous disease. IOP is considered as a risk factor for the advancement of glaucoma even in patients with normal values of IOP, and lowering the IOP often protects the optic nerves (Collaborative Normal Tension Glaucoma Study Group [CNTGSG], 1998). Some optic nerves are more vulnerable even to low levels of IOP than others (Drance et al, 1973). Though many factors have been suspected and investigated, it appears that in addition to variability of the structure of the lamina cribrosa, vascular and genetic factors are most likely involved. Most authors consider normal-tension glaucoma to be a variant of primary open angle glaucoma (POAG) (Caprioli & Spaeth, 1984; Chumbley & Brubaker, 1976); others rely on characteristic clinical features of many normal-tension glaucoma patients to consider it a distinct entity (Caprioli & Spaeth, 1984; Shields, 2008). The debate is ongoing and will probably continue to be the subject of research for many years.

2. Pathogenic theories

The optic nerve damage in normal-tension glaucoma, as in POAG, follows a cascade of pathophysiological events that includes impaired axonal transport, ischemia and free radical formation that leads to apoptosis (Harris et al., 2005). The mechanical theory is based on the assumption that high IOP reduces the axoplasmic axonal flow by causing direct pressure on the axons, resulting in damage to the nerves. Structural differences in the appearance of the optic nerve discs and elastin fibers in glaucoma patients also support the mechanical theory (Dandona et al., 1990; Quigley et al., 1994). The pressure gradient over the optic disc should also be considered, as chronic low intra-cranial pressure may result in a pressure difference that can affect the axoplasmic outflow and lead to glaucomatous progression in normal-tension glaucoma patients.

On the other hand, the vascular ischemic theory suggests that low perfusion to the optic nerve is a major factor in the process of glaucomatous damage. This is supported by many articles that emphasize the importance of low ocular perfusion pressure and blood pressure in the development of POAG (Caprioli & Coleman, 2010). Blood supply to the optic nerve is derived through the ophthalmic artery mainly through the pial system and posterior ciliary arteries, but also from the central retinal artery. Several methods have been used to evaluate the blood flow and resistance of the ophthalmic artery and choroidal vessels, and their relationship with glaucomatous disease progression in POAG and in normal-tension glaucoma patients. Ultrasound Doppler has been used to show correlation between low blood flow and high resistance of the ophthalmic artery, to visual field progression in POAG patients (Galassi et al., 2003). Scanning laser ophthalmoscope demonstrated larger fluorescein filling defects, correlated with low blood flow in the central retinal artery and choroidal vessels of normal-tension glaucoma patients compared with controls (Plange et al., 2003). Heidelberg retinal flowmetry has detected a reduction in neuroretinal rim blood flow in conjunction with visual field defects in normal-tension glaucoma patients (Sato et al., 2006). The future of understanding the ischemic aspect in the development of glaucoma may be by optical measurement of retinal vessel oxygenation. Oxygenation of retinal arteries was found to be lower in normal-tension glaucoma patients than in healthy subjects (Michelson et al., 2006). Other factors influence the perfusion of the optic nerve and participate in the development and progression of the disease. Hypertension leads to a greater resistance in small blood vessels and causes atherosclerotic changes. Hypotension, especially in the presence of insufficient vascular autoregulation, may participate in the development of the ischemia (Goldberg et al., 1981). Circadian fluctuation of mean ocular perfusion pressure was found to be an important clinical risk factor for severity of glaucoma in eyes with normal-tension glaucoma (Choi et al., 2007). Nocturnal dips have also been evaluated and are thought to play a role in the development of normal-tension glaucoma (Bechetoille et al., 1995; Graham et al., 1995). Another observation that indirectly supports the vascular theory is that many normal-tension glaucoma patients suffer from vasospastic diseases such as migraine (Corbett et al., 1985; Phelps & Corbett, 1985) and Raynaud disease (Broadway & Drance, 1998). However, other studies found no difference in the prevalence of atherosclerotic vascular disease in NTG and POAG patients (Klein et al., 1993; Leighton & Phillips, 1972). The role of vascular disease in the pathogenesis of NTG is probably related to the reduction of optic nerve resistance to the IOP and this may precedes changes in vasculature that occur also in POAG. Many believe that both theories have a part in the pathogenesis and their importance in the advancement of the disease varies from patient to patient.

3. Epidemiology

Normal tension glaucoma has been found to be common in many population-based studies, though the numbers vary in different studies and populations. The main reasons for the variation are the difference in normal IOP range in different populations and the difficulty in making the diagnosis. Ruling out high-tension glaucoma by diurnal measurements was not performed in most of these studies. Other causes of "burned out" secondary glaucoma such as steroid-induced or uveitis-related glaucoma were not diagnosed and excluded in some studies. Large epidemiological studies in North America, Europe and Australia estimated the prevalence of normal-tension glaucoma to be up to half that of POAG (Leibowitz et al., 1980; Sommer et al., 1991). The Beaver Dam Eye Study estimated the prevalence of normal-tension glaucoma to be up to 1.6% in patients over 75 years of age

(Klein et al., 1992). In Japan the prevalence is considerably higher. The Tajimi eye study assessed the prevalence of POAG in patients over 40 years and found it to be 3.9%, in 92% the IOP was 21 mmHg or lower (Iwase et al., 2004). A nationwide survey estimated the normal-tension glaucoma with (IOP under 21mmHg) prevalence to be 3.5 times that of POAG, but these numbers are thought to be biased since normal IOP in Japan is lower than in the western population, averaging 10-18 mmHg. The prevalence of normal tension glaucoma is higher in women than in men, this and other risk factors will be discussed later in this chapter. Whatever the prevalence of normal tension glaucoma is in various populations, it is obvious that the numbers are higher than once assumed, and patients are actually diagnosed only when optic disc and visual field abnormalities are already present.

4. Genetic considerations

Family history is a major risk factor in glaucoma ,and genetic mutations related to specific phenotypes of glaucoma are under investigation. Such information can help diagnose and classify subtypes of glaucoma, and perhaps even to clarify the pathogenesis. Research may find ways to repair mutation in utero or early in life, before glaucomatous damage has occurred. Genetic research has found transmission of a NTG phenotype in only a few families, all of them are autosomal dominant (Bennett et al., 1989). Of the seven gene loci that have been linked to POAG, two genes have been identified and named TIGR/ Myocilin and Optineurin (Optic Neuropathy-Inducing Protein - ONTP). A specific mutation GLC1E locus of the ONTP was found in location 10p14-15, with autosomal dominant inheritance as in all POAG locui that were identified (Sarfarazi et al., 1998). ONTP is expressed in the retina and was found to be involved in apoptosis. The Blue Mountains Eye Study in Australia found that the prevalence of mutation in the ONTP gene was higher in POAG than in healthy subjects but the difference was not statistically significant (Baird et al., 2004). Reports found the ONTP mutation associated with high prevalence of POAG and NTG in adult Japanese patients, suggesting it may be involved in the pathogenesis of both entities (Fuse et al., 2004; Umeda et al., 2004). Other reports could not find OPTN mutations in NTG (Toda et al., 2004). Genetic screening for the gene is not an option because of the low incidence of the mutation. Recently another locus GLCA3 was investigated for association with NTG, but no statistically significant relationship was found (Kamio et al., 2009).

5. Diagnosis and differential diagnosis

The diagnosis of normal-tension glaucoma is illusive and requires a high degree of suspicion. Since IOP measurements are usually in the high teens in normal-tension glaucoma, routine IOP screening measurement may be deceiving. Often, the first sign is an abnormal optic disc or disk asymmetry suspicious of glaucomatous damage. In up to half of the patients repeated measurements or daily IOP curve discovers high IOP, and the diagnosis of POAG is made (Ito et al., 1991; Perkins, 1973). The significance of a daily IOP curve in the diagnosis of NTG is crucial. Few other factors must be considered. Pachymetry should be performed to adjust the difference between measured IOP by Goldman tonometry and true IOP. Ocular hypertension study (OHTS) highlighted the importance of thin corneas in the diagnosis of glaucoma. Thinner corneas can lead to underestimation of IOP, and misdiagnosis has occurred in many NTG patients compared with POAG patients (Morad et al., 1998). The effect of corneal hysteresis and scleral rigidity should be considered and Ocular Response Analyzer (ORA) can help in estimating the true IOP (Morita et al.,

2010). Thin corneas following corneal refractive surgery and in patients after penetrating or lamellar keratoplasty can make the task of IOP estimation more challenging (Papastergiou et al., 2010; Sanchez-Naves et al., 2008). Other factors such as refraction and astigmatism should also be considered and ORA may achieve a better estimation of the true IOP in these patients (Hagishima et al., 2010).

The controversy of whether NTG is different from POAG is demonstrated in many articles regarding optic disc appearance. While some studies show no difference in the optic disc appearance between NTG and POAG (Tomita, 2000), others found distinct characteristics such as thin rim that can help distinguish NTG (Caprioli & Spaeth, 1985). OCT plays a major role in the diagnosis and monitoring of glaucoma especially when the diagnosis is not certain. Measuring the RNFL thickness, optic disk cupping and their correlation with visual field abnormalities is a powerful tool. Recently a study comparing the optic discs using optical coherence tomography (OCT) and Heidelberg retina topography (HRT) supports some of the differences (Shin et al., 2008). Disc appearance in NTG is traditionally divided into two sub-groups. The more common is the senile sclerotic group, which is characterized by a pale shallow sloping neuroretinal rim. These patients are often older in age and suffer from vascular diseases. The other group, focal ischemic, is characterized by deep focal notching of the rim. Splinter hemorrhages are a typical finding in NTG and imply in most cases a progressive disease (Drance et al., 2001; Jonas & Xu, 1994). Beta zone peripapillary atrophy has also been suggested related to optic nerve damage in NTG (Xia et al., 2005). The site of the hemorrhage may predict an area of notch development with a correlated visual field loss (Chumbley & Brubaker, 1976; Siegner & Netland, 1996; Tomita, 2000). Visual field patterns in NTG are similar to the ones seen in POAG, still some articles found differences in the distribution and shape of the scotomas. Scotomas observed in NTG visual fields often tend to be deeper, steeper and closer to fixation than in POAG patients (Caprioli & Spaeth, 1984; Harrington, 1960). Some articles mainly from japan found that scotomas in NTG may be more predominant in the lower hemifield (Araie, 1995).

The ophthalmologist should rule out "burned out" secondary glaucoma and other misleading diagnosis. Careful history and meticulous ophthalmic examination should look for previous trauma, uveitis, glaucomatocyclitic crisis, pigmentary glaucoma, previous topical or systemic steroid treatment, previous acute angle closure attack and the use of systemic medication that lowers IOP (e.g., beta-blockers). Compliance should be appreciated to rule out the possibility that the patient takes his anti-glaucoma medications only before the ophthalmologist examination in order to "please" their doctor. Non-glaucomatous optic disc abnormalities such as congenital colobomas, optic nerve pit, anterior ischemic optic neuropathy, traumatic optic neuropathy, optic nerve or chiasm compressing lesion, and various retinal abnormalities should be considered and revoked. The diagnosis and follow-up of NTG is more challenging with hypoplastic and myopic tilted discs. Systemic evaluation is advised to identify diseases that are more frequent in NTG patients, and when the diagnosis is difficult. Blood pressure, ischemic vascular disease, perfusion pressure, vasospastic disorders (migraine, Raynaud phenomenon) and obstructive sleep apnea should be assessed in selected cases. Some cases may require neurological evaluation and hematological work-up to search for various neurological conditions or coagulopathies. Generally, systemic evaluation is reserved for atypical cases when the optic disc appearance and visual field do not correlate with glaucomatous damage, when glaucomatous damage is found with IOP lower than the high teens before treatment or when other neurological symptoms are present. Neurological examination is vital in all cases of NTG with atypical clinical manifestation. Lesions such as meningiomas, craniopharingiomas, pituitary adenomas, and compressive vascular lesions such as aneurisms can mimic NTG. Some ophthalmic signs are more suggestive of a neurological disease and should prompt a neurological evaluation. Perhaps the most important of them is a rapid progression of the disease despite low IOP with or without treatment. Other signs that should raise suspicion are pale optic disks and poor best corrected visual acuity. Needless to say any neurologic symptoms prompt neurologic workup. Some authors believe that it is important in all cases of NTG to perform a CT scan (Gutman et al., 1993), though others found no value for a routine neurological examination in NTG patients (Kesler et al., 2010).

Risk factors for the development of NTG in untreated patients that were found in the Collaborative Normal Tension Glaucoma Study (CNTGS) are migraine, female gender and splinter disc hemorrhage at the diagnosis (Drance et al., 2001). Age over 60 years is common (Klein et al., 1992), and a high prevalence was found in Japanese as mentioned earlier (Iwase et al., 2004; Shiose et al., 1991). Other risk factors found to be more prevalent in NTG than in POAG patients were ischemic vascular disease, obstructive sleep apnea, autoimmune diseases, and coagulopathies, but their effect on development of NTG was not consistent.

The progression of glaucomatous damage in NTG is usually very slow. Collaborative Normal Tension Glaucoma Study (CNTGS) showed that half of the untreated patients did not progress in 5 years, and in most cases the progression was slow (Anderson, 2003). In some of these patients a previous hypotensive crisis from a massive bleeding or arrhythmia resulted in optic disk cupping. (Drance, 1977). In patients without a subsequent hypotensive crisis the glaucoma is not expected to progress. Other cases such as steroid responders or "burned out" pigmentary or uveitic glaucoma may not progress at all. Despite their effect as risk factors for the development of NTG, neither age nor untreated level of IOP affected the risk for progression in untreated eyes (Anderson, 2003). Disc hemorrhages, as mentioned earlier, where also found to be related to the progression of glaucomatous damage (Ishida et al., 2000).

6. Practical steps for diagnosis

It is difficult to diagnose NTG if the cup to disc ratio is over 0.5 even if the differences in cupping are 0.2 or higher in the presence of normal IOP. At this stage, the visual fields are usually normal. If the cornea is thin, POAG may be suspected after correction of the IOP according to the corneal thickness. But if the corneal thickness is normal, the diagnosis of NTG cannot be established. Those patients may stay with the diagnosis of glaucoma suspects until new signs of disk abnormalities appear that correlate with the glaucomatous visual field defects. Although these patients may deteriorate slowly, other glaucoma patients may deteriorate rather quickly. Therefore, it is recommended to follow individuals over the age of 40, glaucoma suspects and individuals with family history, at least every 6 months. There have been cases were glaucoma appeared and progressed within less than a year, and this is the reason for a 6 months routine follow-up. Preperimetric normal tension glaucoma should be evaluated using FDT or Swap when available.

The diagnosis is made when optic disc cupping and glaucomatous visual field defects are found in conjunction with normal IOP. POAG should be ruled out by corneal pachymetry and adjustment of the IOP to the corneal thickness. Other causes for optic disc cupping and visual field defects should be ruled out by detailed anamnesis (e.g., episodes of major blood loss) and further analysis (e.g., brain computed tomography to rule out tumors as mentioned earlier).

7. Treatment

The decision to treat a patient suspected with NTG must include the patient's age and all aspects of the disease, its extent, pathogenic factors and especially the rate of progression. If the patient's disease seems not to be progressive, monitoring of the disease is advised. When the disease is bilateral and not severe, treatment in one eye may be suitable. Careful follow-up and comparison of both eyes for progression is essential. Some patients suffer from visual field loss and disc damage and require prompt therapy. As in POAG, it is customary to begin with medical therapy, but laser and even surgical treatment should be considered for advanced cases. The target IOP was recommended to be 30% reduction by CNTGS and this reduces the progression from 35% in untreated patients to 12% in the treated group. Approximately two-thirds of the patients that did not receive any therapy did not progress (Drance et al., 2001). Target IOP was reached with medication and laser trabeculoplasty in half of CNTGS patients. This was achieved without beta-blockers or prostaglandin analogs. Currently the available drugs are thought to produce better effects on lowering the IOP, better compliance and better results in preventing disease progression. Still some patients continue to deteriorate after proper IOP reduction.

Some drops especially brimonidine were found to have neuroprotective effects in animal models (Vidal et al., 2010; Wolde Mussie et al., 2001). The research to achieve better control of glaucoma using a mechanism other than lowering IOP is promising. Unfortunately, neuroprotection by preventing the death of retinal ganglion cells, and vision preservation have not yet been proven in humans (Saylor et al., 2009). Long-term follow-up should determine whether or not neuroprotective agents may be beneficial for glaucoma patients (Sena et al., 2010). A low-tension glaucoma study LoGTS is currently underway comparing timolol and brimonidine treatment in NTG patients. The authors believe the neuroprotective effect of brimonidine will provide better results in preventing the disease progression. Dorzolamide, betaxolol, and latanaprost were considered to increase blood flow around the optic nerve (Harris et al., 1996, 2000), but newer published studies suggest that the effect, if exists at all, is minor (Bergstrand et al., 2002; Harris et al., 2003). Calcium channel blockers treatment was proved to be beneficial (Koseki et al., 2008; Netland et al., 1993). The treatment is recommended especially if a vasospastic disorder is diagnosed. Systemic side effects of calcium channel blockers such as flushing, edema, hypotension, headaches and reflex tachycardia requires careful selection of patients for this therapy.

In patients with low compliance or troubling side effects, laser treatment should be considered. Selective laser trabeculoplasty has promising results on lowering IOP and is considered a safe and reproducible treatment for NTG (El Mallah et al., 2010; Realini, 2008). Argon laser trabeculoplasty was studied as treatment for normal-tension glaucoma patients. The results varied from little to no effect (Schulzer, 1992; Sharpe & Simmons, 1985). SLT is considered a safe and effective treatment for lowering IOP, especially in noncompliant patient and in patients with severe side effects from topical or systemic drug treatment.

Trabeculectomy was found to lower IOP and slow the progression after long term follow-up (Bhandari et al., 1997; Shigeeda et al., 2002). Both medical and surgical treatments increase the risk for cataract formation. Cataract development was more frequent in patients undergoing trabeculectomy than in patients receiving only medical treatment (Drance et al., 2001). Follow-up and cataract extraction is advisable to improve visual acuity and follow-up reliability. Finally any systemic disease that can affect optic nerve perfusion such as systemic hypertension, congestive heart failure, arrhythmia and anemia, should be treated (Chumbley & Brubaker, 1976).

8. References

Anderson, D.R. Normal Tension Glaucoma Study. (2003). Collaborative Normal Tension Glaucoma Study. *Current Opinion in Ophthalmology*, Vol.14, No.2, pp. 86-90

Araie, M. (1995). Pattern of Visual Field Defects in Normal-Tension and High-Tension Glaucoma. *Current Opinion in Ophthalmology*, Vol.6, No.2, pp. 36-45

Baird, P.N., Richardson, A.J., Craig, J.E., Mackey, D.A., Rochtchina, E., & Mitchell, P. (2004). Analysis of Optineurin (OPTN) Gene Mutations in Subjects With and Without Glaucoma: The Blue Mountains Eye Study. *Clinical and Experimental Ophthalmology*, Vol.32, No.5, pp. 518-522

Bechetoille, A. & Bresson-Dumont, H. (1994). Diurnal and Nocturnal Blood Pressure Drops in Patients with Focal Ischemic Glaucoma. *Graefes' Archive for Clinical and Experimental Ophthalmology*, Vol. 232, No. 11, pp. 675-679

Bennett, S.R., Alward, W.L., & Folberg, R. (1989). An Autosomal Dominant Form of Low Tension Glaucoma. *American Journal of Ophthalmology*, Vol.108, pp. 238–244

Bergstrand, I.C., Heijl, A., & Harris, A. (2002). Dorzolamide and Ocular Blood Flow in Previously Untreated Glaucoma Patients: A Controlled Double-Masked Study. *Acta Ophthalmologica Scandinavica*, Vol.80, No.2, pp. 176-182

Bhandari, A., Crabb, D.P., Poinoosawmy, D., Fitzke, F.W., Hitchings, R.A., & Noureddin, B.N. (1997). Effect of Surgery on Visual Field Progression in Normal-Tension Glaucoma. *Ophthalmology*, Vol.104, No.7, pp. 1131-1137

Broadway, D.C. & Drance, S.M. (1998). Glaucoma and Vasospasm. *British Journal of Ophthalmology*, Vol.82, No.8, pp. 862-870

Caprioli, J. & Spaeth, G.L. (1984). Comparison of Visual Field Defects in the Low-Tension Glaucomas with Those in the High-Tension Glaucomas. *American Journal of Ophthalmology*, Vol.97, No.6, pp. 730-737

Caprioli, J. & Spaeth, G.L. (1985). Comparison of the Optic Nerve Head in High- and Low-Tension Glaucoma. *Archives of Ophthalmology*, Vol.103, No.8, pp. 1145-1149

Caprioli, J. & Coleman, A.L. (2010). Blood Pressure, Perfusion Pressure, and Glaucoma. *American Journal of Ophthalmology*, Vol.149, No.5, pp.704-712

Choi J, Kim, K.H., Jeong, J., Cho, H.S., Lee, C.H., & Kook, M.S. (2007). Circadian Fluctuation of Mean Ocular Perfusion Pressure is a Consistent Risk Factor for Normal-Tension Glaucoma. *Investigative Ophthalmology & Visual Science*, Vol.48, pp. 104-111

Chumbley, L.C. & Brubaker, R.F. (1976). Low-Tension Glaucoma. *American Journal of Ophthalmology*, Vol.81, No.6, pp. 761-767

Collaborative Normal Tension Glaucoma Study Group. (1998). The Effectiveness of Intraocular Pressure Reduction in the Treatment of Normal Tension Glaucoma. *American Journal of Ophthalmology*, Vol.126, pp. 498-505

Corbett, J.J., Phelps, C.D., Eslinger, P., & Montague, P.R. (1985). The Neurologic Evaluation of Patients with Low-Tension Glaucoma. *Investigative Ophthalmology & Visual Sciences*, Vol. 26, No.8, pp. 1101-1104

Dandona, L., Quigley, H.A., Brown, A.E., & Enger, C. (1990). Quantitative Regional Structure of the Normal Human Lamina Cribrosa. A Racial Comparison. *Archives of Ophthalmology*, Vol.108, pp. 393-398

Drance, S.M., Sweeney, V.P., Morgan, R.W., & Feldman, F. (1973). Studies of Factors Involved in the Production of Low Tension Glaucoma. *Archives of Ophthalmology*, Vol. 89, No.6, pp. 457-465

Drance, S.M. (1977). The Visual Field of Low Tension Glaucoma and Shock-Induced Optic Neuropathy. *Archives of Ophthalmology*, Vol. 95, No. 8, pp. 1359-1361

Drance, S., Anderson, D.R., & Schulzer, M. Collaborative Normal-Tension Glaucoma Study Group. (2001). Risk Factors for Progression of Visual Field Abnormalities in Normal-Tension Glaucoma. *American Journal of Ophthalmology*, Vol.131, No.6, pp. 699-708

El Mallah, M.K., Walsh, M.M., Stinnett, S.S., & Asrani, S.G. (2010). Selective Laser Trabeculoplasty Reduces Mean IOP and IOP Variation in Normal Tension Glaucoma Patients. *Clinical Ophthalmology*, Vol. 4, pp. 889-893

Fuse, N., Takahashi, K., Akiyama, H., Nakazawa, T., Seimiya, M., Kuwahara, S., & Tamai, M. (2004). Molecular Genetic Analysis of Optineurin Gene for Primary Open-Angle and Normal Tension Glaucoma in the Japanese Population. *Journal of Glaucoma*, Vol. 13, No. 4, pp. 299-303

Galassi, F., Sodi, A., Ucci, F., Renieri, G., Pieri, B., & Baccini, M. (2003). Ocular Hemodynamic and Glaucoma Prognosis. A Color Doppler Imaging Study. *Archives in Ophthalmology*, Vol. 121, No. 12, pp. 1711-1715

Goldberg, I., Hollows, F.C., Kass, M.A., & Becker, B. (1981). Systemic Factors in Patients with Low Tension Glaucoma. *British Journal of Ophthalmology*, Vol. 65, No. 1, pp. 56-62

Graham, S.L., Drance, S.M., Wijsman, K., Douglas, G.R., & Mikelberg, F.S. (1995). Ambulatory Blood Pressure Monitoring in Glaucoma. The Nocturnal Dip. *Ophthalmology*, Vol.102, No.1, pp.61-69

Gutman I, Melamed S, Ashkenazi I, Blumenthal M. Optic nerve compression by carotid arteries in low-tension glaucoma. *Graefes Arch Clin Exp Ophthalmol*. 1993 Dec; 231(12):711-7.

Hagishima, M., Kamiya, K., Fujimura, F., Morita, T., Shoji, N., & Shimizu, K. (2010). Effect of Corneal Astigmatism on Intraocular Pressure Measurement Using Ocular Response Analyzer and Goldmann Applanation Tonometer. *Graefes Archive in Clinical and Experimental Ophthalmology*, Vol. 248, No. 2, pp. 257-262

Harrington, D.O. (1960). Pathogenesis of the Glaucomatous Visual Field Defects: Individual Variations in Pressure Sensitivity, In: Newell FW, editor: *Conference on Glaucoma. Transactions of the Fifth Josiah Macy Conference*, F.W. Newell, (ed.), Josiah Macy Foundation, New York

Harris, A., Arend, O., Arend, S., & Martin, B. (1996). Effects of Topical Dorzolamide on Retinal and Retrobulbar Hemodynamics. *Acta Ophthalmologica Scandinavica*, Vol. 74, No. 6, pp. 569-572

Harris, A., Arend, O., Chung, H.S., Kagemann, L., Cantor, L., & Martin, B. (2000). A Comparative Study of Betaxolol and Dorzolamide Effect on Ocular Circulation in Normal-Tension Glaucoma Patients. , *Ophthalmology*, 2000, Vol. 107, No. 3, pp. 430-434

Harris, A., Migliardi, R., Rechtman, E., Cole, C.N., Yee, A.B., & Garzozi, H.J. (2003). Comparative Analysis of the Effects of Dorzolamide and Latanoprost on Ocular Hemodynamics in Normal Tension Glaucoma Patients. *European Journal of Ophthalmology*, Vol. 13, No. 1, pp. 24-31

Harris, A., Rechtman, E., Siesky, B., Jonescu-Cuypers, C., McCranor, L., & Garzozi, H.J. (2005). The Role of Optic Nerve Blood Flow in Pathogenesis of Glaucoma. *Ophthalmology Clinics of North America*, Vol. 18, No. 3, pp. 345-353

Ishida, K., Yamamoto, T., Sugiyama, K., & Kitazawa, Y. (2000). Disk Hemorrhage is a Significantly Negative Prognostic Factor in Normal-Tension Glaucoma. *American Journal of Ophthalmology*, Vol. 129, No. 6, pp. 707-714

Ito, M., Sugiura, T., & Mizokami, K. (1991). A Comparative Study on Visual Field Defect in Low-Tension Glaucoma. *Nippon Ganka Gakkai Zasshi*, Vol. 95, pp. 790-794

Iwase, A., Suzuki, Y., Araie, M., Yamamoto, T., Abe, H., Shirato, S., Kuwayama, Y., Mishima, H.K., Shimizu, H., Tomita, G., Inoue, Y., & Kitazawa, Y. Tajimi Study Group, Japan Glaucoma Society. (2004). The Prevalence of Primary Open Angle Glaucoma in Japanese: The Tajimi Study. *Ophthalmology*, Vol. 111, No. 9, pp. 1641-1648

Jonas, J.B. & Xu, L. (1994). Optic Disk Hemorrhages in Glaucoma. *American Journal of Ophthalmology*, Vol. 118, pp. 1-8

Kamio, M., Meguro, A., Ota, M., Nomura, N., Kashiwagi, K., Mabuchi, F., Iijima, H., Kawase, K., Yamamoto, T., Nakamura, M., Negi, A., Sagara, T., Nishida, T., Inatani, M., Tanihara, H., Aihara, M., Araie, M., Fukuchi, T., Abe, H., Higashide, T., Sugiyama, K., Kanamoto, T., Kiuchi, Y., Iwase, A., Ohno, S., Inoko, H., & Mizuki, N. (2009). Investigation of the Association Between the GLC3A Locus and Normal Tension Glaucoma in Japanese Patients by Microsatellite Analysis. *Clinical Ophthalmology*, Vol.3, pp. 183-188

Kesler, A., Haber, I., & Kurtz, S. (2010). Neurologic Evaluations in Normal-Tension Glaucoma Workups: Are They Worth the Effort? *Israel Medical Association Journal*, Vol. 12, No. 5, pp. 287-289

Klein, B., Klein, R., Sponsel, W.E., Franke, T., Cantor, L.B., Martone, J., & Menage, M.J. (1992). Prevalence of Glaucoma: The Beaver Dam Eye Study. *Ophthalmology*, Vol. 99, No. 10, pp. 1499-1504

Klein, B.E., Klein, R., Meuer, S.M., & Goetz, L.A. (1993). Migraine Headache and Its Association with Open-Angle Glaucoma. The Beaver Dam Eye Study. *Investigative Ophthalmology and Visual Sciences*, Vol. 34, No. 10, pp. 3024-3027

Koseki, N., Araie, M., Tomidokoro, A., Nagahara, M., Hasegawa, T., Tamaki, Y., & Yamamoto, S. (2008). A Placebo-Controlled 3-year Study of a Calcium Blocker on Visual Field and ocular Circulation in Glaucoma with Low-Normal Pressure. *Ophthalmology*, Vol. 115, No. 11, pp. 2049-2057

Leighton, D.A. & Phillips, C.I. (1972). Systemic Blood Pressure in Open-Angle Glaucoma, Low Tension Glaucoma and the Normal Eye, *British Journal of Ophthalmology*, Vol. 56, pp. 447-53

Leibowitz, H.M., Krueger, D.E., Maunder, L.R., Milton, R.C., Kini, M.M., Kahn, H.A., Nickerson, R.J., Pool, J., Colton, T.L., Ganley, J.P., Loewenstein, J.I., & Dawber, T.R. (1980). The Framingham Eye Study Monograph: An Ophthalmological and

Epidemiological Study of Cataract, Glaucoma, Diabetic Retinopathy, Macular Degeneration, and Visual Acuity in a General Population of 2631 Adults, 1973-1975. *Survey of Ophthalmology*, Vol. 24 (Suppl), pp. 335-610

Michelson, G. & Scibor, M. (2006). Intravascular Oxygen Saturation in Retinal Vessels in Normal Subjects and Open-Angle Glaucoma Subjects. *Acta Ophthalmologica Scandinavica*, Vol. 84, No. 3, pp. 289-295

Morad, Y., Sharon, E., Hefetz, L., & Nemet, P. (1998). Corneal Thickness and Curvature in normal-Tension Glaucoma. *American Journal of Ophthalmology*, Vol. 125, No. 2, pp. 164-168

Morita, T., Shoji, N., Kamiya, K., Hagishima, M., Fujimura, F., & Shimizu, K. (2010). Intraocular Pressure Measured by Dynamic Contour Tonometer and Ocular Response Analyzer in Normal Tension Glaucoma. *Graefes Archive of Clinical and Experimental Ophthalmology*, Vol. 248, No. 1, pp. 73-77.

Netland, P.A., Chaturvedi, N., & Dreyer, E.B. (1993). Calcium Channel Blockers in the Management of Low-Tension and Open-Angle Glaucoma. *American Journal of Ophthalmology*, Vol. 115, No. 5, pp. 608-613

Papastergiou, G.I., Kozobolis, V., & Siganos, D.S. (2010). Effect of Recipient Corneal Pathology on Pascal Tonometer and Goldmann Tonometer Readings in Eyes after Penetrating Keratoplasty. *European Journal of Ophthalmology*, Vol. 20, No. 1, pp. 29-34

Perkins, E.S. (1973). The Bedford Glaucoma Survey. I. Longterm Followup of Borderline Cases. *British Journal of Ophthalmology*, Vol. 57, No. 3, pp. 179-185

Phelps, C.D. & Corbett, J.J. (1985). Migraine and Low-Tension Glaucoma. A Case-Control Study. *Investigative Ophthalmology and Visual Sciences*, Vol. 26, No. 8, pp. 1105-1108

Plange, N., Remky, A., & Arend, O. (2003). Colour Doppler Imaging and Fluorescein Filling Defects of the Optic Disc in Normal Tension Glaucoma. *British Journal of Ophthalmology*, Vol. 87, No. 6, pp. 731-736.

Quigley, H., Pease, M.E., & Thibault, D. (1994). Change in the Appearance of Elastin in the Lamina Cribrosa of Glaucomatous Optic Nerve Heads. *Graefes Archive of Clinical and Experimental Ophthalmology*, Vol. 232, pp. 257-261

Realini, T. (2008). Selective Laser Trabeculoplasty: A Review. *Journal of Glaucoma*, Vol. 17, No. 6, pp. 497-502.

Sánchez-Navés, J., Furfaro, L., Piro, O., & Balle, S. (2008). Impact and Permanence of LASIK-Induced Structural Changes in the Cornea on Pneumotonometric Measurements: Contributions of Flap Cutting and Stromal Ablation. *Journal of Glaucoma*, Vol. 17, No. 8, pp. 611-618

Sarfarazi, M., Child, A., Stoilova, D., Brice, G., Desai, T., Trifan, O.C., Poinoosawmy, D., & Crick, R.P. (1998). Localization of the Fourth Locus (GLC1E) for Adult-Onset Primary Open-Angle Glaucoma to the 10p15-p14 Region. *American Journal of Human Genetics*, Vol. 62, No. 3, pp. 641-652

Sato, E.A., Ohtake, Y., Shinoda, K., Mashima, Y., & Kimura, I. (2006). Decreased Blood Flow at Neuroretinal Rim of Optic Nerve Head Corresponds with Visual Field Deficit in Eyes with Normal Tension Glaucoma. *Graefes Archive of Clinical and Experimental Ophthalmology*, Vol. 244, No. 7, pp. 795-801

Saylor, M., McLoon, L.K., Harrison, A.R., & Lee, M.S. (2009). Experimental and Clinical Evidence for Brimonidine as an Optic Nerve and Retinal Neuroprotective Agent: An Evidence-Based Review. *Archives of Ophthalmology*, Vol. 127, No. 4, pp. 402-406

Schulzer, M. (1992). The Normal-Tension Glaucoma Study Group: Intraocular Pressure Reduction in Normal-Tension Glaucoma Patients. *Ophthalmology*, Vol. 99, pp. 1468-1470

Sena, D.F., Ramchand, K., & Lindsley, K. (2010). Neuroprotection for Treatment of Glaucoma in Adults. *Cochrane Database of Systematic Reviews*, Vol. 17, CD006539

Shields, M.B. (2008). Normal-Tension Glaucoma: Is It Different From Primary Open-Angle Glaucoma? *Current Opinion in Ophthalmology*, Vol. 19, No. 2, p. 85-88

Sharpe, E.D. & Simmons, R.J. (1985). Argon Laser Trabeculoplasty as a Means of Decreasing Intraocular Pressure from "Normal" Levels in Glaucomatous Eyes. *American Journal of Ophthalmology*, Vol. 99, No. 6, pp. 704-707

Shigeeda, T., Tomidokoro, A., Araie, M., Koseki, N., & Yamamoto, S. (2002). Long-Term Follow-Up of Visual Field Progression After Trabeculectomy in Progressive Normal-Tension Glaucoma. *Ophthalmology*, Vol. 109, No. 4, pp. 766-770

Shin, I.H., Kang, S.Y., Hong, S., Kim, S.K., Seong, G.J., Tak, M.K., & Kim, C.Y. (2008). Comparison of OCT and HRT Findings Among Normal, Normal Tension Glaucoma, and High Tension Glaucoma. *Korean Journal of Ophthalmology*, Vol. 22, No. 4, pp. 236-241

Shiose, Y., Kitazawa, Y., Tsukahara, S., Akamatsu, T., Mizokami, K., Futa, R., Katsushima, H., & Kosaki, H. (1991). Epidemiology of Glaucoma in Japan: A Nationwide Glaucoma Survey, *Japan Journal of Ophthalmology*, Vol. 35, No. 2, pp. 133-155

Siegner, S.W. & Netland, P.A. (1996). Optic Disc Hemorrhages and Progression of Glaucoma. *Ophthalmology*, Vol. 103, No. 7, pp. 1014-1024

Sommer, A., Tielsch, J.M., Katz, J., Quigley, H.A., Gottsch, J.D., Javitt, J., & Singh, K. (1991). Relationship Between Intraocular Pressure and Primary Open Angle Glaucoma among White and Black Americans. The Baltimore Eye Survey. *Archives of Ophthalmology*, Vol. 109, No. 8, pp. 1090-1095

Toda, Y., Tang, S., Kashiwagi, K., Mabuchi, F., Iijima, H., Tsukahara, S., & Yamagata, Z. (2004). Mutations in the Optineurin Gene in Japanese Patients with Primary Open-Angle Glaucoma and Normal Tension Glaucoma. *American Journal of Medical Genetics A*, Vol. 125, No. 1, pp. 1-4

Tomita, G. (2000). The Optic Nerve Head in Normal-Tension Glaucoma. *Current Opinion in Ophthalmology*, Vol. 11, No. 2, pp. 116-120

Umeda, T., Matsuo, T., Nagayama, M., Tamura, N., Tanabe, Y., & Ohtsuki, H. (2004). Clinical Relevance of Optineurin Sequence Alterations in Japanese Glaucoma Patients. *Ophthalmic Genetics*, Vol. 25, pp.:91

Vidal, L., Díaz, F., Villena, A., Moreno, M., Campos, J.G., & Pérez de Vargas, I. (2010). Reaction of Müller Cells in an Experimental Rat Model of Increased Intraocular Pressure Following Timolol, Latanoprost and Brimonidine. *Brain Research Bulletin*, Vol. 82, No. 1-2, pp. 18-24

WoldeMussie, E., Ruiz, G., Wijono, M., & Wheeler, L.A. (2001). Neuroprotection of Retinal Ganglion Cells by Brimonidine in Rats with Laser-Induced Chronic Ocular

Hypertension. *Investigative Ophthalmology and Visual Sciences*, Vol. 42, No. 12, pp. 2849-2855

Xia, C.R., Xu, L., & Yang, Y. (2005). A Comparative Study of Optic Nerve Damage Between Primary Open Angle Glaucoma and Normal Tension Glaucoma. *Zhonghua Yan Ke Za Zhi*, Vol. 41, No. 2, pp. 136-140

12

Plateau Iris

Yoshiaki Kiuchi, Hideki Mochizuki and Kiyoshi Kusanagi
Hiroshima University
Japan

1. Introduction

Primary angle-closure glaucoma (PACG) is a common form of glaucoma in Asia (Foster & Johnson, 2001). It is associated with a high risk of visual loss (Congdon et al., 1992; Foster et al., 1996). PACG was estimated to blind 5 times more people than primary open-angle glaucoma (Quigley et al. 2001). The original concept of primary angle closure glaucoma was a pupil- block angle-closure mechanism occurring in predisposed eyes with shallow anterior chamber angles. Peripheral iridectomy prevents the progression of primary angle closure glaucoma (Lowe, 1964). However, many patients experienced recurrent angle-closure glaucoma attacks after iridectomy (Wand et al., 1977). The occurrence of narrow angle in eyes with relatively normal depth in the anterior chamber and a relatively flat iris plane had been noted as early as 1940 (Gradle & Sugar, 1940). Chandler presented the case of a patient with repeated intermittent angle-closure glaucoma attacks despite a patent iridectomy, who was successfully treated with pilocarpine (Wand et al., 1977). Those cases were considered to be different from ordinary cases of narrow angle glaucoma. They were particularly found

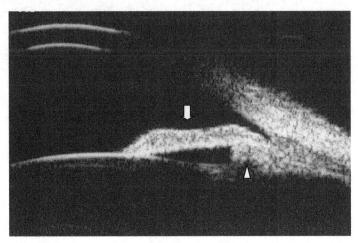

Fig. 1. Plateau iris configuration. Ultrasound biomicroscopy image shows a flat iris plane (⬇) accompanied by a narrow or closed anterior chamber angle. Plateau iris configuration is caused by anteriorly located ciliary processes (Λ), which close the ciliary sulcus and provide support to the peripheral iris

in younger patients in whom a peripheral iridectomy is often ineffective. These patients had a flat iris and a narrow angle secondary to an abrupt angulation at the root of the iris. This iris shape was called a plateau iris configuration.

The concept of the plateau iris was introduced in a publication by Shaffer (Shaffer, 1960). Primary angle closure includes those that are caused by a pupillary block and plateau iris configuration (Tarongoy et al., 2009).

2. Plateau iris configuration and plateau iris syndrome

Wand et al. reported that the plateau iris syndrome should be differentiated from the plateau iris configuration, to avoid confusion. Native plateau iris configuration refers to a preoperative (iridectomy or iridotomy) condition, in which angle-closure glaucoma is confirmed by gonioscopy, but the iris is flat and the anterior chamber is not shallow (Wand et al., 1977). One third of all patients demonstrating primary angle closure were estimated to have plateau iris configuration (Kumar et al., 2009, Mochizuki et al., 2010).

Plateau iris syndrome refers to the development of angle closure in an eye with plateau iris configuration. The intraocular pressure (IOP) increases because of angle closure after pupillary dilation. Plateau iris configuration can be diagnosed before iridotomy. However, plateau iris syndrome is normally diagnosed after laser iridotomy. Plateau iris syndrome is rare. Less than 10 % of all patients with primary angle closure are considered to have plateau iris syndrome.

The prevalence of angle closure attack in plateau iris syndrome is not known.

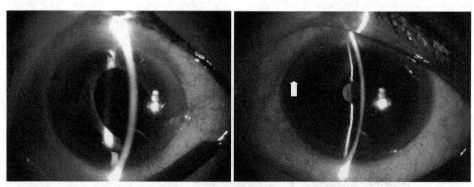

Fig. 2. Slit lamp photograph of an eye with a re-attack of acute closer attack and the patient's opposite eye. Right eye; Pupil is dilated after the second attack. Left eye; The laser iridotomy hole (⬆) is observed at 10 o'clock

The right eye developed acute closed-angle attack on December 2005. After successful treatment by laser iridotomy patients had a re-attack on October 2006. This patient underwent cataract surgery for the relief of the angle closure attack. Cataract surgery stabilized the IOP in the right eye.

Plateau iris syndrome is classified into two groups. Complete syndrome has a high plateau and covers the chamber angle after dilation and causes elevation of the IOP. Incomplete Syndrome partially covers the chamber angle after dilation of the pupil. The IOP will not elevate after dilating the pupil. However, the peripheral anterior synechia (PAS) increases over time (Wand et al., 1977). Many people tend to confuse incomplete plateau syndrome with plateau iris configuration.

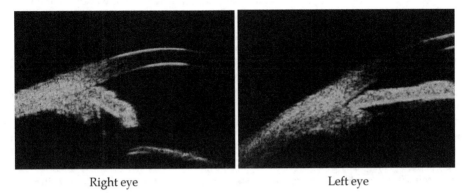

Right eye   Left eye

Fig. 3. Ultrasound biomicroscopy image of Figure 2

3. Diagnosis

3.1 Gonioscopic findings

Generally, the diagnosis of a plateau iris configuration is based on typical gonioscopic findings. A plateau iris configuration is defined as a flat iris plane accompanied by a narrow or closed anterior chamber angle. Some patients with a plateau iris configuration show an increased intraocular pressure after the pupils are dilated by angle closure even after laser iridotomy.

Indentation gonioscopy of eyes with a plateau iris configuration following patent iridotomy reveals a sine-shaped curve of the iris surface. Indentation presses the iris surface backward. The deepest point of indentation is not at the iris periphery, but at approximately two-thirds of the distance between the center of the pupil and the iris root. The iris rises again from this point to the site of appositional closure. This shape is called a double hump sign.

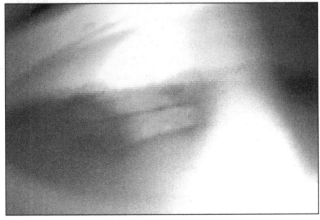

Fig. 4. Double hump sign after indentation

A double hump sign observed on indentation gonioscopy was strongly correlated with the presence of a plateau iris, and is, therefore a useful indicator of a plateau iris configuration. Therefore, a plateau iris configuration can be detected in many cases, without using a UBM (Kiuchi et al., 2009; Ritch, 1992).

3.2 Ultrasound biomicroscopy (UBM) findings

UBM provides detailed sub surface images of the angle region. This method showed that plateau iris configuration is caused by anteriorly located ciliary processes, which close the ciliary sulcus and provide support to the peripheral iris (Roberts et al., 2008). The ciliary processes were situated anteriorly in all the plateau iris configuration patients in comparison to the position in normal subjects and in patients with angle closure caused by pupillary block. The ciliary processes provide structural support beneath the peripheral iris, preventing the iris root from falling away from the trabecular meshwork after iridotomy (Pavlin et al., 1992).

Observation with a slit lamp causes miosis and thus the iris becomes thinner. An unintentional indentation and/or miosis induced by the slit-lamp light might prevent the identification of appositional angle closure during regular gonioscopic examination (Sakata et al., 2006). The importance of the diagnosis of plateau iris configuration by UBM resides in the fact that the plateau iris configuration can be detected without any interference from the effect of the lighting. Provocative tests were not usually helpful for detecting plateau iris syndrome (Ritch et al., 2009).

4. Gender and age

Women from Japan, Israel, Finland, and Thailand showed a consistently more frequent occurrence of PACG (Yamamoto et al., 2005). One study found no sexual predisposition for plateau iris configuration (Ritch, 1992). Others report that most patients with plateau iris were female and younger than those with pupillary block. The average age of the patients studied by Diniz et al. was 60.1 years old (Diniz et al., 2010). This is consistent with the results of the study by Mandell et al (Mandell et al., 2003), in which the plateau iris configuration patients averaged 57.5 years old.

Ritch, et al. evaluated the findings in patients 40 years of age or younger with angle closure. Sixty-seven patients (49 females, 18 males) met the entry criteria. Plateau iris configuration was found in 35 patients (52.2%) (Ritch et al., 2003).

On the other hand, the prevalence of PACG significantly increases with age in population based epidemiological studies (Yamamoto et al., 2005). Pupillary block angle closure is a disease of older persons, peaking in incidence between 55 and 70 years of age (Suzuki et al., 2008).

4.1 Prevalence of plateau iris configuration

Kumar et al. used standardized UBM criteria and found plateau iris in about one third of PACS eyes after laser iridotomy (Kumar et al., 2008, 2009). Mochizuki et al. conducted a study under the same criteria used by Kumar et al. to determine the prevalence of plateau iris configurations in acute angle-closure, chronic angle-closure glaucoma, and open-angle glaucoma eyes using ultrasound biomicroscopy The study included fellow eyes from 27 acute angle-closure patients, 26 open-angle glaucoma patients, and 26 chronic angle-closure glaucoma patients with no history of acute angle-closure. Plateau iris configurations were found in the opposite eyes of 10 (37.0%) of 27 patients with acute angle-closure, 9 (34.6%)of 26 patients with chronic angle-closure glaucoma, and 5 (19.2%) of 26 patients with open-angle glaucoma (Mochizuki et al., 2010). Filho also reported that plateau iris configuration in 10.2% of patients with open-angle glaucoma (Diniz Fiho et al., 2010). The clinical significance of plateau iris configurations in open-angle glaucoma eyes is unclear. Open-angle glaucoma eyes do not have plateau iris configurations high enough to occlude the trabecular meshwork, which is associated with the elevation of IOP or other clinical events. However, lower plateau iris configuration may become higher over time due to increased thickness and anterior movement of the lens, which would consequently result in angle closure.

4.2 Prevalence of plateau iris syndrome

Cases of recurrent angle-closure glaucoma after iridectomy, as a result of plateau iris syndrome are relatively rare. Plateau iris syndrome is believed to constitute a small percentage of eyes with plateau iris configuration. A study of eyes that had experienced angle-closure episodes was conducted to determine the relative frequency of plateau iris syndrome. All of the patients had undergone peripheral iridectomy. The IOP increased more than 8 mmHg after topical application of homatropine in 4 (6.2%)of the 65 eyes. Those 4 eyes were classified as the iris plateau type of angle –closure glaucoma (Godel et al., 1968). Saitoh reported that five of 50 iridectomized PACG eyes developed complete closure of the angle with an increase in the IOP exceeding 10 mmHg following the administration of homatropine which acts on the sphincter muscle located at the pupillary margin. However, those 5 subjects did not show IOP elevation after topical application of phenilephrine hydrochloride (alpha adrenergic stimulator) Phenilephrine acts on the iris dilator muscle which is located just above the iris pigment epithelium. Homatropine and phenilephrine act on different muscles in the iris, and the difference in the distribution of the dilator muscle and the sphincter muscle causes the different morphological changes in the iris after application of the midriatic agents. This may explain the difference in IOP response after dilation of pupil by midriatic agents (Saitoh, 1974).

4.3 Biometrics of plateau iris configuration

Historically, plateau iris configuration is regarded as angle closure with normal anterior chamber depth and flat iris plane. Mandel et al. reported that all plateau iris configuration eyes showed biometric parameters that were completely different for those of normal eyes, except for the peripheral iris thickness at 500 µm from the scleral spur. The eyes with plateau iris configuration showed a shallower anterior chamber depth than normal eyes (Mandell et al., 2003). The mean anterior chamber depth in patients with plateau iris syndrome (2.04 +/- 0.30 mm) was significantly smaller than the hypothesized normal anterior chamber depth (3 mm). The mean anterior chamber depth in patients with pupillary block (2.17 +/- 0.30 mm) was also significantly smaller than the hypothesized normal anterior chamber depth. Although a review of the literature suggested that patients with plateau iris had a normal or deeper axial anterior chamber depth in comparison to those with pupillary block, the mean anterior chamber depth in patients with plateau iris syndrome was significantly smaller than the anterior chamber depth in patients with pupillary block in the report by Mandell et al (Mandell et al., 2003).

There is one more report related to the biometrics of plateau iris configuration. Kiuchi et al. reported that patients with plateau iris configuration had deeper anterior chamber and longer axial length than chronic angle closure patients without plateau iris configuration (Kiuchi et al., 2009). Further study is necessary to clarify this issue.

4.4 Changes in the biometrics of plateau iris configuration after intervention

Palvin et al. used ultrasound biomicroscopy to image angles in the dark, in the light, and following pilocarpine administration to clarify factors that produce angle opening changes in this syndrome. Changes in angle opening in dark and light were solely related to changes in iris thickness. Their results were consistent with the concept that the space between the ciliary processes and trabecular meshwork constitutes a passageway of fixed dimension. An increase in iris thickness resulted in a decrease in angle opening, and a decrease in iris thickness resulted in an increase in angle opening. Angle closure occured if the iris thickness fills the space between the ciliary processes and the trabecular meshwork (Pavlin & Foster, 1999).

5. The cause of plateau iris configuration

The cause of the plateau iris configuration is not known. The anomaly of the pars plicata position could be developmental or acquired. Ciliary processes develop during the 24th week of embryogenesis and initially overlap the trabecular meshwork but later recede to a position behind the scleral spur. This repositioning is thought to be due to a differential growth rate of the various tissue elements. The specific features of the ciliary processes in the eyes with plateau iris might be due to the failure of the ciliary processes to separate from the posterior iris surface. The displacement of the pars plicata from the peripheral iris to the iris root during embryogenesis may be incomplete in eyes with a shorter axial length. However, incomplete cleavage between the iris and ciliary body is unlikely (Razeghinejad & Kamali-Sarvestani, 2007; Tran et al., 2003).

Tran and associates (Tran et al., 2003) examined the anterior segments of 6 patients with plateau iris syndrome before and after cataract surgery. They found that irido-ciliary apposition persisted after extracapsular cataract extraction, thus indicating that the age related growth of the lens (i.e., acquired changes in the zonular fibers stretched by cataract formation) does not induce a reversible anterior pulling and or rotation of the ciliary body processes.

Etter investigated the prevalence of plateau iris syndrome in the first-degree relatives of patients affected with plateau iris syndrome. They found a high prevalence of plateau iris configuration in family members of patients with plateau iris syndrome. Five of the 10 participating patients (50%) were found to have at least 1 first-degree family member with plateau iris configuration. The presence of plateau iris configuration in successive generations, where there was not consanguineous marriage, therefore suggested that it might be inherited in an autosomal dominant manner with incomplete penetrance (Etter et al., 2006).

6. Differential diagnosis

6.1 Iris cyst

Tanihara et al. reported a case of high, broad, peripheral anterior synechiae caused by multiple, bilateral iridociliary cysts. The peripheral anterior synechia extended to the corneal endothelium beyond Schwalbe's line. Ultrasound biomicroscopic imaging showed that multiple, bilateral iridociliary cysts causes elevation of the iris structure (Tanihara et al., 1997). This report showed that an iris cyst could cause the pseudo-plateau configuration. The incidence and sector distribution of ciliary body cysts in normal subjects is not low. A UBM study conducted by Kunimatsu et al. showed that cysts were detected in 63 (54.3%) of the 116 subjects. The number and diameter of the cysts decreased with age. Gender and refractive error did not affect the incidence and distribution. A significant bilateral correlation was found in the number, incidence, and distribution of ciliary body cysts (Kunimatsu et al., 1999). There was a high prevalence of iris cysts in young subjects. Younger subjects with a bumpy peripheral iris have a higher likelihood of a diagnosis of pseudo-plateau iris (Shukla et al., 2008).

6.2 Others
Any disorder that causes swelling of the ciliary body or forward rotation of the ciliary body can create a pseudo-plateau iris configuration. Sulfa based compounds like hydrochlorothiazide, oral acetazolamide, supra ciliary effusions and ciliary body thickening after scleral buckling procedures can cause ciliary swelling and precipitate angle closure glaucoma.(Geason & Perkins, 1995; Palvin et al., 1997; Tripathi et al., 2003)

7. Management

7.1 Miotics
Miotic therapy is one option for plateau iris configuration. One drop of pilocarpine causes significant changes in the anterior eye segment morphology. This decreases the pupillary diameter and the iris thickness (Németh et al., 1996-1997). A single drop of 2% pilocarpine is an effective agent for thinning the iris and opening the angle in plateau iris syndrome. The ability to visualize the degree of angle opening produced by pilocarpine can be helpful in predicting the efficacy of this therapy (Pavlin and Foster, 1999). There are two problems associated with pilocarpine treatment for glaucoma associated with plateau iris configuration. Most patients are relatively young in age in comparison to the usual angle-closure glaucoma patients, and therefore, are unhappy with pilocarpine- induced myopia and miosis. These side effects may decrease the compliance (adherence) to the medical therapy.

Yasuda et al. examined the long-term effects of topical pilocarpine on IOP control in primary angle-closure glaucoma without iridectomy. Six (43%) out of 14 eyes with acute PACG under topical pilocarpine therapy had re-attacks while one eye (7%) developed increased IOP. Twelve of 47 fellow eyes of patients with acute PACG (26%) developed acute attacks while 3 eyes (6%) showed increased IOP. They concluded that long-term medical therapy for PACG is unsatisfactory. A single drop of pilocarpine works only for 6 hours. Short acting duration of pilocarpine and poor compliance (adherence) may play some role in this result. They included all types of angle closure glaucoma in their study. Patients with plateau iris configuration might yield the same results (Yasuda & Kageyama, 1988).

7.2 Laser treatment
7.2.1 Laser iridotomy
Laser iridotomy (LI) is the appropriate treatment for angle closure glaucoma due to primary pupillary block. UBM studies in patients with pupillary block glaucoma post-LI

demonstrated substantial increases in the anterior chamber angle aperture following laser iridotomy. Previous studies have also shown that in eyes with an acute attack, the angle widened in the first 2 weeks after LI, but did not change thereafter over 1 year, and the amount of peripheral anterior synechia (PAS) remained stable throughout. The results indicate the effectiveness of LI in preventing progressive closure of the angle in the first year after the angle closure attack (Porikoff et al., 2005). However, laser iridotomy is insufficient to treat glaucoma associated with plateau iris. Many patients with a patent iridotomy hole experienced acute angle-closed attacks. Polikoff et al. also examined the effect of laser iridotomy on anterior segment anatomy of patients with plateau iris configuration. Iridotomy will remove any contribution from pupillary block in these patients, but the angle will remain narrow because the anteriorly positioned ciliary processes prevent the peripheral iris from moving posteriorly. This report also showed that pupil block and plateau iris configuration coexists in many cases (Polikoff et al., 2005). Approximately one of three of the eyes showed PAS progression during a 3-year follow-up period after LI. The probability of progression was found to be high in the eyes that exhibited plateau iris (Choi & Kim, 2005). These data show that laser iridotomy alone is not an effective treatment for glaucoma with plateau iris configuration.

7.2.2 Argon laser peripheral iridoplasty

Argon laser peripheral iridoplasty can effectively eliminate residual appositional closure after laser iridotomy caused by plateau iris syndrome, and the effect is maintained for years. Argon laser iridoplasty may also prove valuable in the treatment of plateau-like iris configuration resulting from iridociliary cysts (Crowston et al., 2005). Rich et al. documented the long-term effect of argon laser iridoplasty in patients with plateau iris syndrome. A total of 26 argon laser iridoplasty procedures were performed in 23 eyes of 14 patients. The angle remained open in 20 of 23 (87.0%) eyes after only 1 treatment with Argon laser iridoplasty over a follow-up period of 78.9 ± 8.0 months (range, 72–188 months). They concluded that Argon laser iridoplasty could effectively eliminate residual appositional closure after laser iridotomy caused by plateau iris syndrome (Ritch et al., 2004). However, there are no other reports that indicate the effectiveness of laser peripheral iridoplasty.

7.2.3 Cataract surgery

Hayashi showed that the anterior chamber depth and angle width in angle closure glaucoma eyes approximates that of POAG eyes and control eyes without glaucoma after phaco-emulsification and posterior chamber intraocular lens implantation (Hayashi et al., 2000). They thought that these changes contribute to the significant IOP reduction seen in the postoperative follow-up period of 12 months. Tran et al. evaluated the ultrasound biomicroscopic appearance of the anterior segment before and after cataract extraction in eyes with plateau iris syndrome. None of the six eyes with plateau iris syndrome in their study showed a change in the configuration of the ciliary body after IOL implantation. However, the anterior chamber depth increased and the angle opened further after cataract surgery. The persistent iridociliary apposition after cataract surgery suggests that the iris and pars plicata appear to move together (Tran et al., 2003). Nonaka et al. reported cataract surgery for angle closure including plateau configuration opened the angle concomitant with attenuation of the anterior positioning of the ciliary processes. Cataract surgery would contribute to postoperative widening of the angle not only by completely removing the lens volume and pupillary block, but also by attenuating the anterior positioning of the ciliary processes in eyes with primary angle closed eyes (Nonaka et al., 2006). There are currently no randomized controlled trials supporting the use of clear lens extraction as the treatment of choice for PACG. However, the potential of obtaining some benefit from this procedure is considered to be biologically plausible (Thomas et al., 2011).

Phacoemulsification and goniosynechialysis (PEGS) is also effective in managing acute and subacute primary angle closure including patients plateau iris (Harasymowycz et al., 2005).

Topical application of miotic agents, laser peripheral iridoplasty and cataract surgery seem to be effective for glaucoma with plateau iris configuration. There is a lack of well-designed, randomized, controlled trials to assess the effect as a therapeutic modality for glaucoma with plateau iris configuration, because the occurrence of plateau iris is relatively rare.

8. Conclusions

A plateau iris configuration is defined as a flat iris plane accompanied by a narrow or closed anterior chamber angle. Pathological and physiological data of plateau iris configuration and plateau iris syndrome are increasing. However, we do not have enough information related to plateau iris configuration and syndrome to manage them. The prognosis of this disorder compared to pupillary block angle closure glaucoma also remains to be elucidated. There are no quantitative diagnosis criteria, yet. This condition confuse the interpretation of the data appeared at the journals. The best therapeutic protocol should be established in future. New imaging technology will help us to obtain the new information.

9. References

Choi, JS. & Kim, YY. (2005). Progression of peripheral anterior synechiae after laser iridotomy., American Journal of Ophthalmology, Vol.140, No.6, (2005), pp.1125–1127

Congdon, N., Wang, F., & Tielsch, JM. (1992). Issues in the epidemiology and population-based screening of primary angle-closure glaucoma, Survey of Ophthalmology, Vol.36, No.11, (1992), pp.411–423

Crowston, JG., Medeiros, FA. Mosaed, S., & Weinreb, RN. (2005). Argon laser iridoplasty in the treatment of plateau-like iris configuration as result of numerous ciliary body cysts, American Journal of Ophthalmology, Vol.139, No.2, (2005), pp.381–383

Diniz Filho, A., Cronemberger, S., Ferreira, DM., Mérula, RV., & Calixto, N. (2010). Plateau iris configuration in eyes with narrow-angle: an ultrasound biomicroscopic study, Arquivos brasileiros de oftalmologia, Vol.73, No.2, (2010), pp.155-160

Etter, JR., Affel, EL., & Rhee, DJ. (2006). High prevalence of plateau iris configuration in family members of patients with plateau iris syndrome, Journal of Glaucoma, Vol.15, No.5 (2006), pp.394–398

Foster, PJ., Baasanhu, J., Alsbirk, PH., Munkhbayar, D., Uranchimeg, D., & Johnson, J. (1996). Glaucoma in Mongolia: a population-based survey in Hovsgol province, northern Mongolia, Archives of Ophthalmology, Vol.114, No.10, (1996), pp.1235–1241

Foster, PJ. & Johnson, GJ. (2001). Glaucoma in China: how big is the problem?, British Journal of Ophthalmology, Vol.85, No.11, (2001), pp.1277–1282

Geanon, JD. & Perkins, TW.(1995). Bilateral acute angle-closure glaucoma associated with drug sensitivity to hydrochlorothiazide, Archives of Ophthalmology, Vol.113, No.10, (1995), pp.1231–1232

Godel, V., Stein, R., & Feiler-Ofry, V. (1968). Angle-closure glaucoma: following peripheral iridectomy and mydriasis, *American Journal of Ophthalmology*, Vol.65, No.4, (1968), pp.555-560

Gradle, HS. & Sugar, HS. (1940). Concerning the chamber angle. III. A clinical method of goniometry, *American Journal of Ophthalmology*, Vol.23, (1940), pp.1135-1139

Harasymowycz, PJ., Papamatheakis, DG., Ahmed, I., Assalian, A., Lesk, M., Al-Zafiri, Y., Kranemann, C., & Hutnik, C. (2005). Phacoemulsification and goniosynechialysis in the management of unresponsive primary angle closure, *Journal of Glaucoma*, (2005), pp.186-189

Hayashi, K., Hayashi, H., Nakao, F., & Hayashi, F. (2000). Changes in anterior chamber angle width and depth after intraocular lens implantation in eyes with glaucoma, *Ophthalmology*, Vol.107, No.4, (2000), pp.698-703

Kiuchi, Y., Kanamoto, T., & Nakamura, T. (2009). Double hump sign in indentation gonioscopy is correlated with presence of plateau iris configuration regardless of patent iridotomy, *Journal of Glaucoma*, Vol.18, No.2, (2009), pp.161-164

Kumar, RS., Baskaran, M., Chew, PT., Friedman, DS., Handa, S., Lavanya, R., Sakata, LM., Wong, HT., & Aung ,T.(2008) . Prevalence of plateau iris in primary angle closure suspects an ultrasound biomicroscopy study, *Ophthalmology*, Vol.115, No.3, (2008), pp.430-434

Kumar, RS., Tantisevi, V., Wong, MH., Laohapojanart, K., Chansanti, O., Quek, DT., Koh, VT., MohanRam, LS., Lee, KY., Rojanapongpun, P., & Aung, T. (2009). Plateau iris in Asian subjects with primary angle closure glaucoma, *Archives of Ophthalmology*, Vol.127, No.10, (2009), pp.1269-1272

Kunimatsu, S., Araie, M., Ohara, K., & Hamada, C. (1999). Ultrasound biomicroscopy of ciliary body cysts, *American Journal of Ophthalmology*, Vol.127, No.1, (1999), pp.48-55

Lim, LS., Aung, T., Husain, R., Wu, YJ., Gazzard, G., & Seah, SK. (2004). Acute primary angle closure: configuration of the drainage angle in the first year after laser peripheral iridotomy, *Ophthalmology*, Vol.111, No.8, (2004), pp.1470-1474

Lowe, RF. (1964). Primary angle-closure glaucoma. Investigation after surgery for pupil block, *American Journal of Ophthalmology*, Vol.57, (1964), pp.931-938

Mandell, MA., Pavlin, CJ., Weisbrod, DJ., & Simpson, ER. (2003). Anterior Chamber Depth in Plateau Iris Syndrome and Pupillary Block as Measured by Ultrasound Biomicroscopy, *American Journal of Ophthalmology*, Vol.136, No.5, (2003), pp.900-903

Mochizuki, H., Takenaka, J., Sugimoto, Y., Takamatsu, M., & Kiuchi, Y. (2010). Comparison of the Prevalence of Plateau Iris Configurations Between Angle-closure Glaucoma and Open-angle Glaucoma Using Ultrasound Biomicroscopy, *Journal of Glaucoma*, (2010)

Németh, J., Csákány, B., & Pregun, T. (1996-1997). Ultrasound biomicroscopic morphometry of the anterior eye segment before and after one drop of pilocarpine, *International Ophthalmoogyl*, Vol.20, No.1-3,(1996-1997), pp.39-42

Nonaka, A., Kondo, T., Kikuchi, M., Yamashiro, K., Fujihara, M., Iwawaki ,T., Yamamoto, K., & Kurimoto, Y. (2006). Angle widening and alteration of ciliary process configuration after cataract surgery for primary angle closure. *Ophthalmology*, Vol.113, No.3, (2006), pp.437-441

Pavlin,CJ & Foster, FS.(1999). Plateau iris syndrome: changes in angle opening associated with dark, light, and pilocarpine administration, *American Journal of Ophthalmology*, Vol.128, No.3, (1999), pp.288-291

Pavlin, CJ., Ritch R., & Foster, FS. (1992). Ultrasound biomicroscopy in plateau iris syndrome, *American Journal of Ophthalmology*, Vol.113, No. 4, (1992), pp.390-395

Pavlin, CJ., Rutnin, SS., Deveny R., Wand, M. & Foster, FS.(1997). Supraciliary effusions and ciliary body thickening after scleral buckling procedures, *Ophthalmology*, Vol.104, No. 3, (1997), pp.433-438

Polikoff, LA., Chanis, RA., Toor, A., Ramos-Esteban, JC., Fahim, MM., Gagliuso, DJ., & Serle, JB. (2005). The effect of laser iridotomy on the anterior segment anatomy of patients with plateau iris configuration, *Journal of Glaucoma*, Vol.14, No.2, (2005), pp.109-113

Quigley, HA., Congdon, NG., & Friedman, DG. (2001). Glaucoma in China (and worldwide): changes in established thinkingwill decrease preventable blindness, *British Journal of Ophthalmology*; Vol.85, No.11, (2001), pp.1271–1272

Razeghinejad, MR. & Kamali-Sarvestani,E. (2007). The plateau iris component of primary angle closure glaucoma: developmental or acquired, *Medical Hypotheses*, Vol. 69, No.31, (2007), pp.95–98

Ritch, R. (1992). Plateau iris is caused by abnormally positioned ciliary processes, *Journal of Glaucoma*, Vol.1, (1992), pp.23-26

Ritch, R., Aung, T., & Lam, DS. (2009). Angle-closure Glaucoma, *Journal of Glaucoma*, Vol.18, No.7, (2009), pp.567-570

Ritch, R., Chang, BM., & Liebmann, JM. (2003). Angle closure in younger patients, *Ophthalmology*, Vol.110, No.10, (2003), pp.1880–1889

Ritch, R., Tham, CC., & Lam DS (2004). Long-term success of argon laser peripheral iridoplasty in the management of plateau iris syndrome, *Ophthalmology*, Vol.111, No.1, (2004), pp.104–108

Roberts, DK., Ayyagari, R., & Moroi, SE. (2008). Possible association between long anterior lens zonules and plateau iris configuration, *Journal of Glaucoma*, Vol.17, No.5, (2008), pp.393–396

Saitoh, S. (1974). Midriasis test in primary angle-closure glaucoma, *Nippon Ganka Gakkai Zasshi*, Vol.78, No.11, (1974), pp.1179-1185

Sakata, LM., Sakata, K.,& Susanna, R Jr. (2006). Long ciliary processes with no ciliary sulcus and appositional angle closure assessed by ultrasound biomicroscopy, *Journal of Glaucoma*, Vol. 15, No.5, (2006), pp.371–379

Shaffer, RN. (1960). Primary Glaucomas. Gonioscopy, ophthalmoscopy and perimetry, *Transactions - American Academy of Ophthalmology and Otolaryngology*, Vol.64, (1960), pp.112-127

Shukla, S., Damji, KF., Harasymowycz, P., Chialant, D., Kent, JS., Chevrier, R., Buhrmann, R., Marshall, D., Pan, Y., & Hodge, W. (2008). Clinical features distinguishing angle closure from pseudoplateau versus plateau iris, *British Journal of Ophthalmology*, Vol. 92, No.3, (2008), pp.340-344

Suzuki, Y., Yamamoto, T., Araie, M., Iwase, A., Tomidokoro, A., Abe, H., Shirato, S., Kuwayama, Y., Mishima, HK., Shimizu, H., Tomita, G., Inoue, Y., & Kitazawa, Y. (2008). Tajimi Study review, *Nippon Ganka Gakkai Zasshi*, Vol.112, No.12, (2008), pp.1039-1058

Tanihara, H., Akita, J., Honjo, M., & Honda, Y. (1997). Angle closure caused by multiple bilateral iridociliary cysts, *Acta ophthalmologica Scandinavica*, Vol. 75, No.2, (1997), pp.216–217

Tarongoy, P., Ho, CL., & Walton, DS. (2009). Angle-closure glaucoma: the role of the lens in the pathogenesis, prevention, and treatment, *Survey of Ophthalmology*, Vol.54, No. 2, (2009), pp.211--225

Tran, HV., Liebmann, JM., & Ritch, R. (2003). Iridociliary apposition in plateau iris syndrome persists after cataract extraction, *American Journal of Ophthalmology*, Vol.135, No.1, (2003), pp.40–43

Tripathi, RC., Tripathi, BJ., Haggerty C. (2003). Drug-induced glaucomas: mechanism and management, *Drug safety*, Vol. 26, No.11, (2003), pp.749–767

Wand, M., Grant, WM., Simmons, RJ., & Hutchinson, BT. (1977). Plateau iris syndrome, *Transactions. Section on Ophthalmology. American Academy of Ophthalmology and Otolaryngology*, Vol. 83, No. 1, (1977), pp.122-130

Yamamoto, T., Iwase, A., Araie, M., Suzuki, Y., Abe, H., & Shirato, S. (2005). The Tajimi Study report 2: prevalence of primary angle closure and secondary glaucoma in a Japanese population, *Ophthalmology*, Vol. 112, No.10,(2005), pp.1661–1669

Yasuda, N. & Kageyama, M. (1988). The long-term effects of local medication on intraocular pressure control in primary angle-closure glaucoma, *Nippon Ganka Gakkai Zasshi*, Vol.92, No.10, (1988), pp.1644-1649

13

Drug-Induced Glaucoma (Glaucoma Secondary to Systemic Medications)

Eitan Z. Rath

Department of Ophthalmology, Western Galilee – Nahariya Medical Center, Israel

1. Introduction

Glaucoma comprises a group of diseases that have in common a characteristic optic nerve and visual field damage and elevated intraocular pressure (IOP) is the main risk factor. The IOP depends on the balance between the formation and drainage of aqueous humor. The glaucoma can be classified into four main groups: open-angle (OAG), acute angle-closure (ACG), secondary and developmental glaucoma. The first two refer to the pathophysiology of the disease.

Drug-induced glaucoma is a form of secondary glaucoma induced by topical and systemic medications. The most common one is glucorticoid OAG. Several drugs like antidepressants, anticoagulants, adrenergic antagonists, sulpha -based drugs and antiepileptic dugs have been reported to produce an acute ACG and especially in those with predisposed angle closure.

Bilateral simultaneous ACG is extremely a rare entity. Drug-induced uveal effusion causing secondary ACG have been reported[1-9] involving medications such as topiramate,[2,4,6,9] trimethoprin[1] and venlafaxine.[3] The mechanism of secondary OAG is usually the microscopic obstruction of the trabecular meshwork whereas ACG is induced by uveal effusion. The treatment of these two entities is similar to OAG and, it could be medically as well as surgical.

The differential diagnosis, prognosis and several future directions for research will be discussed.

Ophthalmologists should be aware of these types of glaucoma, which to my opinion are becoming more common in a busy glaucoma clinic.

2. Epidemiology

Armaly as shown that within the general population 5 to 6 % of the healthy subjects will develop marked elevation of IOP, 4 to 6 weeks after administration of topical dexamethasone or betamethasone eye drops.[12] These studies have also shown that these numbers are directly related to the frequency of the administration and duration of usage of this medication. Increasing usage is related to the increased risk for elevated IOP. At higher risk are patients with primary open-angle glaucoma, their first-degree relatives, diabetic patients, highly myopic individuals, and patients with connective tissue disease, specifically rheumatoid arthritis. In addition, patients with angle recession glaucoma are more susceptible to corticosteroid-induced glaucoma.

3. Mechanisms of IOP elevation in drug-induced glaucoma

3.1 Open-angle

Corticosteroid is a group of drugs that may produce IOP elevation by open-angle mechanism. Not all the patients taking steroid will develop this glaucoma. The risk factors include preexisting primary open-angle glaucoma, a family history of glaucoma, high myopia, diabetes mellitus and young age.[13] It has been shown that 18-36% of the general population and 46–92% of patients with primary open-angle glaucoma respond to topical ocular administration of corticosteroids with an elevation of IOP, usually within 2–4 weeks after therapy has been instituted.

Topically applied eye drops and creams to the periorbital area and intravitreal injections are more likely to cause IOP elevation than intravenous, parenteral and inhaled forms. Since IOP elevation can be gradual and asymptomatic, patients on chronic corticosteroid therapy may remain undiagnosed, which can result in glaucomatous optic nerve damage. Steroid-induced IOP elevation typically occurs within a few weeks after commencing steroid therapy. In most cases, IOP returns spontaneously to the baseline within a few weeks to months upon discontinuing the steroid (steroid responders). In rare situations, the IOP remains high (steroid-induced glaucoma) that may require prolonged glaucoma medication or even surgery. This subject is discussed in details in the chapter on steroid-induced glaucoma.

3.2 Closed-angle

Some drugs have contraindications or adverse effects that are related to acute angle-closure glaucoma. These drugs will incite an attack in individuals with very narrow anterior chamber angles that are prone to occlusion, especially when the pupils are dilated. The classes of medications that have the potential to induce angle-closure are topical anticholinergic or sympathomimetic pupil dilating drops, tricyclic antidepressants, monoamine oxidase inhibitors, antihistamines, anti-Parkinson drugs, antipsychotic medications and antispasmolytic agents.

Sulfonamide-containing medications may induce an ACG by a different mechanism, involving the anterior rotation of the cilliary-body. Typically, the angle-closure is bilateral and occurs within the first few doses. Patients with narrow or wide open angles are potentially susceptible to this rare and idiosyncratic reaction.

4. Pathophysiology of drug-induced glaucoma

4.1 Open-angle

The exact pathophysiology of steroid-induced glaucoma is unknown. It is known that steroid-induced IOP elevation is secondary to increased resistance to aqueous outflow. Some evidence shows that there could be an increased accumulation of glycosaminoglycans or increased production of trabecular meshwork-inducible glucocorticoid response (TIGR) protein, which could mechanically at microscopic level obstruct the aqueous outflow. Other evidence suggests that the corticosteroid-induced cytoskeletal changes could inhibit pinocytosis of aqueous humour or inhibit the clearing of glycosaminoglycans, resulting in the accumulation of this substance and blockage of the aqueous outflow.

4.2 Closed-angle

Aqueous humor is secreted by the ciliary body and circulates through the pupil to reach the anterior chamber angle. (Fig. 1) The pathophysiology of angle-closure glaucoma is usually due to pupillary block, i.e. iris-lens contact at the pupillary border resulting from pupillary dilation.

People at risk for Angle Closure Glaucoma (ACG) are those with hypermetropia, microphthalmus and nanophthalmos. Medications have a direct or indirect effect, either in stimulating sympathetic or inhibiting parasympathetic activation causing pupillary dilation, which can precipitate an acute angle-closure in patients with occludable anterior chamber angles. These agents include adrenergic agonists (e.g. β2-specific adrenergic agonists (e.g. salbutamol), non-catecholamine adrenergic agonists (e.g. amphetamine, dextroamphetamine, methamphetamine and phendimetrazine) and anticholinergics (e.g. tropicamide). Histamine H1receptor antagonists (antihistamines) and histamine H2 receptor antagonists (e.g. cimetidine and ranitidine) have weak anticholinergic adverse effects. Antidepressants such as fluoxetine, paroxetine, fluvoxamine and venlafaxine also have been associated with acute angle-closures, which is believed to be induced by either the anticholinergic adverse effects or the increased level of serotonin that cause mydriasis.

Sulfa-containing medications may result in acute angle-closures by a different mechanism. This involves the anterior rotation of the ciliary body with or without choroidal effusions, resulting in a shallow anterior chamber and blockage of the trabecular meshwork by the iris. Pupillary dilation and a preexisting shallow anterior chamber angle are not necessary. The exact reason for ciliary body swelling is unknown but it occurs in susceptible individuals. Topiramate is a sulfa-containing anticonvulsant. There were reports about patients on topiramate developing acute angle-closure. However, a pilot study was conducted in the Hong Kong Eye Hospital and the Prince of Wales Hospital recently, which showed that short-term use of topiramate, did not induce an asymptomatic angle narrowing. Therefore, it was suggested that topiramate induced secondary angle-closure glaucoma may be an all-or-none phenomenon.

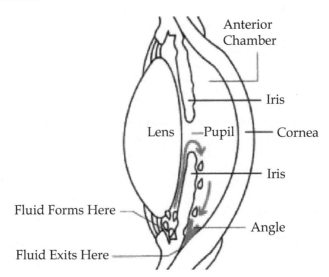

Fig. 1. Aqueous humor flow

Carbamazepine is also an anticonvulsive medication and a mood stabilizer and is primarily used in treating of epilepsy, bipolar disorders and trigeminal neuralgia.[10] It stabilizes and inactivates the sodium Chan resulting in fewer active channels and fewer excited brain cells. It was only reported once as causing this disorder.[8]

We had two cases that developed simultaneously acute angle-closure glaucoma 4-6 weeks after intake of PO carbamazepine.

Case no. 1

A 58-year-old woman presented with a bilateral acute ACG. Her medical history included epilepsy treated with carbamazepine (Novartis Pharma BU (Novolog), Basel, Switzerland) 200 mg once a day for 4 weeks to stabilize her medical status. Eleven years earlier she underwent thyroidectomy due to hyperthyroidism.

The best-corrected visual acuity (BCVA) was 20/80 (with +3.75D) OD and 20/100 (with +4.25D) OS. The intraocular pressure (IOP) was 54 OD and 46mmHg OS. Both corneas were edematous and the anterior chambers were shallow. Gonioscopy revealed angle closure in both eyes and fixed, mid-dilated pupils. Ultrasound biomicroscopy (UBM) showed an anterior displaced crystalline lens with extensive irido-lenticular contact and peripheral anterior synechiae OU. The axial length was 21.35 mm OD and 21.30 mm OS. B-Scan ultrasound showed normal posterior segment OU.

The patient was treated systemically with PO acetazolamide 250mg, topical timolol maleate – dorzolamide HCl and brimonidine tartrate twice a day and the IOP decreased to 18mmHg OD and 16mmHg OS .Neodymium: Yttrium-Aluminum-Garnet (Nd: YAG) laser iridotomy was successfully performed OU. A week later, the BCVA improved to 20/80 OD and 20/60 OS, on ocular examination, potent iridotomies, mid dilated pupils with sphincter atrophy, mild nuclear sclerosis and normal optic discs were noted. The anterior chamber depth measured by Scheimpflug imaging (Pentacam®, Oculus Optikgerate GmbH, Wetzlar, Germany) was 1.54mm OD and 1.67mm OS and the volume was 90mm³ and 76mm³ respectively. The pachymetry was 572μm OD and 568μm. The visual fields 30-2 (Humphrey II® automatic perimeter, Allergan-Humphrey, San Leandro, CA) performed two months later showed inferior nasal step OU.

Case no. 2

A 53-year-old female was admitted due to high IOP simultaneously in both eyes. She was hypermetropic since childhood and had amblyopic OS. She suffered from epilepsy and had two attacks four and six weeks before being hospitalized for which she received PO carbamazepine 200mg/d for five weeks. A day before admission, she experienced severe bilateral ocular pain, vomiting and decrease in visual acuity OU.

Her BCVA was 20/40 with +5.50D OD and 20/100 with + 7.50D OS. The IOP was 54 mmHg OD and 49 mmHg OS. Both eyes had edematous cornea, very shallow anterior chamber, iris bombe and mid-dilated pupil that were not reacting to light. The anterior chamber had a narrow angle 360 degrees OU on UBM (Fig. 2). The posterior poles were normal. The patient was treated with topical pilocarpine 2% qid and PO acetazolamide 250mg bid.

The patient underwent Nd: YAG laser iridotomy OU. Three days later, the BCVA improved to 20/25 OD and 20/60 OS. The IOP decreased to 8mmHg OD and 6mmHg OS. The anterior chambers' depth was deepened and patent iridotomies, mild-dilated pupil, clear lens and posterior pole with normal optic discs were observed.

The mechanism of these agents causing bilateral AACG has been attributed to ciliochoroidal effusion, which causes forward rotation of the lens–iris diaphragm resulting in a secondary angle-closure and increased IOP. This medication and others can produce an excessive amount of aqueous production as well as causing culinary body edema. The common denominator to our patients was hypermetropia. Indeed, patients with short axial length, such as nanophthalmos and hyperopia have a tendency to develop thickened uvea, which can be aggravated by intraocular procedures such as cataract surgery resulting in acute ACG.[11]

5. Non-steroidal agents associated with glaucoma

Unlike corticosteroid agents, the list of non-steroidal agents associated with glaucoma is wide and diverse (Table 1). [14] The causes of glaucoma associated with these agents are also varied. The largest single cause of glaucoma in these patients appears to be an atropine-like effect, eliciting pupillary dilatation. This class of agents includes antipsychotropics, antidepressants, monoamine oxidase (MAO) inhibitors, antihistamines, antiparkinsonian agents, antispasmolytic agents, mydriatic agents, sympathetic agents, and botulinum toxin. The pupillary dilatation seen in these cases may be enough to precipitate an attack of angle-closure glaucoma in patients with narrow angles.

Concerning open-angle glaucoma, the causes of elevated IOP are much more varied, including the release of pigment during the pupillary dilation with subsequent obstruction of the trabecular meshwork, and a possible increase of inflow during papillary dilation. As an alternative, some agents have been documented to produce an idiopathic swelling of the lens, associated with angle closure glaucoma. These agents include the antibiotics sulfa, quinine, and aspirin. Some agents directly obstruct the trabecular meshwork, such as the viscoelastic agents and silicone oil.

5.1 The role of psychotropic agents

Of the antipsychotropic agents on the market today, only perphenazine (Trilafon®) and fluphenazine decanoate (Prolixin®) have been documented to cause glaucoma. In both instances these were attacks of angle-closure glaucoma. These episodes were felt to reflect the anticholinergic effect of these agents on the eyes.

5.2 The role of antidepressant agents

Amitryptiline (Elavil® and Amitril®) and imipramine (Tofranil®), which are antidepressant tricyclic agents, have been shown to produce attacks of an angle-closure glaucoma. Of the non-tricyclic drugs, fluoxetine (Prozac®) and mianserin hydrochloride (Bolvidon®) [15] have been documented to be associated with attacks of angle-closure glaucoma.

5.3 The role of mood-altering agents, such as minor tranquilizers, sedatives, and stimulants

This is a rather diverse class of agents including sedatives such as diazepam (Valium®), morphine, barbiturates, and stimulants such as amphetamine and methylxanthines such as caffeine and theophylline. Diazepam has been reported to be taken by some patient having an attack of angle-closure glaucoma, in the literature there it is believed that this drug accentuate the anti cholinergic action on the eye in some rare cases with predisposed ACG . Barbiturates, morphine, para-aldehyde, meperidine, reserpine, and phenytoin have not been reported to produce an elevated IOP. The amphetamines have not been documented to produce an elevated IOP in any patient.

5.4 The role of antibiotics

Sulfa drugs

Agents that contain sulfa have been well documented to produce an idiosyncratic swelling of the lens associated with shallowing of the anterior chamber, retinal edema, and elevated IOP. These episodes do not involve the pupil and are not responding to cycloplegic agents. This observation has been confirmed by A-scan measurements of the eye during such an attack[16].

Antipsychotropic agents
Phenothiazines
Perphenazine (Trilafon), fluphenazine decanoate (Prolixin)

Antidepressants
Tricyclic agents
Amitryptiline (Elavil), imipramine (Tofranil)
Nontricyclic agents
Fluoxetine (Prozac), mianserin HC1 (Bolvidin)

Monoamine oxidase (MAO) inhibitors
Phenylzine sulfate (Nardil)
Tranylcypromine sulfate (Parnate)

Antihistamines
Ethanolamines
Orphenadrine citrate (Norgesic)

Antiparkinsonian agents
Trihexyphenidyl HC1 (Artane)

Antispasmolytic agents
Propantheline bromide (Pro-Banthine)
Dicydomine HC1 (Bentyl)

Antibiotics
Sulfa, quinine

Sympathomimetic agents
Epinephrine, ephedrine
Phenylephrine
Amphetamine
Hydroxyamphetamine

Mydriatic agents
All agents
Surgical agents
Viscoelastic agents, silicone oil

Botulin toxin
Cardiac agents
Disopyramide phosphate (Norpace)

Table 1. Non-steroidal agents

5.5 The role of antiparkinsonian agents

The anti-Parkinson agents act through two mechanisms: (1) Replenishing diminished stores of dopamine in the corpus striatum, and (2) Acting as a strong anticholinergic. Indeed, trihexyphenidyl

HCl (Artane)[17] has been documented to precipitate angle-closure glaucoma. This finding is felt to reflect the anticholinergic effect of this agent.

5.6 The role of antispasmolytic agents

These agents act to reduce both the gastrsecretion and the motility of the stomach. Their effect directly reflects their anticholinergic power. Although no attacks of angle-closure glaucoma are documented with these agents, propantheline bromide (Pro-Banthine®) and dicyclomine HCl (Bentyl®) [18] have been documented to raise the IOP in patients with open-angle glaucoma probably because of their anticholinergic effect.

5.7 The role of anesthetic agents

General anesthesia has always entailed an increased risks to the patient, including the risk of elevated IOP and glaucoma. It has always been difficult to separate the various risk factors to the patient undergoing general anesthesia. The induction of general anesthesia itself may be associated with an elevated IOP from laryngeal spasm, coughing, and wheezing associated with endotracheal intubation. Specifically, succinylcholine, ketamine and chloral hydrate have been well documented to raise IOP. This effect is felt to be due to an increased extra-ocular muscle tone from these agents. [19] The preoperative use of atropine, scopalmine, and ephedrine associated with attacks of angle-closure glaucoma following general anesthesia.

5.8 The role of antihistamines in inducing glaucoma

The antihistamines are a diverse group of agents that can be divided into two classes the H1 and the H2 antihistamines. The H1 antihistamines block the action of histamine on capillary permeability and vascular, bronchial, and other smooth muscles.[20] The H2 antihistamines block the effect of histamine on the smooth muscle in peripheral blood vessels and secretion of gastric acid. This group is important because of their anticholinergic effect of these agents. Although the anticholinergic action is mild, orphenadrine citrate (Norgesic®), an H1 antihistamine, has been documented to precipitate an attack of angle-closure glaucoma. It should also be noted that the H1 antihistamine promethazine HCl (Phenergan®) has been shown to produce an idiopathic swelling of the lens as documented with the sulfa agents. These agents exert only a weak response but should be approached with caution in the patient at risk for glaucoma.

5.9 The role of inhalation agents in inducing glaucoma

As mentioned above ,a wide variety of agents are found as inhalation products, including sympathomimetic and parasympathomimeric agents. Salbutamol and ipratropium (used in combination for chronic obstructive airway) have also been documented to precipitate attacks of angle-closure glaucoma due to the anticholinergic effect of ipratropium in combination with the effect of salbutamol (a β2 adreno receptor agonist) on increrasing aqueous humor production.[21] Therefore, these agents should be used with caution in patients at risk for such an attack of glaucoma.

5.10 The role of cardiac agents in inducing glaucoma

The traditional cardiac agents including digitalis and quinidine do not appear to have any effect on the IOP. However, disopyramide phosphate (Norpace®) does appear to have some anticholinergic activity and has indeed been documented to produce an attack of angle-closure glaucoma.[22]

5.11 The role of botulinum toxin (Oculinum)

Botulinum toxin has become popular for the treatment of essential blepharo-spasm and extraocular muscle palsy; this injectable agent has been documented to produce an acute attack of angle closure glaucoma. The effect of this drug is on the ciliary ganglion, producing pupillarymydriasis.[23]

5.12 The role of avastin and lucentis

A series of patients that developed sustained elevation of intraocular pressure (IOP) after intravitreal anti-VEGF injection for the treatment of neovascular age-related macular degeneration (AMD) is presented un numerous of recent publications[24] IOP reflects a balance between the rate that fluid flows into the eye and the rate that it exits the eye. If inflow increases or outflow decreases, then IOP will go up. Intravitreal injection of drugs, such as Lucentis (ranibizumab) or Avastin (bevacizumab), increases the amount of fluid within the eye, and hence will increase IOP. Normally, as the excess fluid gradually exits the eye over a period of time, the IOP returns to normal. However, there are a growing number of cases of patients undergoing Lucentis and Avastin therapy that develop elevation of IOP that does not return to normal.

In a recent study four out of 116 patients with AMD (3.45%) developed sustained elevated intraocular pressure (IOP) after multiple intravitreal injections of Avastin (1.5 mg/0.06 mL) and/or Lucentis (0.5 mg/0.05 mL). An analysis of 4 cases revealed: None of the patients had a previous diagnosis or family history of glaucoma/OHT. Two patients had both bevacizumab and ranibizumab injections. Two patients developed OHT after recent intravitreal ranibizumab and 2 patients after recent intravitreal Avastin injection. It appears that anti-VEGF drugs may, in some persons, lead to sustained elevation of IOP and possible glaucoma. It is not clear why this occurs, nor have any risk factors for this adverse effect, such as family history of glaucoma, been identified. Nor is it clear whether the IOP elevation is permanent, or whether IOP may return to normal after cessation of anti-VEGF injections. Glaucoma medications can lower IOP after it has been elevated by anti-VEGF drug use.

There are some publictions[25] which describe the decrease of rubeosis iridis in patients with neo-vascular after intra- vitreal Avastin injection and can lead to decrease in IOP within 48 hours.

6. Treatment of drug-induced glaucoma

6.1 Medical: Open-angle

If the patient's underlying medical condition can tolerate discontinuation of corticosteroids, then its discontinuation will usually result in normalization of IOP. In case of topical corticosteroid drops, using a lower potency steroid medication, such as the phosphate forms of prednisolone and dexamethasone, loteprednol etabonate or fluorometholone should be considered. These drugs have a lesser chance to increase the IOP, but they are usually not as effective as others. Topical non-steroidal anti-inflammatory medications (e.g., diclofenac, ketorolac) are other alternatives do not cause IOP elevation, but they have only a limited anti-inflammatory activity to treat the patient's underlying condition. In the occasional cases in which the patient's IOP does not normalize upon the cessation of the steroid or in those patients who must continue with treatment, topical anti-glaucoma medications are considered.

6.2 Medical: Closed-angle
If the etiology of closed angle glaucoma is sulfa containing medications, the increase in IOP generally will resolve upon discontinuing the agent. However, severe cases of sulfonamide-induced angle-closure (i.e. IOP >45 mm Hg) may not respond to discontinuing the offending agent. They may respond to intravenous mannitol. Other etiologies of drug-induced angle-closure are treated similar to primary acute angle-closure glaucoma with topical beta-blockers, prostaglandin analogues, cholinergic agonists and often oral acetazolamide.

6.3 Laser treatment
For open-angle steroid-induced glaucoma, selective laser trabeculoplasty or Argon laser trabeculoplasty (Fig. 3) can be applied in the absence of intraocular inflammation if the IOP is suboptimal with medication.

In closed-angle glaucoma, an Argon laser peripheral iridoplasty or YAG laser iridotomy may be performed to widen the angle and deepen the anterior chamber. Laser iridotomy can be performed to reverse pupillary block or to prevent further pupillary block. Laser Irididotomies can be performed as a preventive procedure in hepermetropic naophthalmic and microphthalmic eyes. Fig. 4 shows the effect of Argon laser laser iridotomy. When medical and laser therapy are ineffective in lowering the IOP to target pressure or the patient is intolerant to medical therapy, surgical therapy is indicated. Usually, trabeculectomy, a guarded filtration procedure, with or without intraoperative anti-metabolites, is the primary procedure. In cases of eyes with active neovascularization or inflammation, a glaucoma drainage implant may be used as the primary procedure.

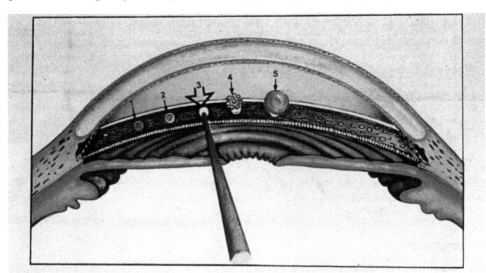

Fig. 2. ALT Argon Laser Trabeculoplasy

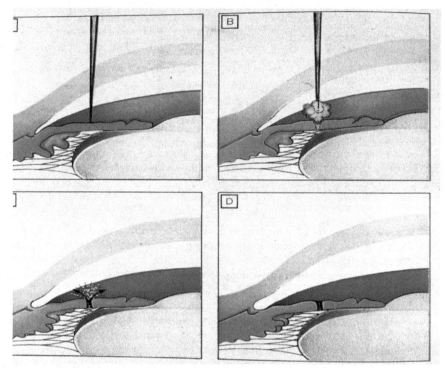

Fig. 3. LI Laser Iridotomy

6.4 Surgical: Closed-angle

Trabeculectomy can also be performed with similar indications as open-angle glaucoma. However, the surgery is more difficult since the anterior chamber is shallower and the cornea is usually hazier due to the acute IOP rise.

7. Prevention of drug induced glaucoma

7.1 Open-angle

Unnecessary prolonged use of cortcosteroid should be avoided. Ophthalmic evaluation is recommended for patients treated with long-term steroids especially with risk factors such as family history of primary open-angle glaucoma.

7.2 Closed-angle

Prophylactic laser iridotomy may be performed in patients requiring frequent mydriasis such as frequent fundus examinations for diabetic retinopathy. Agents causing secondary angle-closure should be avoided in susceptible individuals as far as possible.

8. Conclusion

Drugs that cause or exacerbate open-angle glaucoma are mostly glucocorticoids. Several classes of drugs, including adrenergic agonists, cholinergics, anticholinergics, sulpha-based drugs, selective serotonin reuptake inhibitors, tricyclic and tetracyclic antidepressants, anticoagulants and histamine H(1) and H(2) receptor antagonists, have been reported to induce or precipitate acute angle-closure glaucoma, especially in individuals predisposed with narrow angles of the anterior chamber. In some instances, bilateral simultaneous development of acute ACG occurs after carbamazepine and topiramate intake may occur especially in eyes with short axial length such as hypermetropia, microphthalmia and nanophthalmos. Clinicians should be mindful of the possibility of drug-induced glaucoma, whether or not the drug is listed as a contraindication and if in doubt, consult an ophthalmologist. Patients should visit an ophthalmologist routinely twice a year after the age of 40 and inform him about their different medications.

9. Acknowledgment

I acknowledge the support of Tradis Gat Ltd. in publication of this chapter.

10. References

[1] Matz T, Abbott L. Bilateral acute angle-closure glaucoma. *Resident and Staff Physician* 2008; 54:3.

[2] Kakaria V, Chalam, Tillis T, Farhana S, Brar SA. Acute bilateral simultaneous angle closure glaucoma Topiramate administration: a case report. *J Med Case Reports* 2008; 2:1.

[3] GuMHP, Thiagalingam S, Ong P, Goldberg I. Bilateral acute angle closure caused by supraciliary effusion associated with Velafaxine intake. *MJA* 2005; 182:121-123.

[4] Nemet A, Nesher R, Almog Y, Assia E. Bilateral acute angle closure glaucoma following Topiramate treatment. *Harefuah* 2002; 141:597-9.

[5] Ates H.; Kay O., Lu K., Andac K. Bilateral angel closure glaucoma following general anesthesia: *International Ophthalmology* 1999; 23:129-30.

[6] Singh SK, Thapa SS, Badhu BP. Topiramate induced bilateral angle-closure glaucoma. *Kathmandu University Medical Journal* 2007; 5:234-.

[7] Lachkar Y, Bouassida W. Drug-induced acute angle closure glaucoma. *Curr Opin Ophthalmol* 2007; 18:129-33.

[8] Chan KCY, Sachdev N, Wells AP. Bilateral acute angle closure secondary to uveal effusions associated with Flucloxacillin and Carbamazepine. *Br J Ophthalmol* 2008; 92:428-430.

[9] Levy J, Yagev R, Petrova A, Lifshitz T. Topiramate – induced bilateral angle-closure glaucoma. *Can J Ophthalmol* 2006; 41:221-5.

[10] Sean Sweetman (Ed.). Martindale-the complete drug reference, 36th edition, 471-477.

[11] Brockhurst RJ. Nanophthalmos with uveal effusion: A new clinical entity. *Trans Am Ophthalmol Soc* 1974; 72:371-403.

[12] Arrnaly MF. Statistical attributes of the steroid hypertensive response in the clinically normal eye. I. the demonstration of three levels of response. *Invest Ophthalmol* 1965; 4:187.

[13] Stewart RH, Kimbrough RL .Intraocular pressure response to topically administered fluorometholone. *Arch. Ophthalmol* 1979; 97:2139.

[14] Mandelkom R. Drug induced Glaucoma, clinical pathway in glaucoma, in :Zimmerman and Kooner, New York: Thieme Medical Publishers inc. 2001 350-333

[15] Kinek M .Glaucoma following the antidepressant mianserin. Harefuah 1990:118-699.

[16] Hook SR, Holladay JI, Perager TC, Goosey JD. Transient myopia induced by sulphonamides. *Am J Ophthalmol* 1986; 101:495.

[17] Friedman Z, Neuman E. Benzhexalol induced blindness in Parkinson's disease. *Br Med J* 1972; 1:605.

[18] Mody MV, Keeney AH. Propantheline (probanthine) bromide in relation to normal and glaucomatous eyes: effects on intraocular tension and pupillary size. *JAMA* 1955; 159:1113.

[19] Katz RI, Eakins KB. Mode of action of succinylcholine on intraocular pressure. *J Pharmacol Exp Ther* 1968; 162:1.

[20] Bard L.A. Transient myopia associated with promethazine (phenergan) therapy: report of a case. *Am J Ophthalmol* 1964; 58:682?

[21] Malawi JT, Rhobinson GM, Seneviratne H. Ipratropium bromide induced angle closure glaucoma (letter). *NZ Med J* 1982; 95:759.

[22] Monica ML, Hesse RJ, Messerli FH .The effect of a calcium channel blocking agent on intraocular pressure. *AM J Ophthalmol* 1983; 96:814.

[23] Kupfer C. Selective block of synaptic transmission in ciliary ganglion by type A botulinum toxin in Rabbits. *Proc Soc Exp Biol Med* 1958; 99:474.

[24] Adelman RA, Zheng Q. Mayer HR. Persistent ocular hypertension following intravitreal bevacizumab and ranibizumab injections. *J Ocul Pharmacol Ther*. 2010 Feb; 26(1):105-10.

[25] Milko E. Iliev, Diego Doming, Ute , Sebastin Wolf, Intravitreal Bevacizumab (Avastin®) in the Treatment of Neovascular Glaucoma. *AJO* Volume 142, Pages 1054-56, Dec. 2006.

14

Glaucoma in Cases of Penetrating Keratoplasty, Lamellar Procedures and Keratoprosthesis

Shimon Rumelt
Department of Ophthalmology,
Western Galilee – Nahariya Medical Center, Nahariya,
Israel

1. Introduction

The two main issues that concern glaucoma patients before and after penetrating keratoplasty and posterior lamellar procedures and patients that develop glaucoma after surgery are the risks of graft failure and the aggravation of the glaucoma. Failure of the corneal graft may require regrafting, which increases the risk of developing or aggravating glaucoma, while uncontrolled glaucoma may result in graft failure and further damage to the optic disc and visual field. These two problems may lead to each other creating a vicious circle. They should be treated by glaucoma and corneal specialists or by someone who is expert with both.

Glaucoma was found in 10-42% of the patients with a single corneal transplantation, 0-27% of them had preoperative glaucoma.[1-6] Preexisting glaucoma was usually a result of an initial insult such as chemical burn or secondary glaucoma. In repeated corneal transplantation, the incidence of postoperative glaucoma was higher (14-47%) than in primary transplantation.[7-12] It increases with increased number of regrafts and in aphakia. Corneal graft failure 3 years after keratoplasty occurred in 29-47% when glaucoma was present, compared with 9-30% when it was absent.[13,14]

Patients requiring penetrating keratoplasty and lamellar procedures (deep lamellar keratoplasty, Descemet's stripping (automated) endothelial keratoplasty, Descemet's membrane endothelial keratoplasty) may suffer from preexisting various types of open and closed angle glaucomas, which may be primary or secondary. Primary open angle and primary closed angle glaucomas may preexist and corneal surgery may be required for unrelated disorders such as Fuchs' corneal dystrophy. Secondary glaucomas may occur due to open and closed globe injuries. In those injuries, the glaucoma may be of open angle and caused by obstruction of the trabecular meshwork by red blood cells (from hyphema), ghost cells (ghost cell glaucoma) or tearing of the meshwork (angle recession). It may also be closed-angle caused by peripheral anterior synechiae. Corneal transplantation may also be required in chemical burns especially alkali. In these cases, the cornea may be opaque because of chronic edema and scarring. Secondary glaucoma may also be associated with corneal abnormalities such as anterior mesenchymal dysgenesis (e.g., Peter's and Axenfeld-Rieger's anomalies). In these disorders, in addition to corneal opacity due to scarring, the angle may be poorly formed. The common features for all these conditions are persistent corneal edema and scarring due to endothelial decompensation. The decompensation is a result of a combination of damaged or compromised endothelium (whether by trauma or other corneal disorders) and increased intraocular pressure (IOP) that contributes to egress of aqueous humor into the corneal layers. Corneal opacity due to persistent edema and scarring is more common in these conditions than in normal population.

Repeated or even primary corneal transplantation may also result in secondary glaucoma. The attributing factors for secondary glaucoma include 1. Donors button undersizing, which results in corneal graft over-stretching, causing corneal flattening and angle closure. 2. Trauma to the angle by the inadvertent touch by surgical instruments. The damage might be micro or macroscopic. 3. Corticosteroid-induced glaucoma, since topical and sometimes systemic corticosteroids are being frequently use after transplantation to decrease the risk for corneal graft rejection or to treat it. 4. Posterior synechiae that may develop due to postoperative intraocular inflammation especially if the angle is traumatized or becomes shallow. The most common forms of post-keratoplasty glaucoma in single and repeated corneal transplantation are chronic angle closure followed by steroid-induced glaucoma.

2. Assessment of patients requiring penetrating keratoplasty

The preoperative office evaluation of patients requiring penetrating keratoplasty or lamellar procedure whether or not having glaucoma includes defining the primary indication for surgery. Certain indications may require certain precautions or additional treatment to prevent loss of the graft clarity. For example, corneal transplantation for infectious diseases such as herpetic, fungal or acanthamebic keratitis require prolonged postoperative anti-herpetic, fungal or acanthamebic treatment to prevent reactivation. Defining the associated ocular disorders of the recipient and donor is paramount.[12] Corneal vascularization increases the risk of corneal graft rejection especially if involves three or more quadrants and requires prolonged use of corticosteroids as well as immuno-suppressants. Ocular surface disorders such as entropion and trichiasis also increase the likelihood of graft loss due to persistent rubbing of the ocular surface that results in corneal epithelial defects and ulcers that may lead to perforation.[15] Limbal cell deficiency in corneal cicatricial disorders such as ocular cicatricial pemphigoid and erythema multiforme (Steven Johnson disease) provides poor supporting environment to the graft, while dry eyes do both (poor supporting and increased friction upon blinking). Poor blinking and lagophthalmos may also cause dryness of the ocular surface resulting in persistent epithelial defects, ulcers and even perforation. These findings should be pretreated.

Cataract, glaucoma and retinal disorders may be associated with poor visual prognosis despite of clear corneal graft and should be evaluated before any corneal procedure. Defining the associated systemic disorders in recipient and donor are also essential. Diabetes mellitus is also manifested as fragile epithelium and slow epithelial healing, which could endanger the corneal graft.

Before any corneal surgery, best-corrected visual acuity of each eye should be obtained and recorded. This will assist in surgery decision making. Ultrasound is part of the evaluation if the cornea is severely opaque and fundus cannot be evaluated. It is used to rule out retinal detachment and intraocular masses (e.g., choroidal melanoma). When ocular disorders other than corneal disease exist, such as glaucoma and retinal disorders, they should be evaluated for their contribution to visual acuity. The evaluation includes potential acuity meter (PAM), Lambda and laser interferometry. With these instruments, if the visual acuity is improved, the eye has a potential for visual recovery and a corneal surgery should be attempted. In non-verbal patients as children or in patients with mental retardation, a less accurate method to evaluate the potential for visual recovery is electroretinography (ERG). When anamnesis cannot be obtained, poor prognostic factors for visual improvement are nystagmus, which develops in the first 3 postnatal months, and esotropia that develop in the first 6 postnatal months and indicate severe irreversible amblyopia. Exotropia on the other hand may be acquired at older age and therefore, with poor anamnesis is not a poor prognostic factor for visual recovery.

The preoperative evaluation should include a complete ocular examination including examining the anterior chamber angle, especially following ocular trauma, burns, preexisting glaucoma and candidates for large diameter grafts. If the cornea is opaque, ultrasound biomicroscopy (UBM) is a good alternative for gonioscopy. In presence of shallow anterior chamber, peripheral anterior synechiae or partially closed angle even with normal IOP, placement of anterior chamber IOL is contraindicated in triple procedures, because it may result in the development of secondary glaucoma.

3. Preoperative tips

Consider alternative treatment options for penetrating keratoplasty, especially if glaucoma exists. If the corneal opacity is central and localized (e.g., in Peter's anomaly), optical iridectomy may be a better surgical alternative. Rotational autokeratoplasty is an alternative for eccentric. If the corneal opacity is minimal, surgery may not be warranted. It is always imperative to consider whether the expected visual acuity will be better than the preoperative visual acuity. If not, it is better to avoid surgery.

It is important to perform complicated surgical procedures such as filtration surgery in uncontrolled and controlled glaucoma patients before corneal transplantation or posterior lamellar procedures. The IOP should be controlled at time of the penetrating keratoplasty or posterior lamellar procedures. Otherwise, the graft may become edematous and lost. In patients with glaucoma, any procedure should spare the limbus and conjunctiva as much as possible to allow glaucoma filtration surgery.

4. Surgical steps of penetrating keratoplasty to increase the success rate

Oversized donor corneal button is always required to decrease the risk for development of secondary glaucoma and aggravating a preexisting one. The details for oversizing are described below.

Specular microscopy of the donor button to ensure an endothelial cell count of more than 2,000 mm^2 without endothelial polymegatism or pleomorphism will at least guarantee that the corneal graft has safety margins and that the risk of endothelial decompensation will be decreased.

Pretreatment of preexisting glaucoma is a crucial step in successful penetrating and posterior lamellar procedures. Therefore, it is important recognizing the type and the etiology of preexisting glaucoma. Surgical pretreatment should be considered even in medically controlled glaucoma, because these patients may become uncontrolled after surgery and this may endanger the transparency of the corneal graft. Trabeculectomy is the treatment of choice for primary open angle glaucoma. Antimetabolites such as mitomycin-C (MMC) are indicated for all patients under the age of 55 even in primary surgery, for repeated surgery and for combined procedures. Trabeculectomy should be preferred over glaucoma drainage devices in triple procedures and in the presence of corneal graft. MMC should be applied in all cases of secondary glaucomas, triple procedure or in the presence of corneal graft although potential diffusion of the drug may endanger the endothelium. MMC 0.04% is soaked by a small piece of sponge and is placed under the scleral flap before penetrating into the anterior chamber or under the conjunctival flap for 2min avoiding its edges. It should not be placed over corneal button–recipient bed interface. Such a low concentration and short exposure minimize the risks for complications such as poor healing, scleral melting, anterior chamber reaction and increased IOP.

In angle closure glaucoma, laser iridotomy and laser iridoplasty or synechiolysis are warranted. Laser iridotomy may facilitate aqueous flow from the posterior into the anterior chamber and deepen the anterior chamber. Laser iridoplasty causes shrinkage of the peripheral iris and retracts the base of the iris to open the angle, while, synechiolysis has a similar effect by breaking peripheral anterior synechiae and opening the angle. The last two procedures are beneficial if peripheral anterior synechiae have been present for less than 6 months. Peripheral iridectomy may replace laser iridotomy only if iridotomy cannot be performed due to corneal opacity, thick iris or when laser in unavailable. The procedures are described below.

Penetrating keratoplasty should be delayed until the intraocular inflammation subsides and the IOP is stable within the target pressure range. This should be at least 3 months after any intraocular surgery.

5. Prevention of secondary glaucoma

Several precautions should be employed to prevent a secondary glaucoma. As mentioned, preoperative evaluation of the anterior chamber angle is essential especially in patients with preexisting glaucoma. If the angle is already compromised (close, narrow or has peripheral anterior synechiae), the risks of development of glaucoma or aggravation of preexisting one increase. It is important to oversize corneal donor button by 0.5-0.75 mm. In keratoconus or keratoglobus, an over-sizing of 0.25 mm is sufficient to decrease the risk of postoperative angle closure, while preventing too steep postoperative graft. For large graft diameter (8.0-9.5 mm) that is required sometimes for corneal perforations, large descematocele or widespread disease, an over-sizing of 0.75-1.0 mm is advocated. Avoiding manipulations near the angle with surgical instruments is important. The only exception is when synechiolysis is performed. The angle may also be filled with viscoelastic agent to protect it during the procedure, but the viscoelastic material should be aspirated at the conclusion of the surgery to prevent postoperative high IOP. To decrease damage to the trabecular meshwork, preoperative and postoperative intraocular inflammation should be controlled. This may be done by topical corticosteroids with high corneal penetrance such as prednisolone acetate (Pred Forte®). The frequency of drop instillation depends on the degree of inflammation and it is tapered gradually according to the response. Additional systemic corticosteroids may be employed for severe or recurrent sterile uveitis. Usually, 1 gr/kg/day of prednisone is sufficient.

6. Post-keratoplasty glaucoma

If glaucoma develops after corneal surgery, a distinction between immediate postoperative and late postoperative glaucoma should be made. Immediate postoperative glaucoma develops within a week after surgery in 42-55% of the primary keratoplasties. The causes for its development include viscoelastic agent left in the anterior chamber and blocking the drainage of the aqueous humor through the angle and corticosteroid-induced glaucoma. The later develops after the initiation of corticosteroid treatment and occurs at least in 20-30% of the patients. It can occur with any form of corticosteroid although it occurs more often after topical use. The increase in IOP in these cases is usually reversible if diagnosed early and if corticosteroids are discontinued. Therefore, topical and if necessary systemic corticosteroids should be replaced immediately with non-steroidal anti-inflammatory (NSAID) medications. Corticosteroid-induced glaucoma may be avoided by employment of topical NSAID such as ketorolac tromethamine 0.5% (Acular® or Tradol®), diclofenac sodium (Voltaren® (0.1%), Solaraze® (3%)) or indomethacin 1% (Indoptic®). Its incidence is also lowered with IOP sparing corticosteroids such as loteprednol etabonate 0.5% (Lotemax®) or rimexolone 1% (Vexol®) but because of their low potency, they may be more frequently required.

Late postoperative glaucoma may develop weeks or months after surgery. The incidence of this complication is 10-42% after primary keratoplasty. The risk factors for its development include preexisting glaucoma in 27-80% of the cases, aphakia in 20-39%, semi-flexible, closed-loop anterior chamber IOL in 23-50%, regrafting in 43% and wound dehiscence in 50%. Anterior mesenchymal disorders are risk factors for glaucoma in 50-90% of the patients, while open or closed globe injury in 31-77%. Glaucoma may be encountered in up to 47% of the patients with pseudophakic or aphakic bullous keratopathy, and the corneal edema may be a result of it. Certain old types of IOLs have also been associated with late postoperative glaucoma including iris-fixed anterior chamber IOL due to uveitis-glaucoma-hyphema (UGH) syndrome, caused by rubbing of the IOL against the iris. Large corneal grafts and posterior lamellar grafts may also increase the risk for glaucoma development because they may interfere with the angle. The same may occur from the sutures if they are long, tight and full thickness The causes for late postoperative glaucoma include synechial angle closure, changes in angle ultrastructure, direct mechanical damage to angle by surgical instruments, chronic postoperative inflammation causing toxic effects and presence of vitreous in the angle. Immune graft rejection was found to be more common in patients developing postoperative glaucoma than in those who did not develop it.[16,17] The glaucoma also increases with the number of corneal transplantation procedures.[17]

7. Post-keratoplasty evaluation of preexisting and secondary glaucoma

The evaluation of the anterior chamber is important not only before corneal transplantation and other posterior lamellar procedures but also after surgery, because if there is a progressive closure of the angle or formation of peripheral anterior synechiae, they may be treated before the development of glaucoma or to prevent its worsening. Periodic gonioscopy for development of anterior chamber angle closure is performed with gonioscopic lens when the peripheral cornea is clear. A 4 mirror hand-held lens has the advantages of avoiding viscoelastic material and of short diameter that allow indentation of the cornea. This allows distinguishing between apposition of the iris against the angle and true closure. It also allows breaking of fresh anterior synechiae if present. Indentation should be performed cautiously immediately after surgery, because it can result in wound dehiscence. Other gonioscopic lenses include the Goldman three and four mirror lenses, which have a broader base (diameter) and cannot indent only the cornea. They also require viscoelastic agent. Newer imaging modalities of the anterior chamber angle include the anterior segment optical coherence tomography (OCT) using 1310nm wavelength, which has a resolution of 10μm and Scheimpflug camera (Pentacam®) that has UV-free blue light source of 475nm with a similar resolution. Scheimpflug camera requires a clear cornea and direct visualization of the angle is still a better choice. When the peripheral cornea is opaque, ultrasound biomicroscopy (UBM) is the imaging of choice. It may also assists in evaluation of the ciliary body for congestion as part of uveal effusion syndrome and for aqueous misdirection. Thus, it may elucidate the mechanism of closed angle glaucomas.

Periodic IOP measurements are essential to disclose the development of glaucoma or aggravation of preexisting one. They should be performed in scheduled meetings during different hours of the day to reveal high IOP spikes in patients with high diurnal variations. In cases of doubt, a diurnal IOP curve is indicated and is usually performed every 4 hours between 8:00 and 20:00, but may be performed more frequently (i.e., every 2 hours) and during nighttime as well. IOP measurements should be especially performed when a patient is treated with topical and/or systemic corticosteroids or receives corticosteroid in other forms (e.g., inhalations). If newly IOP elevation is disclosed, recognizing the type of secondary glaucoma is important in treatment decision making (see above). IOP measurements of with Goldmann applanation tonometry may be challenging, because of corneal graft edema, which underestimate the real IOP and corneal graft astigmatism that distorts the image. When measured with Goldmann, the prism may be rotated to aim the red mark on it to the least curved corneal meridian (the negative axis). To overcome the astigmatism, the IOP may be measured twice, one in 90 degrees from the other, and the mean IOP may be calculated from these two measurements. IOP measurements may be performed by pneumatic tonometer, Tono-Pen or Mackay-Marg tonometer if they are impossible to be obtained with Goldmann. Alternatively, the IOP may be qualitatively estimated with a glass rod or by digital palpation. In eyes with corneal scarring, the IOP is overestimated.

When the diagnosis of postoperative or secondary glaucoma is established and the patient is being treated, it is important to avoid discontinuation of the anti-glaucoma medications, unless the patient is closely being followed-up. The course of postoperative glaucoma may be unpredictable and unstable. There might be high long-term fluctuations; i.e. cycles of normal IOP may alternate with increased IOP and the ophthalmologist may mislead to think that the glaucoma has resolved.

Actually, when a diagnosis of secondary glaucoma is made, the patient should always be on anti-glaucoma medications, unless he/ she develops excessive low IOP or intermittent ocular hypotony. In such cases, the anti-glaucoma medications should be discontinued while the patient is followed- up closely. These cases may represent a transition to phthisis bulbi. In cases of ocular hypotony, corticosteroids either topically or systemically may induce some IOP elevation, but if this does not result, pars plana vitrectomy with silicone oil injection into the vitreous might prevent phthisis. Pars plana vitrectomy with silicone oil injection is indicated for chronic ocular hypotony even if the visual acuity is no light perception, because it may prevent phthisis bulbi.

8. Treatment of progressive angle closure

The treatment of postoperative progressive angle closure even with normal IOP includes peripheral laser iridotomy and topical corticosteroids to control anterior chamber inflammation. If the IOP increases, a prompt surgical synechiolysis is warranted.

9. Treatment of secondary glaucoma

Open angle glaucoma is treated in the following order. The first line of treatment is medical with alpha-agonists (brimonidine tartrate) and beta-blockers (timolol maleate, betaxolol). In phakic eyes, prostaglandin analogs (latanoprost) and adrenergic agents (dipivefrin, epinephrine) may be added. In aphakic and pseudophakic eyes, prostaglandin analogs and adrenergic agents may induce cystoid macular edema (CME), which may result in a decrease in visual acuity, and therefore should be avoided. Topical carbonic anhydrase inhibitors (dorzolamide, brinzolamide) may cause graft failure due to toxicity to endothelial cells. Miotics may initiate intraocular inflammation by breaking the blood-aqueous barrier and may increase the likelihood of corneal graft rejection. In aphakic eyes, the risk of retinal detachment also increases. Therefore, these agents should be spared if possible.

The adverse effects of beta-blockers include superficial punctate keratopathy, corneal anesthesia and dry eyes. Alpha-adrenergic agents may also cause superficial punctate keratopathy and dry eyes.

If medical treatment fails, trabeculectomy with MMC (option for two such procedures) should be considered (Figure 1). However, some authors suggested that the prognosis might be poorer than for placement of a glaucoma drainage implant. If a trabeculectomy is performed, a soaked sponge (WekCel) of MMC 0.2-0.4 mg/ml under the scleral flap before penetrating the anterior chamber (or under the conjunctiva avoiding its edge) for 2-3 min should be added. The MMC should not be placed over corneal button–recipient bed interface. Then the area should be copiously irrigated with balanced salt solution or saline. This procedure may be repeated if it failed once. In some cases, the filtration procedure may be functioning well causing a decrease in IOP, but to insufficient level (above the target pressure). In such a case, an additional trabeculectomy rather than anti-glaucoma medications may be successful decreasing further the IOP to the desired level because they may diminish the filtration through the trabeculectomy resulting in its failure for long term. Also, with a successful second trabeculectomy, the patient may not need long-term topical medications, which are a burden. An alternative for MMC is 5-fluorouracil (5FU). Five-mg may be injected subconjunctivally before or at intervals after surgery, but is less potent. Another option is to place 50mg/ml of 5-FU over or under the scleral flap intraoperatively. It inhibits epithelial proliferation, while MMC is better against fibrous proliferation. Both drugs may be injected in conjunction.

The complications of trabeculectomy with MMC in the presence of corneal graft are similar to those without a graft, but in addition, damage to the endothelium may be caused by the MMC, if it penetrates into anterior chamber. The same precautions that apply for placing MMC during surgery for primary open angle glaucoma should be applied here.

If one or two trabeculectomies with MMC have been failed or as a first surgical option, glaucoma shunt tube may be performed. Anterior or posterior drainage devices are available. Anterior drainage devices connect the anterior chamber with the subconjunctival space. Schlemm's canal or suprachoroidal space are easier to implant and require only limited healthy conjunctiva to function. Among the anterior drainage devices are Ex-Press,

Solx Gold shunt and iStent. Posterior drainage devices also drain the anterior chamber through a silastic tube, but the tube is connected to a plate that is placed under the conjunctiva posteriorly. This is the reason that they are called posterior devices. Two types of posterior shunt tubes exist. The first type is with control of the flow (with a "valve" or flow resistance) includes Ahmed (New World Medical, Rancho Cucamonga, CA) and Krupin-Denver (Hood Laboratories, Pembroke, MA) drainage implants. The second type is without pressure control and includes Molteno single or double plate (IOP, Inc., Costa Mesa, CA, USA, and Molteno Ophthalmic Limited, Dunedin, New Zealand), Baerveldt (Advanced Medical Optics, Santa Ana, California, USA), Shocket (self-assembled) and Eagle Vision (Eagle Vision, Inc. Memphis, TN, USA) implants. The later require blocking the aqueous flow for a few days externally by temporary suture or internally by passing a suture through the lumen of the tube or injecting viscoelastic agent. The implantation may also be performed as a two-stage implantation, to decrease the risk for postoperative hypotony. Ahmed and Krupin implants should be preferred over the implants without a valve, because the risk for postoperative overflow and hypotony that may result in endothelial-iris and lens touch is decreased. Ahmed has a convenient plate to implant and suture in variable sizes including for pediatric population.

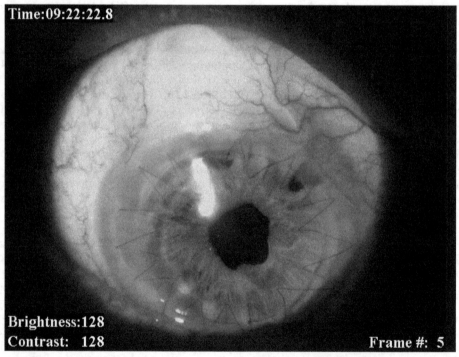

Fig. 1. Trabeculectomy in presence of clear corneal graft in a pseudophakic eye. Note the two patent peripheral iridectomies

The experience with anterior drainage devises is limited to a short follow-up, since they are relatively new. Results with Ex-press are promising.[18] The success rate defined as IOP below 21mmHG in 15 corneal transplanted eyes with closed angle glaucoma was 87% over a mean follow-up of 12 months, but a longer follow-up is required. The implantation is performed under 5x5mm partial thickness scleral flap similar to limbal-based trabeculectomy and MMC 0.05% is applied for 3min and rinsed after it. No data exist yet concerning the other anterior devices. In cases of corneal transplantation or posterior lamellar procedure, the position of the shunt tube may play a critical role in preservation of clear graft. In phakic eyes, the tube is usually placed through the anterior chamber angle. This results in control of the glaucoma in 68-96%.[19-25] However, placement of the tube into the anterior chamber may endanger the transparency of the graft due to tube-endothelial touch or turbulent flow of aqueous through the tip even in the absence of touch. Additional causes include eye rubbing and pressure on the cornea on sleeping. This complication is unique for corneal grafts and for compromised corneas (e.g., in Fuchs' endothelial dystrophy), since it has been demonstrated that progressive endothelial cell lost is observed after placement of glaucoma drainage tube into the anterior chamber angle, and this may occur even in the absence of endothelial-tube touch. Forty-two percent of the eyes with corneal transplants develop corneal decompensation.[23]

It is possible to redirect the tube placed into the anterior chamber angle through an existing iridectomy to the posterior chamber in aphakic or pseudophakic eyes as long as the iris would not block it. Another alternative in pseudophakic or aphakic eyes, is to place the tube into the posterior chamber through the ciliary sulcus, by an incision made 1mm posterior to the limbus.[26] This procedure is especially advantageous in eyes with corneal transplants or which are candidates for corneal transplantation or posterior lamellar grafts, Fuchs' corneal dystrophy, shallow anterior chamber and extensive synechial angle closure. A meticulous anterior vitrectomy is required if cases of vitreous loss.

For placement of glaucoma shunt tube into the ciliary sulcus, limbal peritomy is performed in the upper temporal (or if not feasible, inferonasal) quadrant and dissection is carried posteriorly over the sclera. The drainage plate is secured to the sclera with 6-0 polyester sutures 8 to 10mm posterior to the limbus between the superior and the horizontal recti muscles. A 2 to 5mm-long scleral tunnel is fashioned with angled crescent knife and the drainage tube is passed beneath it. Alternatively, the tube may be covered with scleral, corneal, pericardial or dural patch adjacent to the external sclerostomy. The tube is passed into the ciliary sulcus through a sclerostomy performed 1mm posterior to the limbus at 11 or 1 o'clock position under a half-thickness, limbal based scleral flap of 3x3mm. The sclerostomy is performed with a myringotomy blade that is inserted with its shaft perpendicular to the limbus and beveled parallel to the iris plane (as performed for scleral-fixated intraocular lens). The position of the tip of the blade is observed through the dilated pupil to confirm its position and avoid ciliary body separation. The edge of the tube is protruding 3mm into the posterior chamber. It should not exceed the dilated pupil margin to avoid glare and should not be too short to avoid blockage by ciliary processes. The fornix-based conjunctival flap is secured to the limbus with 7-0 polygalactin sutures (Figures 2,3). At the conclusion of the surgery betamethasone acetate 3mg and gentamicin sulfate 20mg are injected subconjunctivally 180° away from the implant plate. Topical corticosteroid, antibiotic and cycloplegic are prescribed and tapered gradually. The main potential complications include ciliary body separation and suprachoroidal hemorrhage. These were not observed in a series of patients that underwent this procedure.[26-28] The corneal grafts remained clear for years of follow-up and the glaucoma was controlled following this procedure. Placement of the shunt tube into the posterior chamber through the ciliary sulcus is contraindicated in phakic eyes because it may endanger the integrity of the crystalline lens.

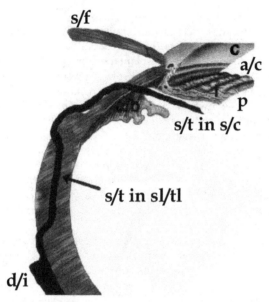

Fig. 2. A diagram showing a side view of placement of a glaucoma drainage device in the ciliary sulcus. c – cornea, a/c – anterior chamber, I – iris, p – pupil, s/f – scleral flap, c/b – ciliary body, s/t in c/s – shunt tube in the ciliary sulcus, s/t in sl/tl – shunt tube in scleral tunnel, d/i – implant disc

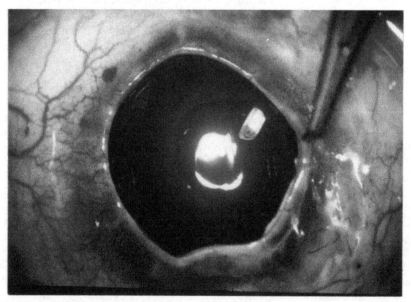

Fig. 3. The tip of ciliary sulcus glaucoma shunt tube behind the iris during surgery before placing a corneal graft

In cases of posterior segment disorders, when pars plana vitrectomy is required, the tube may be placed into the vitreous cavity through it.[30,31] A meticulous vitrectomy is a prerequisite so vitreous strands will not block the tube. The common feature for placement of the shunt tube into the posterior chamber through the ciliary sulcus or into the vitreous cavity through the pars plana is placing the tip of the tube away from the corneal graft, which decreases the risk of endothelial cell loss and corneal graft decompensation.

For pars plana placement of glaucoma drainage device, a limbal peritomy is performed and the lateral and superior rectus muscles are engaged by 4-0 silk traction sutures. The sclera is exposed further back by elevating the conjunctiva and Tenon's capsule with blunt dissection. The plate is secured to the superotemporal sclera with 6-0 polyester sutures. Then a three-port pars plana vitrectomy is performed through sclerostomies 3.5mm from the limbus. The tube is introduced 5mm into the vitreous through the superotemporal sclerostomy. A sclera, corneal, dural or pericardial patch may be used to cover the tube and the conjunctival-Tenon flap is sutured to the limbus with 7-0 polygalactin sutures. A Pars Plana Clip (Model PC,New World M, Inc., Rancho Cucamonga, CA, USA), which can be used with any drainage device, or Hoffman elbow, which is mounted on a Baerveldt 350-mm2 implant (Advanced Medical Optics, Inc., Santa Ana, CA, USA) may be used. New pars plana Ahmed and Baeverdlt implants are also available and the procedure may be performed using even the regular glaucoma setones, preferably those with a "valve". Fluid-gas exchange provides a temporary tamponade and prevents postoperative hypotony. Pars plana vitrectomy and placement of glaucoma shunt device may be performed endoscopically in eyes with media opacity such as corneal opacity.[32] This procedure allows controlling the glaucoma first and then performing corneal surgery later to improve visual acuity. Possible unique complications for this procedure include vitreous hemorrhage, retinal detachment and choroidal detachment. Although corneal graft failure is reduced if the glaucoma drainage device is placed through the ciliary sulcus or pars plana and if the glaucoma is controlled, it should be remembered that there are other causes that may result in graft failure.

In posterior lamellar grafts, if a glaucoma shunt tube is introduced into the anterior chamber, the graft may block the tip of the tube resulting in increased IOP. It can be avoided by trimming the tip of the tube, so it will not be blocked. It is also possible to pre-plane the corneal surgery and to prepare a thin lamellar graft or perform a DMEK rather than DSAEK (Figures 4,5).[29] Tube-endothelial touch without blockage may also occur and is manifested as corneal edema. It may increase the risk for corneal graft rejection. If tube-endothelial touch or tube blockage is suspected, the diagnosis may be confirmed by direct visualization with slit lamp biomicroscopy or indirectly with UBM, Scheimpflug camera (Pentacam) or anterior segment OCT. When tube-endothelial touch or tube blockage is confirmed, the tube should be trimmed. The trimming should be performed so that the opening of the tip would not face the corneal graft, because turbulence at the tip may cause progressive loss of endothelial cells and corneal decompensation that will require a new transplant. The opening should not face the iris as well because it may be blocked. The tip may also be redirected if long and mobile enough. This can be done by retrieving the tube from the anterior chamber, creating a new passage into the chamber and suturing the old route. Just moving the tube in the existing route is usually unhelpful. If the graft is edematous at the time of managing the tube, regrafting may be performed later when the IOP is stable and the eye is quiet, if the edema has not been resolved.

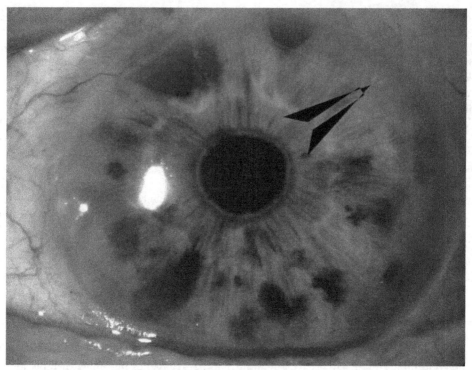

Fig. 4. Glaucoma shunt tube (arrow) in an eye after Descemet's membrane - endothelial keratoplasty (DMEK). Note the clear lamellar graft

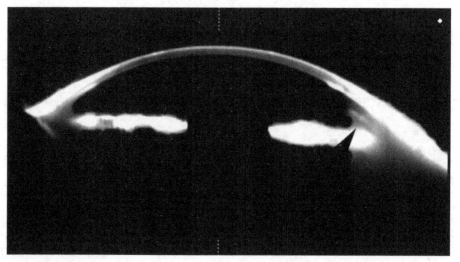

Fig. 5. Pentacam image of the same eye as in figure 4 showing the position of the tube in the anterior chamber (arrow)

Laser procedures for the angle such as selective trabeculoplasty have a limited value in the long-term treatment of secondary open angle glaucomas and therefore, were not included in the sequence of treatment. The main reason is their limited effect in this type of glaucoma. Even in primary open angle glaucoma, where it is more effective, the success rate is only 50% 5 years after the procedure.

10. Closed angle glaucoma

Closed angle glaucoma should be confirmed by gonioscopy or UBM or with other imaging techniques (anterior segment OCT or Scheimpflug camera). The first treatment modality, which is usually simplest, if the cornea is clear, is peripheral laser iridotomy. This is usually performed with Neodymium: Yttrium-Aluminum-Garnet (Nd:YAG) laser. After instillation of topical pilocarpine 2% or 4% and topical analgesic (e.g., oxybuprocaine HCl 0.4% or proparacaine HCl 0.5%) eye drop, a spot of 10mJ is placed over the peripheral iris. Two pulses may be used simultaneously. The size of the spot is constant depending on the instrument (50-70μm). The spot is placed at the periphery of the iris in the superior half to avoid glare and over a thin part of the iris (usually a crypt) avoiding blood vessels. If bleeding occurs, the cornea is pressed by a contact lens until bleeding ceases. The procedure may be performed with contact lens such as Abraham (+66D), Wise (+103D), CGI or without it. The advantages of a contact lens are additional magnification, focusing the beam, absorbing part of the heat, stabilizing the eye and maintaining the eyelids open. Topical glycerin may be placed over the cornea before the procedure if it is edematous. Topical apraclonidine (Iopidine®) 0.5%-1.0% or other alpha 2 agonist (e.g., brimonidine tartrate) is administered following the procedure to decrease IOP spikes and corticosteroids such as prednisolone acetate 1% qid are prescribed of a week to decrease intraocular inflammation and risk for synechiae formation. Additional anti-glaucoma medications may be added. This procedure facilitates aqueous flow from the posterior into the anterior chamber and may result in deepening of the anterior chamber and lowering the IOP. The major complication is acceleration of cataract. If Nd:YAG laser is unavailable, Argon laser iridotomy may be performed. The parameters for this procedure depend on the iris pigmentation. For brighter iris, the power is lower than for darker ones. The preparatory stretch burns are of 200-600mW, 0.2-0.6 sec, 200-500μm. The penetration burns are of 800-1000mW, 0.2 sec, 50μm. The iridotomy size should be increased to 150-500μm. The position of the Argon iridotomy in this case is preferably supero-nasal to prevent injury to the macula. The treatment before and after the procedure is identical to Nd:YAG laser iridotomy. Perforation of the iris is obtained when aqueous mixed with pigment is flowing from the posterior to the anterior chamber through the iridotomy. The lens should be visible through the iridotomy, since positive transillumination is not reliable. When laser iridotomy is not feasible, surgical peripheral iridectomy should be performed. Complications include visual disturbances such as halo and glare, development and progression of cataract, corneal burns that are usually transient, temporary increase in IOP, intraocular inflammation and rarely retinal injury, CME and malignant glaucoma.

If laser iridotomy does not result in decrease in IOP, surgical peripheral goniosynechiolysis or laser peripheral iridoplasty may be performed. This should be performed as earlier as possible and preferably if the angle closure is of less than 6 months. Otherwise, it is usually useless, because of scarring. Peripheral goniosynechiolysis is performed through a paracentesis. It may be performed under viscoelastic material or with anterior chamber maintainer. A spatula is transferred along the peripheral iris to withdraw it from the angle.

Goniosynechiolysis may be performed in a similar way with viscoelastic agent injected toward the angle to open it. However, the viscoelastic material should be removed at the conclusion of the procedure to prevent postoperative high IOP. Laser iridoplasty is performed after instillation of topical anesthetic eye drop with Argon laser, 200-400mW, 0.3-0.6 sec, 500 μm, 20-40 burns in a row with 2-beam diameter space between each spot over 360° peripheral iris avoiding blood vessels. The procedure is performed with a contact lens such as the Abraham (+66D), Wise (+103D), CGI or Goldmann three-mirror lens (through the center, non-mirror part) or without it. The preparations before and the management following the procedure are similar to this described above for Nd:YAG laser iridotomy. The procedure is aimed to contract the peripheral iris away from the angle. The contraindications for the procedure include extensive synechial closure and flat anterior chamber. The complications of the procedure include corneal burns, increased IOP, iritis, new synechiae formation and mydriasis.

If the IOP did not decrease substantially to the target level following these two procedures, medical treatment with anti-glaucoma medications including pilocarpine 2% four times a day may be added. If pilocarpine is added, it is worthwhile to have two consecutive days off this medication every month. This decreases the probability to have fixed small pupil, which may be an obstacle if cataract extraction is required.

If the IOP remained high or becoming high despite of medical treatment, other surgical procedures may be performed. The usual approach is to have trabeculectomy first. Trabeculectomy in this case may require a long tunnel (or sclerostomy) that will penetrate the peripheral cornea anterior to the peripheral anterior synechiae.

When a trabeculectomy is failed, a glaucoma shunt tube may be placed as mentioned earlier. In aphakic and pseudophakic eyes it may be placed into the ciliary sulcus.

11. Steroid-induced glaucoma

Steroid-induced glaucoma is defined as elevation of IOP following administration of topical and/or systemic corticosteroids that remains high after their discontinuation. Steroid responder is a patient in whom the IOP returns to normal after discontinuation of the steroids. These medications are often used after corneal transplantation to prevent or treat corneal graft rejection. They are also used to treat postoperative intraocular inflammation. Differentiation between steroid-induced glaucoma and inflammatory (uveitic) glaucoma may be performed by increasing the topical corticosteroid dosage for several days. If IOP remains high despite decreased intraocular inflammation, a corticosteroid-induced glaucoma is most reasonable.

In cases of steroid responders or steroid-induced glaucoma, discontinuation of the corticosteroids is mandatory. Patients, who are steroid responders, should be aware that they are "allergic" to steroid in the specific form that causes their IOP to increase. This should be written in their medical chart and added to a note (or a card) for the patient, specify that he should not receive this type of drug. For episodes of graft immune rejection, a combination of topical NSAID (sodium diclofenac 0.1% or ketorolac tromethamine 0.5%) and topical cyclosporine-A may be employed. Systemic cyclosporine-A or other drugs such as PO tacrolimus 0.1mg/kg/day may be added. Another option is to use IOP-sparing corticosteroids such as loteprednol etabonate 0.5% (Lotemax®) or rimexolone 1% (Vexol®). Judicious use of systemic corticosteroids instead of topical corticosteroids may be adopted if they do not cause an increase in IOP.

The treatment of steroid-induced glaucoma follows the same principles applied for primary open-angle glaucoma (see above).

12. Glaucoma in patients with corneal and posterior segment disorders

Glaucoma in cases of posterior segment disorders (e.g. proliferative diabetic retinopathy, neovascular glaucoma, uveitic glaucoma) along with corneal disorders are more challenging to treat. Pars plana vitrectomy may require a temporary keratoprosthesis for visualization of the posterior segment. Following which, a corneal transplantation is being performed. Otherwise, pars plana vitrectomy may be performed endoscopically. In both instances, if the glaucoma is refractory to medical treatment, a pars plana implantation of glaucoma drainage implant is advised.

Cyclodestructive procedures should be avoided if possible, because the degree of IOP reduction and intraocular inflammation are unpredictable. Excessive intraocular inflammation may cause intense pain, CME and hypotony that may result in phthisis bulbi. External inflammation may cause excessive scarring of the conjunctiva, preventing other procedures such as trabeculectomy to be performed. The corneal graft may also fail. Cyclodestructive procedures should be reserved only for painful eyes with no potential for visual rehabilitation. If cyclodestructive procedures are employed, transscleral cyclophotocoagulation (contact or non-contact, Nd:YAG or diode laser) or transcorneal ciliary processes photocoagulation should be preferred over cyclocryoablation. The former causes less postoperative pain, postoperative inflammatory reaction and phthisis bulbi than cyclocryoablation. Even when transscleral cyclophotocoagulation (contact or non-contact, Nd:YAG or diode laser) or transcorneal ciliary processes photocoagulation is being performed, it may be applied to half to two thirds of the ciliary body to prevent these complications. This book contains a chapter on controlled cyclophotocoagulation to decrease complications.

For cyclodestructive procedures, sub-Tenon, peribulbar or retrobulbar anesthesia with 2% lidocaine (or a 1:1 mixture with 0.75% bupivicaine) is used. Transscleral Nd:YAG (1064nm) may be contact or non-contact, continuous or pulsed. Eight to 25 applications of 1.5-10J are placed 2-3mm beyond the limbus over 180°. This position corresponds to the location of the ciliary body and is confirmed by transillumination. Trans scleral Diode (810nm), 10-20 applications of 5-6mJ over 180-270° is performed 2mm posterior to the limbus. Following the procedure, topical corticosteroids such as prednisolone acetate 1% qid or more and atropine sulfate 1% tid for a few weeks are warranted. Analgesia may also be required. The anti-glaucoma medications are tapered gradually according to the decrease in IOP. The success of the procedure is usually assessed 4 weeks after treatment. The complications include hyphema, corneal decompensation, chronic intraocular inflammation, CME, epiretinal membranes, chronic hypotony and even phthisis bulbi. They may be fewer with Diode laser with G-probe.[33]

13. Prognosis

The prognosis of preexisting glaucoma depends on its type.[17] It is usually more favorable for primary open angle glaucoma as long as precautions have been taken during the penetrating keratoplasty or the lamellar grafting. The prognosis for graft survival is also better than with other types of preexisting glaucoma, as long as the IOP is well controlled and the corneal graft has a healthy endothelium.

The prognosis for secondary open angle glaucoma is similar. If the IOP is poorly controlled, there are increased risks for corneal decompensation and development of bullous keratopathy that may require additional grafting. However, performing corneal transplantation in an eye with uncontrolled glaucoma is inadvisable. Resolution of post-keratoplasty glaucoma has been observed in chronic angle closure glaucoma after an additional corneal transplantation probably due to changes in the angle configuration by applying the above advises. In steroid responders, the IOP returns to normal following discontinuation of the corticosteroids.

With the approaches described in this chapter, it would be possible to improve the outcomes of patients with corneal transplants and coexisting glaucoma.

13.1 Follow-up

Patients undergoing corneal surgery and having or developing glaucoma usually have concurrent disorders and are more challenging to treat. These patients should be followed-up regularly at least every 3 months for their lifetime. If they experience ocular pain, decrease in vision or redness of the eye, they should immediately report to their ophthalmologist. It is essential not to postpone the next step in treatment if the current one is not sufficient to abolish the risk of further deterioration.

14. Controversies in management of glaucoma in patients with corneal grafts

Whether trabeculectomy with MMC or glaucoma drainage implant is the surgical treatment of choice for glaucoma in patients with corneal grafts is still controversial. Different authors have reported comparable results with both. At present, it is up to the decision of the surgeon according to his experience. Comparative studies are required for a definite answer. Such studies will be required also to decide whether simultaneous procedures have the same success rate as separate procedures and whether the new anterior glaucoma devices such as Solx gold shunt or iStent, will have a benefit over the posterior ones.

15. Glaucoma in cases of permanent keratoprosthesis

Several types of keratoprosthesis are available including one that pass through the cornea and fused eyelids (type II) and the more common ones through the cornea only (type I, e.g., Boston and osteo-odonto-keratoprosthesis) (Figures 6,7). Keratoprosthesis is usually reserved for eyes in which other corneal procedures have failed and the prognosis for additional ones is poor. A publication on repeated corneal transplantation demonstrated that as the number of repeated corneal grafts is increased, the prognosis for long-term survival of the regraft decreases.[12] Most of the regrafts do fail due to graft rejection, glaucoma and other complications. These findings have led keratoprosthesis specialists to advocate keratoprosthesis. However, the publication was intended to elaborate the importance of proper preventive measures and early and correct treatment of corneal transplantation complications of rather than to advocate the use of keratoprosthesis. With better preventive measures and treatments, it will be possible to decrease the necessity for repeated transplantation and of course to avoid keratoprosthesis.

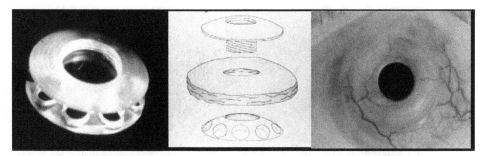

Fig. 6. Type I keratoprosthesis (courtesy of Peter Rubin, MD)

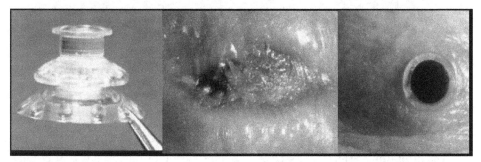

Fig. 7. Type II keratoprosthesis (courtesy of Peter Rubin, MD)

Many of the patients undergoing keratoprosthesis have multiple ocular pathologies and glaucoma is one of them. Between 36-76% of the eyes with keratoprosthesis have glaucoma.[34-39] Of these, about 2-28% develop glaucoma after the implantation of keratoprosthesis, usually because of progressive angle closure. This may be caused because of inadvertent injury to the angle and postoperative intraocular inflammation. A peripheral iridectomy may decrease the risk of postoperative angle closure. The prosthesis may also serve as a scaffold for retoprosthetic membrane that may cover the angle. The use of corticosteroids for prolonged period may also cause corticosteroid-induced glaucoma in susceptible patients.

Glaucoma is more frequent in keratopsrosthetic patients than in repeated corneal transplantation. One of the most challenging situations in the presence of keratoprosthesis is to detect and follow-up glaucoma, because it is impossible to check the IOP using the standard methods such as Goldmann applanation tonometry or Schiotz indentation tonometry. These instruments are employed through normal cornea and not through a keratoprosthesis, which cannot be indent. In many cases, visualization of the optic disc may be difficult and therefore, changes in cupping are difficult to observe or document directly, or indirectly using Heidelberg Retinal Tomography (HRT), scanning laser polarimeter (GDx) or OCT. Reliable visual fields may also be difficult to obtain and the maximal field that may be obtained is 60° with type I and 40° with type II.

It is paramount to obtain the history of glaucoma in patients with keratoprosthesis and to document it. In presence of keratoprosthesis, IOP qualitative estimation may be performed by digital palpation over the sclera. It should not be performed over the keratoprosthesis or the glaucoma shunt plate. Qualitative estimation with glass rod over the conjunctiva is

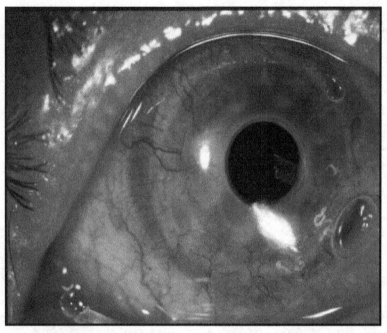

Fig. 8. The tip of Ahmed shunt tube seen through type I keratoprosthesis. It was placed into the vitreous though the pars plana (courtesy of Peter Rubin, MD)

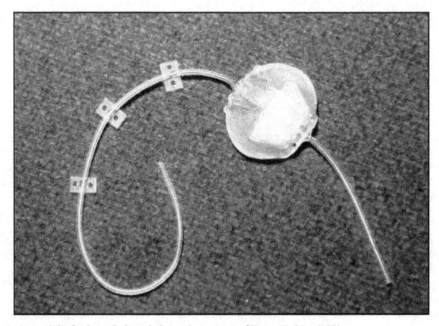

Fig. 9. A modified Ahmed closed shunt (courtesy of Peter Rubin, MD)

more challenging as quantitative estimation of the IOP by Tonopen or Schiotz indentation tonometry through the limbal area. If the IOP cannot be estimated in follow-up visits, it is also possible to follow patients by observing the optic disc and visual fields for deterioration as is done with some patients without keratoprosthesis who do not allow checking their IOP. New transducers are being developed to allow IOP measurements in patients with keratoprosthesis.

In patients who are candidate for keratoprosthesis, it is preferable to implant glaucoma drainage device and to wait for 3-6 months before placing the keratoprosthesis especially when the IOP is refractory to medical treatment or the damage to the optic disc is advanced. This period would allow the postoperative intraocular inflammation to subside and to the IOP to stabilized.

The respond to medical treatment in patients with keratoprosthesis is limited because there is no absorption area in patients with type II and limited absorption area with type I keratoprosthesis and the glaucoma is usually more severe compared with glaucoma in penetrating keratoplasty. The next step is introducing a glaucoma drainage device (Figure 8). A placement of glaucoma shunt tube into the vitreous through the pars plana may be better than into the anterior chamber that is already crowded because of the back-plate of the prosthesis. In aphakic eyes, it is mandatory to ascertain that no vitreous remains in the anterior chamber, by meticulous anterior vitrectomy. Since the patients are either aphakic or pseudophakic, the tube may be inserted through the ciliary sulcus. Recently, it was suggested to place the valved drainage tube such as Ahmed valve in the lacrimal sac, ethmoid or maxillary sinuses and to avoid the subconjunctival plate.[38,39] The shunt tube was modified for this purpose (Figure 9) and was placed into the lacrimal sac or the ethmoid sinus through an external dacryocystorhinostomy incision although it may be placed in a similar manner as a Pyrex tube in conjunctivo-dacryo-cystorhinostomy. Placement into the maxillary sinus was performed through a lower eyelid crease or subciliary incision but it is also possible to go through the inferior fornix. Penetration may be performed with intravenous catheter and the tube may be passed through it after removing the catheter hub. These procedures may decrease the failure of glaucoma shunt tube from fibrosis around the subconjunctival plate. The main risk in these cases is endophthalmitis. Therefore, I would not advocate these procedures if the lacrimal sac or the sinus is not sterile. Therefore, such a procedure should be avoided in patients with active sinusitis or history of this disorder. In one series of 37 patients, one (3%) developed endophthalmitis.[38] Cyclophotocoagulation may be employed as an adjunct treatment to glaucoma drainage implants for painful eyes with no potential for visual rehabilitation.[42,43]

16. References

[1] Thoft RA, Gardon JM, Dohlman CH. Glaucoma following penetrating keratoplasty. *Trans Am Acad Ophthalmol Otolaryngol* 1974;78:352-64.

[2] Polack FM. Keratoplasty in aphakic eyes with corneal edema: results in 100 cases with 10-year follow-up. *Ophthalmic Surg* 1980;11:701-7.

[3] Goldberg DB, Schanzlin DJ, Brown SI. Incidence of increased intraocular pressure after keratoplasty. *Am J Ophthalmol* 1981;92:372-7.

[4] Foulks GN. Glaucoma associated with penetrating keratoplasty. *Ophthalmology* 1987; 94:871-4.

[5] Polack FM. Glaucoma in keratoplasty. *Cornea* 1988;7:67-9.

[6] Simmons RB, Stern RA, Teekhasaenee C, Kenyon KR. Elevated intraocular pressure following penetrating keratoplasty. *Trans Am Ophthalmol Soc* 1989;87:79-91.

[7] Cowden J, Kaufman HE, Polack FM. The prognosis of keratoplasty after previous graft failures. *Am J Ophthalmol* 1974;78:523-5.

[8] Robinson CH. Indications, complications and prognosis for repeated penetrating keratoplasty. *Ophthalmic Surg* 1979;10:27-34.

[9] Insler MS, Pechous B. Visual results in repeat penetrating keratoplasty. *Am J Ophthalmol* 1986;102:371-5.

[10] MacEwen CJ, Khan ZUH, Anderson E, MacEwen CG. Corneal re-graft: indications and outcome. *Ophthalmic Surg* 1988;19:706-12.

[11] Rapuano CJ, Cohen EJ, Brady SE et al. Indications and outcomes of repeat penetrating keratoplasty. *Am J Ophthalmol* 1990;109:689-95.

[12] Bersudsky V, Blum-Hareuveni T, Rehany U, Rumelt S. The profile of repeated corneal transplantation. *Ophthalmology* 2001;108:461-9.

[13] Sugar A. An analysis of corneal endothelial and graft survival in pseudophakic bullous keratopathy. *Trans Am Ophthalmol Soc* 1989;87:762-801.

[14] Byrd S, Tayeri T. Glaucoma associated with penetrating keratoplasty. *Clin Ophthalmol* 1999;39:17-28.

[15] Rumelt S, Blum-Hareuveni T, Bersudsky V, Rehany U. Persistent epithelial defects and ulcers in repeated corneal transplantation: incidence, causative agents, predisposing factors and treatment outcomes. *Eye*, 2008;246:1139-1145.

[16] Aldave AJ, Rudd JC, Cohen EJ et al. The role of glaucoma therapy in the need for repeat penetrating keratoplasty. *Cornea* 2000, 19:772-6.

[17] Rumelt S, Bersudsky V, Blum-Hereuveni T, Rehany U. Preexisting and postoperative glaucoma in repeated corneal transplantation. *Cornea*, 2002;21:759-765.

[18] Kirkness CM. Penetrating keratoplasty, glaucoma, and silicone drainage tubing. *Dev Ophthalmol* 1987;14:161-5.

[19] Ates H, Palamar M, Yagci A, Egrilmez S. Evaluation of mini Ex-Press glaucoma shunt implantation in refractory penetrating glaucoma. *J Glaucoma* 2010;19:556-60.

[20] McDonnell PJ, Robin JB, Schanzlin DJ et al. Molteno implant for control of glaucoma in eyes after penetrating keratoplasty. *Ophthalmology* 1988;95:364-9.

[21] Kirkness CM, Ling Y, Rice NSC. The use of silicone drainage tubing to control postkeratoplasty glaucoma. *Eye* 1988;2:583-90.

[22] Beebe WE, Starita RJ, Fellman RL, Lynn JR, Gelender H. The use of Molteno implant and anterior chamber tube shunt to encycling band (ACTSEB) for treatment of glaucoma in penetrating keratoplasty. *Ophthalmology* 1990;97:1414-22.

[23] Sherwood MB, Smith MF, Driebe WT Jr et al. Drainage tube implants in the treatment of glaucoma following penetrating keratoplasty. *Ophthalmic Surg* 1993;24:185-9.

[24] Rapuano CJ, Schmidt CM, Cohen EJ, et al. Results of alloplastic tube shunt procedures before, during, oafter penetratikeratoplasty. *Cornea* 1995;14:26-32.

[25] Coleman AL, Mondino BJ, Wilson MR, Casey R. Clinical experience with the Ahmed glaucoma valve implant in eyes with prior or concurrent penetrating keratoplasties. *Am J Ophthalmol* 1997;123:54-61.

[26] Rumelt S. Rehany U. Implantation of glaucoma drainage implant tuinto the ciliary sulcuin patients with corneal transplants. *Arch Ophthalmol* 1998;116:685-7.

[27] Tello C, Espana EM, Mora R, et al. Baerveldt glaucoma implant insertion in the posterior chamber sulcus. *Br J Ophthalmol* 2007;91:739-42.

[28] Weiner A, Cohn AD, Balasubramaniam M, Weiner AJ. Glaucoma tube shunt implantation through the ciliary sulcus in pseudophakic eyes with high risk of corneal decompensation. *J Glaucoma* 2010;19:405-11.

[29] Bersudsky V, Treviño A, Rumelt S. Management of endothelial decompensation because of glaucoma shunt tube touch by Descemet membrane endothelial keratoplasty and tube revision. *Cornea* 2011;30:709-11.

[30] Gandham SB, Costa VP, Katz LJ, Wilson RP, SA, Belmont J, Smith M. Aqueous tube-shunt implantation and pars plana vitrectomy in eyes with refractory glaucoma. *Am J Ophthalmol* 1993;116:189-95.

[31] Ritterband DC, Shapiro D, Trubnik V, et al. Cornea Glaucoma Implant Study Group (COGIS). Penetrating keratoplasty with pars plana glaucoma drainage devices. *Cornea* 2007;26:1060-6.

[32] Tarantola RM, Agarwal A, Lu P, Joos KM. Long-term results of combined endoscope-assisted pars plana vitrectomy and glaucoma tube shunt surgery. *Retina* 2011; 31:275-83.

[33] Fishbaugh G. Overview and new technology in cyclodestructive procedures. *Insight* 1999;19:26-9.

[34] Netland PA, Terada H, Dohlman CH. Glaucoma associated with keratoprosthesis. *Ophthalmology* 1998;105:751-7.

[35] Zerbe BL, Belin MW, Ciolino JB. Boston Type 1 Keratoprosthesis Study Group. Results from the multicenter Boston Type 1 Keratoprosthesis Study. *Ophthalmology* 2006; 113:1779.

[36] Aldave AJ, Kamal KM, Vo RC, Yu F. The Boston type I keratoprosthesis: improving outcomes and expanding indications. *Ophthalmology* 2009;116:640-51.

[37] Bradley JC, Hernandez EG, Schwab IR, Mannis MJ. Boston type 1 keratoprosthesis: the university of California Davis experience. *Cornea* 2009;28:321-7.

[38] Chew HF, Ayres BD, Hammersmith KM, et al. Boston keratoprosthesis outcomes and complications. *Cornea* 2009;28:989-96.

[39] Rivier D, Paula JS, Kim E, Dohlman CH, Grosskreutz CL. Glaucoma and keratoprosthesis surgery: role of adjunctive cyclophotocoagulation. *J Glaucoma* 2009;18:321-4.

[40] Rubin PA, Chang E, Bernardino CR, Hatton MP, Dohlman CH. Oculoplastic technique of connecting a glaucoma valve shunt to extraorbital locations in cases of severe glaucoma. *Ophthal Plast Reconstr Surg* 2004;20:362-7.

[41] Dohlman CH, Grosskreutz CL, Chen TC, et al. Shunts to divert aqueous humor to distant epithelialized cavities after keratoprosthesis surgery. *J Glaucoma* 2010; 19:111-5.

[42] Rivier D, Paula JS, Kim E, Dohlman CH, Grosskreutz CL. Glaucoma and keratoprosthesis surgery: role of adjunctive cyclophotocoagulation. *J Glaucoma* 2009;18:321-4.

[43] Parthasarathy A, Aung T, Oen FT, Tan DT. Endoscopic cyclophotocoagulation for the management of advanced glaucoma after osteo-odonto-keratoprosthesis surgery. *Clin Experiment Ophthalmol* 2008;36:93-4.

15

Steroid Induced Glaucoma

Avraham Cohen
Western Galilee Hospital,
Department Of Ophthalmology
Israel

1. Introduction

Increased intraocular pressure and glaucoma following corticosteroid therapy are well known issues for the ophthalmologist for more than 50 years. Corticosteroids use has gained popularity in ophthalmology as anti-inflammatory and anti-allergic agents but can have important consequences and should be used only with judicious monitoring. The therapeutic use of corticosteroids can lead to the development of ocular hypertension and iatrogenic open-angle glaucoma in susceptible individuals. It can occur in any age group, either gender and from steroid therapy for any ocular or systemic disease and by any route of administration: topical, systemic or inhaled.

2. Epidemiology

About one in every three people is considered a potential "steroid responder", but only a small percentage will have a clinically significant elevation in intraocular pressure. 5-6% of the normal population develops a marked increase in intraocular pressure of more than 31 mmHg after 4-6 weeks of topical corticosteroids therapy. 33% are moderate responders (elevation of 6-15 mmHg) and the remaining are considered non responreds (less than 6mmHg of elevation in intraocular pressure). Although approximately 30%–40% of the normal population are "steroid responders" (i.e., develop reversible steroid-induced ocular hypertension), most of primary open angle glaucoma patients or with a family history are steroid responders. Normal individuals who are steroid responders are at higher risk for subsequently developing primary open angle glaucoma. In one study, high corticosteroid responders (intraocular pressure greater than 31 mm Hg during dexamethasone administration qid for 6 weeks), 13.0% developed glaucomatous visual field loss during the follow-up period of 5 years. In steroid induced glaucoma patients, glaucoma is triggered by steroid treatment, and intraocular pressure will not decrease after cessation of steroid application. Thus, steroid induced glaucoma patients necessitate anti-glaucoma medications to control intraocular pressure. Steroid responsiveness appears to be heritable, however low concordance of pressure response in monozygotic twins to topical testing may indicate a limited role for a genetic basis. In addition highly myopic patients and diabetic patients have a higher rate of elevated intraocular pressure response to topical steroids.

Age is also an important factor. In pediatric patients taking oral prednisone for inflammatory bowel disease 32% were steroid responders. When children younger than 10 years of age where treated with topical instillation of dexamethasone, marked elevation in intraocular pressure was noted. A dose-dependent hypertensive pressure response occurs more frequently, more severely and more rapidly in children than in adults.

3. Pathophysiology

There have been reports suggesting that endogenous cortisol may play a role in the pathogenesis of primary open angle glaucoma. Excess endogenous production of glucocorticosteroids (Cushing's syndrome) can also cause increase in intraocular pressure. Glucocorticosteroids alter several trabecular meshwork cellular functions including inhibition of cellular proliferation, migration, phagocytosis, and increased cell and nucleus size. Glucocorticosteroids also increase extracellular matrix synthesis and decrease its turnover.

Many mechanisms have been proposed to explain the elevated intraocular pressure in response to glucocorticosteroids. One hypothesis is that glucocorticosteroids protect the lysosomal membrane and thus inhibit release of hydrolases responsible of depolimerization of glycosaminoglycans. Accumulated glycosaminoglycans in the ground substance of the outflow pathways retain water and narrow the trabecular spaces, causing increase in outflow resistance. In steroid-induced glaucoma there is also an increase in fine fibrillar material in the subendothelial region of Schlemm's cannal. These fibrils are deposited underneath the inner wall endothelium. The main finding in steroid-induced glaucoma is an accumulation of basement membrane-like material staining for type IV collagen. These accumulations are found throughout all layers of the trabecular meshwork.

There are multiple isoforms of the glucocorticoid receptor (GR) a ligand-dependent transcriptional factor that activates or represses gene transcription. GRα is the ligand binding form of the receptor that is responsible for the physiologic and pharmacological effects of glucocorticosteroids. Most of the physiological and pharmacological effects of glucocorticosteroids are directly mediated by GRα. GRα resides predominantly in the cytoplasm in the absence of ligand as a multiprotein heterocomplex that contains Hsp 90, Hsp 70 and other proteins. Steroid binding to GRα causes a conformation change and activation of the receptor. Activated GRα can alter gene expression via GRE-dependent (classical) and GRE-independent (nonclassical) mechanisms. In the GRE-dependent pathway activated GRα translocates to the nucleus along microtubules. GRα bind to specific palindromic DNA sequence (GRE) as a homodimer on the promoter region of target genes to induce transcription. In addition, GRα functions as a negative regulator of transcription in a specific subset of genes that contains a negative GRE. The GRE-independent pathway is an additional way to inhibit gene expression. GRα physically interacts with other transcription factors to prevent them from binding to their response elements of genes that encode for proinflammatory cytokines. The anti-inflammatory and immune suppression are mediated via this GRE-independent pathway. GRβ is an alternatively spliced form of the receptor, that resides in the nucleus, which lacks the conventional ligand binding domain, does not bind glucocorticosteroids, and acts as a dominant negative regulator of glucocorticosteroids activity. Increased expression of GRβ appears to be responsible for unresponsiveness to anti-inflammatory therapy for asthma, inflammatory bowel disease rheumatoid arthritis and ulcerative colitis. Recent work has shown that glaucomatous trabecular meshwork cells have lower levels of GRβ compared with normal trabecular meshwork cells, and this appears to be responsible for increased glucocorticosteroids sensitivity in the glaucomatous trabecular meshwork cells. In primary open angle glaucoma an abnormal accumulation of dihydrocortisol may potentiate exogenous glucocorticosteroids activity and increased intraocular pressure.

Changes in protein synthesis have also been implicated in steroid induced glaucoma. *MYOC* gene, located on chromosome 1, encodes a secretory glycoprotein of 504 amino acids named Myocilin, and is the first gene to be linked to juvenile open-angle glaucoma and some forms of adult-onset primary open-angle glaucoma. The gene was identified as an up regulated molecule in cultured trabecular meshwork cells after treatment with dexamethasone and was originally referred to as trabecular meshwork-inducible glucocorticoid response (*TIGR*). Interestingly, the profile of *MYOC* up regulation by dexamethasone is in a dose- and time-dependent manner very similar to the course of development of steroid induced glaucoma. This led many investigators to believe that an increased *MYOC* level is a cause of glaucoma. However, a putative association between *MYOC* induction and primary open angle glaucoma has not been firmly established.

Glucocorticosteroids inhibit prostaglandin synthesis by trabecular cells. Prostaglandins E_2 and F_{2a} normal function is to lower the intraocular pressure by increasing the outflow facility. Endothelial cells of the trabecular meshwork can act as phagocytes of debris. Glucocorticosteroids can suppress phagocytic activity causing accumulation of debris in the trabecular meshwork and decrease in outflow facility.

In a study on rabbit eyes, after topical treatment with dexamethasone, Transmission electron microscopy showed increased abnormality of nucleus of the trabecular meshwork cells, microfilament and microtubules among interstitial cells also increased, cytoplasmic vacuolation, rough endoplasmic reticulum expansion, as well as an increase in intercellular amorphous material. The mechanism of elevated intraocular pressure is thought to be increased aqueous outflow resistance owing to an accumulation of extracellular matrix material in the trabecular meshwork (fig 1).

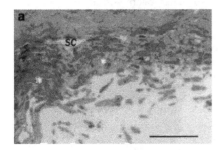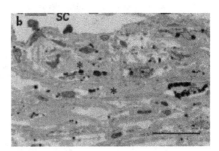

Fig. 1. Light microscopic pictures of the trabecular meshwork from steroid-induced glaucoma (SG). a) (Right eye in case 1), b) (Case 2): Schlemm's canal (SC) is open. The intertrabescular spaces in the outer part of the TM are filled with the homogeneous extracellular matrix (ECM) (asterisks). Azure II staining. Scale bars indicate 50 µm for a) and 20 µm for b)

Effects of Glucocorticosteroids are mediated by the Glucocorticosteroids receptor, which is a ligand-dependent transcription factor altering the expression of trabecular meshwork genes. Glucocorticosteroids increase the expression of extracellular matrix (collagen, fibronectin, laminin), proteinase inhibitor genes (Serpina3) and decreased expression of proteinase genes (MMP1, TPA). Altered expression of cytoskeletal genes (ACTA2, FLNB, and NEBL) may be associated with Glucocorticosteroids mediated reorganization of trabecular meshwork cell microfibrils and microtubules. Glucocorticosteroids reorganizes the actin cytoskeleton to form cross-linked actin networks (CLANs) in cultured trabecular meshwork cells, and is reversible after Glucocorticosteroids withdrawel. In addition Glucocorticosteroids alters microtubules to form microtubule tangles.

4. Routes of corticosteroid administration

4.1 Topical route
Topical route includes ocular drops and ointments. Of various routes of administration, topical therapy most commonly induces elevated intraocular pressure and correlates with the duration and frequency of administration. Dexamethasone and prednisolone increase intraocular pressure more frequently than loteprendol (Lotemax), fluorometholone (FML), rimexolone (Vexol) or hydrocortisone. Fluorometholone (FML) in particular is less likely to increase intraocular pressure but is also a less potent steroid (table 1). Rimexolone has a low intraocular pressure elevating potential comparable to that of fluorometholone in adults. The chemical structure is responsible to the lower propensity to increase intraocular pressure of some steroids. Loteprendol is a site-active steroid that contains an ester rather than a ketone group at the C-20 position, rendering de-esterification to an inactive metabolite. It is highly lipid-soluble, with enhanced penetration into cells. Loteprendol appears to have an improved safety profile compared with ketone corticosteroids. Fluorometholone is deoxygenized at the C-21 position. Rimexolone lacks a hydroxyl substituent at the C-21 position. It has lower aqueous solubility and increased lipophilicity. It appears that the potency of topical steroids is directly correlated with the propensity to elevate intraocular pressure. Intraocular pressure elevation almost never occurs in less than 5 days and rarely in less than 2 weeks of steroid treatment. However, late rise in ocular pressure is not uncommon, even if intraocular pressure has been within normal limits during a treatment course of 6 weeks.

4.2 Intraocular route
Before the advent of anti VEGF, intravitreal steroid injections have been used largely in the treatment of exudative age related macular degeneration, chronic cystoid macular edema, proliferative diabetic vitreoretinopathy, retinal vascular occlusion and chronic uveitis. Rise in intraocular pressure is dependent on dose, presence of aphakia or pseudophkaia and a history of vitrectomy, facilitating penetration of the drug into the anterior segment. Intraocular pressure may rise in 30-50 % of patients as soon as 1-4 weeks after intravitreal injection of triamcinolone acetonide (Kenalog) and often returns to baseline several months after injection. It is advisable to perform a trial of topical prednisolone acetate before intravitreal triamcinolone acetonide injection is performed.
Fluocinolone acetonide intravitreal implants are an effective therapy for non-infectious posterior uveitis. However, patients receiving this treatment are at high risk for development of vision-threatening increased intraocular pressure. Therefore, patients treated with these implants should have frequent intraocular pressure monitoring. Intractable glaucoma may necessitate removal of the depot by pars plana vitrectomy to lower intraoculare pressure. In the SCORE study grid photocoagulation and repeated injections of triamcinolone acetonide 1 or 4 mg seemed to be equally effective in producing improvements in best corrected visual acuity in patients with macular edema due to branch retinal vein occlusion. 41% of patients treated with triamcinolone acetonide 4 mg initiated

intraocular pressure lowering medications during the 12 months study. In patient with central retinal vein occlusion 35% of the patients receiving 4 mg triamcinolone acetonide initiated glaucoma medications. Ozurdex is a slow release intravitreal implant of dexamethasone currently under clinical trials for the treatment of macular edema in retinal vein occlusion disease. It appears that the dexamethasone implant is well tolerated, producing transient, moderate and readily managed increase in intraocular pressure in less than 16% of eyes.

4.3 Periocular route
Subconjunctival, sub-Tenon and retrobulbar injections of triamcinolone acetonide may cause dangerous and prolonged elevation of intraocular pressure because of their long duration of action. Surgical excision of sub-Tenon triamcinolone acetonide deposit should be considered if the primary treatment for steroid-induced glaucoma is refractory to medical treatment.
The application of topical corticosteroids to the eyelids and periorbital region, in the treatment of atopic dermatitis, even over long periods of time, was not related to the development of glaucoma or cataracts.

4.4 Systemic route
Systemic administration includes ingestion, inhalation and nasal spray. It is less likely to cause intraocular elevation. However, intraocular pressure may rise weeks to years after treatment. When administrated concurrently with topical steroids it may have an additive effect and higher intraocular pressure than a single route.
Intranasal corticosteroids have become a gold standard in therapy for allergic rhinoconjunctivitis and recent evidence indicates that may be effective at alleviating ocular symptoms as well. Intranasal corticosteroids are absorbed systemically in small measurable amounts. Some studies suggest a relationship between intranasal steroids and increased intraocular pressure.
Aerosolized drugs delivered with a facemask may inadvertently deposit in the eyes, raising concerns about ocular side effects. Inhaled corticosteroids have been associated with an increased risk of skin thinning, bruising, cataracts and possibly glaucoma in adults. The risks increase with advanced age, higher doses, and longer duration of use. In children, the risks of cataracts and glaucoma were negligible with inhaled corticosteroids, whether a mouthpiece or a mask interface was used. It is not known whether exposed children will have increased risks from inhaled corticosteroids later in life. Therefore, it is wise to avoid face and eye deposition when possible, to use the minimally effective dose and a regular follow up of intraocular pressure.

4.5 Endogenous route
Elevated blood levels of corticosteroids of endogenous production, as seen in adrenal hyperplasia or neoplasia (Cushing syndrome) can also cause increase in the intraocular pressure. After adrenalectomy, increased intraocular pressure may retune to normal values

5. Clinical course

An increase in intraocular pressure may occur days to weeks and even months after the administration of steroids. The increase in intraocular pressure depends on potency, penetration, frequency and route of administration. Individual susceptibility, older age and ocular disease are also important factors. An acute presentation may occur after intense systemic steroid therapy. Patient may complain on pain, decreased vision and conjunctival hyperemia. In infants the clinical picture may resemble that of congenital glaucoma. Signs are tearing, Descement's membrane breaks, corneal edema, enlarged corneal diameter, elevated intraocular pressure and optic disc cupping. Unlike congenital glaucoma, the anterior chamber angle is normal.

Potency	Steroid	Glaucoma risk
High	Betamethasone Clobetasol propionate Dexamethasone Flucinonide	
Medium	Triamcinolone acetonide Loteprendole etabonate Dexamethasone sodium phosphate Fluormethalone	
Low	Hydrocortisone Rimexolone Medrisone	

Table 1. Comparison of anti-inflamatory and intraocular pressure elevating potencies

Additional ocular findings from topical steroids include corneal ulcers, exacerbation of bacterial and viral infections, posterior subcapsular cataracts, mydriasis, delayed wound healing, scleral melting ptosis and skin atrophy and depigmentation of the eyelids. Systemic steroids side effects are suppression of the pituitary-adrenal axis, Cushinoid facies, buffalo hump, truncal obesity, hirsutism, cutaneous striae, easy bruisability, delayed wound healing, osteoporosis, aseptic necrosis of the hip, peptic ulcers, diabetes, hypertension, insomnia and psychiatric disorders.

6. Management

This secondary glaucoma clinically mimics many features of primary open angle glaucoma. Currently, the propensity to develop steroid-induced ocular hypertension must be determined empirically. Therefore, all patients on protracted steroid therapy should have their intraocular pressure monitored periodically.

Steroid induced glaucoma usually responds to cessation of steroid therapy and to topical anti-glaucoma medication. In steroid responders the intraocular pressure generally returns to normal within few days to weeks after discontinuation of steroids. Rarely, intraocular pressure remains elevated despite steroid cessation and may result from damage to outflow channels. In these cases management is similar to that of open angle glaucoma patients.

If anti-inflammatory therapy is needed in known steroid responders or glaucoma patients, treatment with FML 0.1% or medrisone (MHS) are possible options. Loteprendol (Lotemax) and Rimexolone (Velox) are potent anti-inflammatory corticosteroids with reduced propensity to raise intraocular pressure.

Alternative topical anti-inflammatory agents are the nonsteroidal anti-inflammatory agents (NSAIDs), such as diclofenac (Voltaren), ketorolac tromethamine (Acular LS) and bromfenac (Xibrom). NSAIDs do not induce increase in intraocular pressure but their anti-inflammatory potential is lower than that of corticosteroids.

When indicated, topical anti-glaucoma medications should be used. Prostaglandins should be used with caution as they may have pro-inflammatory effect. If intraocular pressure remains intractable despite maximal tolerated medical therapy, Argon laser trabeculoplasty and Nd:YAG laser selective trabeculoplasty (SLT) have variable success and patients required additional surgical procedures. Repeat SLT treatments may be necessary. SLT is a temporizing procedure to consider in patients with steroid-induced elevated IOP.

A possible new treatment under investigation is anecortave acetate injection into the anterior sub-Tenon space in eye with uncontrolled steroid-related ocular hypertension following intravitreal or sub-Tenon injections of triamcinolone acetonide. Anecortave acetate is a synthetic molecule derived from cortisol. The resulting molecule is referred to as a cortisene. The modification renders the molecule free of all glucocorticoid and mineralocorticoid activity. Anecortave acetate possesses antiangiogenic activity via inhibition of the proteases necessary for vascular endothelial cell migration and has been evaluated as a potential therapy for neovascular age-related macular degeneration. In one preliminary, uncontrolled study a rapid and sustained reduction of intraocular pressure was noted as soon as 1 week after treatment. The mechanism by which anecortave acetate lowers intraocular pressure in eyes with steroid-related ocular hypertension is unknown. With glucocorticoid treatment, trabecular meshwork cells increases the expression of plasminogen activator inhibitor-1, a protein that inhibits activation of extracellular proteinases and leads to enhanced extracellular matrix deposition. Recent studies have shown that anecortave acetate blocks glucocorticoid induction of plasminogen activator inhibitor-1, which may be partially responsible for anecortave acetate's intraocular pressure lowering activity.

Surgical treatments include filtration surgery, tube shunt, excision of the sub-Tenon steroid depot, explantation of steroid implant and pars plana vitrectomyfor the removal of the intravitreal depot.

7. References

Armaly MF. The heritable nature of dexamethasone-induced ocular hypertension. Arch Ophthalmol. 1966; 75:32–5.

Bamberger CM, Bamberger AM, de Castro M, Chrousos GP. Glucocorticoid receptor beta, a potential endogenous inhibitor of glucocorticoid action in humans. J Clin Invest. 1995; 95:2435–41.

Bartlett JD, Woolley TW, Adams CM. Identification of high intraocular pressure responders to topical ophthalmic corticosteroids. J Ocul Pharmacol. 1993; 9:35–45.

Becker B, Chevrette L. Topical corticosteroid testing in glaucoma siblings. Arch Ophthalmol. 1966; 76:484–7.

Becker B. Diabetes mellitus and and primary open angle glaucoma. Am J Opphthalmol. 1971; 71:1.

Bregmann J, Witmer MT, Slonim CB. The relationship of intranasal steroids to intraocular pressure. Curr Allergy Asthma Rep. 2009 Jul; 9(4):311-5.

Duma D, Jewell CM, Cidlowski JA. Multiple glucocorticoid receptor isoforms and mechanisms of post-translational modification. J Steroid Biochem Mol Biol. 2006; 102:11–21.

Fautsch MP, Bahler CK, Jewison DJ, et al. Recombinant TIGR/MYOC increases outflow resistance in the human anterior segment. Invest Ophthalmol Vis Sci 2000; 41:4163–8.

Gould DB, Miceli-Libby L, Savinova OV, et al. Genetically increasing MYOC expression supports a necessary pathologic role of abnormal proteins in glaucoma. Mol Cell Biol 2004; 24:9019–25.

Haeck IM, Rouwen TJ, Timmer-de Mik L, de Bruin-Weller MS, Bruijnzeel-Koomen CA. Topical corticosteroids in atopic dermatitis and the risk of glaucoma and cataracts. J Am Acad Dermatol. 2011 Feb; 64(2):275-81.

Hass JS, NootensRH: Glaucoma secondary to benigne adrenal adenoma. Am J Ophthalmol 1974; 78:497.

Jilani FA, Khan AM, Kesharwani RK: Study of topical corticosteroid response in glaucoma suspects and family members of established glaucoma patients. Indian J Ophthalmol 1987; 35:141.

Jonas JB, Degenring RF, Kreissig I, Akkoyun I, Kamppeter BA. Intraocular pressure elevation after intravitreal triamcinolone acetonide injection. Ophthalmology. 2005;112(4):593-598.

Jonas JB. Intravitreal triamcinolone acetonide: a change in a paradigm. Ophthalmic Res. 2006;38(4):218-245.

Jones R 3rd, Rhee DJ. Corticosteroid-induced ocular hypertension and glaucoma: a brief review and update of the literature. . Curr Opin Ophthalmol. 2006 Apr; 17(2):163-7.

Julia A. Haller et al for the OZURDEX GENEVA Study Group. Randomized, sham controlled trial of dexamethasone intravitreal implant in patients with macular edema due to retinal vein occlusion. Ophthalmology 2010;117:1134-46.

Kitazawa Y, Horie T. The prognosis of corticosteroid-responsive individuals. Arch Ophthalmol. 1981; 99:819–23.

Kwok AK, Lam DS, Fan DS, et al. Ocular hypertensive response totopical steroids in children. Ophthalmol1997; 104:2112.

Lewis JM, Priddy T, Judd J, Gordon MO, Kass MA, Kolker AE, Becker B. Intraocular pressure response to topical dexamethasone as a predictor for the development of primary open-angle glaucoma. Am J Ophthalmol. 1988; 106:607–12.

Lutjen-Drecoll E, May CA, Polansky JR, et al. Localization of the stress proteins alpha B-crystallin and trabecular meshwork inducible glucocorticoid response protein in normal and glaucomatous trabecular meshwork. Invest Ophthalmol Vis Sci 1998; 39:517–25.

McCarty GR, Schwartz B. Increased plasma noncortisol glucocorticoid activity in open-angle glaucoma. Invest Ophthalmol Vis Sci. 1991; 32:1600–8.

Mindel JS, Tavitian HO, Smith H, Jr, et al. Comparative ocular pressure elevation by medrysone, fluorometholone, and dexamethasone phosphate. Arch Ophthalmol 1980; 98:1577–8.

NG JS, Fan DS, young AL et al,Ocular hypertensive response to topical dexamethasone in children: a dose-dependent phenomenon. Ophthalmol 2000; 107:2097.

Nguyen TD, Chen P, Huang WD, et al. Gene structure and properties of TIGR, an olfactomedin-related glycoprotein cloned from glucocorticoid-induced trabecular meshwork cells. J Biol Chem 1998; 273:6341-50.

Oakley RH, Sar M, Cidlowski JA. The human glucocorticoid receptor beta isoform. Expression, biochemical properties, and putative function. J Biol Chem. 1996; 271:9550-9.

Ohji M, Kinoshita S, Ohmi E, Kuwayama Y. marked intraocular response to instillation of corticosteroids in children. Am J Ophthalmol 1191; 112:450.

Okka M, Bozkurt B, Kerimoglu H, Ozturk BT, Gunduz K, Yılmaz M, Okudan S. Control of steroid-induced glaucoma with surgical excision of sub-Tenon triamcinolone acetonide deposits: a clinical and biochemical approach. Can J Ophthalmol. 2010 Dec; 45(6):621-6.

Robin AL, Suan EP, Sjaarda RN, Callanan DG, Defaller J; Alcon Anecortave Acetate for IOP Research Team. Reduction of intraocular pressure with anecortave acetate in eyes with ocular steroid injection-related glaucoma. Arch Ophthalmol. 2009 Feb; 127(2):173-8.

Rozsival P, Hampl R, Obenberger J, Starka L, Rehak S. Aqueous humour and plasma cortisol levels in glaucoma and cataract patients. Curr Eye Res. 1981; 1:391–6.

Rubin B, Taglienti A, Rothman RF, Marcus CH, Serle JB. The effect of selective laser trabeculoplasty on intraocular pressure in patients with intravitreal steroid-induced elevated intraocular pressure. J Glaucoma. 2008 Jun-Jul;17(4):287-92.

Schwartz JT, Reuling FH, Feinlieb M et al. Twin study on ocular pressure after topical dexamethasone. I. frequency distribution of pressure response. Am J Ophthalmol 1973; 76:126.

Schwartz JT, Reuling FH, Feinlieb M et al. Twin study on ocular pressure folliing topically applied dexamethasone. II. Inheritance of variation in pressure response. Arch Ophthalmol 1973; 90:281.

SCORE Study Research Group. A randomiezed trial compering the efficacy and safety of intravitreal triamcinolone with standard care to treat vision loss associated with macular edema secondary to central retinal vein occlution: the Standard Care vs Corticosteroid for Retinal Vein Occlusion (SCORE) Study report 5. Arch Ophthalmol 2009;127:1101-14.

SCORE Study Research Group. A randomiezed trial compering the efficacy and safety of intravitreal triamcinolone with standard care to treat vision loss associated with macular edema secondary to branch retinal vein occlution: the Standard Care vs Corticosteroid for Retinal Vein Occlusion (SCORE) Study report 6. Arch Ophthalmol 2009;127:1115-28.

Smithen LM, Ober MD, Maranan L, Spaide RF. Intravitreal triamcinolone acetonide and intraocular pressure. Am J Ophthalmol. 2004;138(5):740-743.

Southren AL, Gordon GG, Weinstein BI. Genetic defect in cortisol metabolism in primary open angle glaucoma. Trans Assoc Am Physicians. 1985; 98:361–9.

Stone EM, Fingert JH, Alward WL, et al. Identification of a gene that causes primary open angle glaucoma. Science 1997; 275:668–70.

Tawara A, Tou N, Kubota T, Harada Y, Yokota K. Immunohistochemical evaluation of the extracellular matrix in trabecular meshwork in steroid-induced glaucoma. Graefes Arch Clin Exp Ophthalmol. 2008 Jul;246(7):1021-8.

Tektas OY, Lütjen-Drecoll E. Structural changes of the trabecular meshwork in different kinds of glaucoma. Exp Eye Res. 2009 Apr;88(4):769-75.

Tripathi RC, Kirschner BS. Kipp M. et al. corticosteroid treatment for inflammatory bowel disease in pediatric patients increases intraocular pressure. Gastroenterology 1992; 102:1957.

Wang RF, Guo BK. Steroid-induced ocular hypertention in high myopia. Chin Med J 1984; 97:24.

Wang X, Johnson DH. mRNA in situ hybridization of TIGR/MYOC in human trabecular meshwork. Invest Ophthalmol Vis Sci 2000; 41:1724-9.

Zhang X, Clark AF, Yorio T. Regulation of glucocorticoid responsiveness in glaucomatous trabecular meshwork cells by glucocorticoid receptor-beta. Invest Ophthalmol Vis Sci. 2005; 46:4607-16.

Zhang X, Ognibene CM, Clark AF, Yorio T. Dexamethasone inhibition of trabecular meshwork cell phagocytosis and its modulation by glucocorticoid receptor beta. Exp Eye Res. 2007;84(2):275-284.

Zhao J, Zhang Q. Ultrastructural changes of the trabecular meshwork in glucocorticoid induced glaucoma. Yan Ke Xue Bao. 2010 Nov; 25(2):119-124.

Zillig M, Wurm A, Grehn FJ, et al. Overexpression and properties of wild-type and Tyr437His mutated myocilin in the eyes of transgenic mice. Invest Ophthalmol Vis Sci 2005; 46:223-34.

Permissions

The contributors of this book come from diverse backgrounds, making this book a truly international effort. This book will bring forth new frontiers with its revolutionizing research information and detailed analysis of the nascent developments around the world.

We would like to thank Shimon Rumelt, MD, MPA, for lending his expertise to make the book truly unique. He has played a crucial role in the development of this book. Without his invaluable contribution this book wouldn't have been possible. He has made vital efforts to compile up to date information on the varied aspects of this subject to make this book a valuable addition to the collection of many professionals and students.

This book was conceptualized with the vision of imparting up-to-date information and advanced data in this field. To ensure the same, a matchless editorial board was set up. Every individual on the board went through rigorous rounds of assessment to prove their worth. After which they invested a large part of their time researching and compiling the most relevant data for our readers. Conferences and sessions were held from time to time between the editorial board and the contributing authors to present the data in the most comprehensible form. The editorial team has worked tirelessly to provide valuable and valid information to help people across the globe.

Every chapter published in this book has been scrutinized by our experts. Their significance has been extensively debated. The topics covered herein carry significant findings which will fuel the growth of the discipline. They may even be implemented as practical applications or may be referred to as a beginning point for another development. Chapters in this book were first published by InTech; hereby published with permission under the Creative Commons Attribution License or equivalent.

The editorial board has been involved in producing this book since its inception. They have spent rigorous hours researching and exploring the diverse topics which have resulted in the successful publishing of this book. They have passed on their knowledge of decades through this book. To expedite this challenging task, the publisher supported the team at every step. A small team of assistant editors was also appointed to further simplify the editing procedure and attain best results for the readers.

Our editorial team has been hand-picked from every corner of the world. Their multi-ethnicity adds dynamic inputs to the discussions which result in innovative outcomes. These outcomes are then further discussed with the researchers and contributors who give their valuable feedback and opinion regarding the same. The feedback is then collaborated with the researches and they are edited in a comprehensive manner to aid the understanding of the subject.

Apart from the editorial board, the designing team has also invested a significant amount of their time in understanding the subject and creating the most relevant covers. They scrutinized every image to scout for the most suitable representation of the subject and create an appropriate cover for the book.

The publishing team has been involved in this book since its early stages. They were actively engaged in every process, be it collecting the data, connecting with the contributors or procuring relevant information. The team has been an ardent support to the editorial, designing and production team. Their endless efforts to recruit the best for this project, has resulted in the accomplishment of this book. They are a veteran in the field of academics and their pool of knowledge is as vast as their experience in printing. Their expertise and guidance has proved useful at every step. Their uncompromising quality standards have made this book an exceptional effort. Their encouragement from time to time has been an inspiration for everyone.

The publisher and the editorial board hope that this book will prove to be a valuable piece of knowledge for researchers, students, practitioners and scholars across the globe.

List of Contributors

Claudio Campa, Luisa Pierro, Paolo Bettin and Francesco Bandello
Department of Ophthalmology, University Vita-Salute, Scientific Institute San Raffaele, Milan, Italy

Anurag Shrivastava and Umar Mian
Montefiore Medical Center, Albert Einstein COM, U.S.A.

Tharwat H. Mokbel
Mansoura University Mansoura, Egypt

Hosam Sheha
Ocular Surface Center & Tissue Tech Inc., Miami, Florida, United States

Parul Ichhpujani
Glaucoma Facility, Department of Ophthalmology, Government Medical College and Hospital, Chandigarh, India

Marlene R. Moster
Anne and William Goldberg Glaucoma Service, Wills Eye Institute, Philadelphia, PA, USA

Sima Sayyahmelli and Rakhshandeh Alipanahi
From the Glaucoma Division, Tabriz Medical Sciences University, Tabriz, Iran

Paul-Rolf Preußner
University Eye Hospital, Langenbeckstr, Germany

Antonio Fea, Dario Damato, Umberto Lorenzi and Federico M. Grignolo
Dipartimento di Fisiopatologia Clinica- Clinica Oculistica, University of Torino, Italy

Jair Giampani Junior and Adriana Silva Borges Giampani
Federal University of Mato Grosso, Brazil

Michael B. Rumelt
Washington University Deparament of Ophthalmology and Visual Sciences, St. Louis, Missouri, USA

Tsvi Sheleg
Department of Ophthalmology, Western Galilee – Nahariya Medical Center, Nahariya, Israel

Yoshiaki Kiuchi, Hideki Mochizuki and Kiyoshi Kusanagi
Hiroshima University, Japan

Eitan Z. Rath
Department of Ophthalmology, Western Galilee – Nahariya Medical Center, Israel

Shimon Rumelt
Department of Ophthalmology, Western Galilee – Nahariya Medical Center, Nahariya, Israel

Avraham Cohen
Western Galilee Hospital, Department Of Ophthalmology, Israel

Printed in the USA
CPSIA information can be obtained
at www.ICGtesting.com
JSHW011443221024
72173JS00004B/925